Our Symphony with Animals

Our Symphony with Animals

ON HEALTH, EMPATHY, AND OUR SHARED DESTINIES

Aysha Akhtar, M.D.

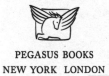

PEGASUS BOOKS
NEW YORK LONDON

OUR SYMPHONY WITH ANIMALS

Pegasus Books Ltd.
148 W 37th Street, 13th Floor
New York, NY 10018

First Pegasus Books edition May 2019

Interior design by Maria Fernandez

The views presented in this book are those of the author and
do not necessarily represent the views of the Department of Defense,
the U.S. Public Health Service, or the U.S. Army Medical Department.

Library of Congress Cataloging-in-Publication Data is available.

ISBN: 978-1-64313-070-5

10 9 8 7 6 5 4 3 2 1

Printed in the United States of America
Distributed by W. W. Norton & Company

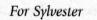

For Sylvester

Contents

Foreword
by Carl Safina

At five today as every day, an hour before dawn I felt our dogs jump onto the bed. They curled up by our feet and we all dozed a bit until my wife said "Good morning." Our first words are their cue to start the day's greeting and the licking. It's a custom they started; we didn't train it. And then it's time to hit the floor and start the day. Every day they get us out of bed at dawn. And though that's not always my favorite idea—if I've had a late night of writing or we've been out—dawn is always my favorite time of day. So I'm always grateful that they get us going. Downstairs they get let out; the coffee goes on. They get let in and fed. Right after they eat they seek us out and seem to thank us, and then they rest while I fill the bird feeders, feed our rescued parrot. Then we usually make breakfast, often sharing a bit with them or letting them lick up leftovers. And by then it's time to let our chickens out. The chickens are not in a rush to venture out at dawn; that's when the hawks hunt and the last fox goes to sleep. So they wait inside, and when I see them appear in their screen coop the dogs and I all go out, I open the coop, and our hens scurry to the back porch steps, where I feed them while the dogs take in the scene. In some years we've had added duties: an orphaned squirrel or raccoon, or a baby owl found fallen and near death. Healing them, their need and seeming appreciation of our care, their feeling comfortable and safe in our presence; this is a great honor and a daily lesson.

The lesson they refresh for me daily is: we are alive, now. They remind me to live present and ready to appreciate what comes our way. They break us through the hurt and grief and gloom that humans create for ourselves, the disappointments and disillusionments. They, like we, come into the world with none of it. In your opportunity to be kind to them, they repay with daily reminding of how pure and innocent living beings can be with each other. If we choose.

After everyone is fed we may take the dogs to the beach—they love that—before we get to work. I love it too. Watching them run and chase and swim, getting wet and sandy, I realize afresh that they get us smiling more times a day than any single aspect of our life. They bless us with their mess. I often think of the words of my friend and hero Peter Matthiessen, who wrote in *The Snow Leopard*, "And it is a profound consolation, perhaps the only one, to this haunted animal that wastes most of a long and ghostly life wandering the future and the past on its hind legs, looking for meanings, only to see in the eyes of others of its kind that it must die." What I see in the eyes of others *not* of my kind is: let's live. Let's just live.

In a world of wounds, the invitation into compassion is the greatest gift a human can be offered. The symphony that is the controlled chaos of our morning, whether it is the noise of the chickens or a sandy snout against my hip, awakens and lifts my spirit like music. It is our best route out of grief.

I am a scientist, but many scientists have long wrongly believed that only humans are conscious and can feel anything. That belief is unscientific. It is also an excuse for humans to abuse the non-humans among us. There is far too much of this. And of course there is far too much abuse of other people. Other animals are considered "brutes," or "savage beasts." But as Herman Melville noted in his great psychological classic, *Moby-Dick*, "There is no folly of the beasts of the earth which is not infinitely outdone by the madness of men." Abuse of animals often goes hand in hand with abusive behavior toward people. Learning to treat animals with gentleness gentles people toward people too. Humaneness is good for humans and humanity as a whole.

The organizing principle of all biology is that all life is kin, related and genetically connected down through billions of years of unbroken chains of ancestors and living descendants. Many of our genes have been on Earth for hundreds of millions of years. Think of it this way: the physical similarities you see in other species—eyes, ears, skeletons, organs, heartbeats—carry into similarities we can't see in brains and their functioning. But you can see the functioning of minds in the logic of behaviors. And more formally, behavioral neuroscience has come light-years. Researchers in these branches of science have looked at brains as they function, in MRI machines and using other modern techniques. They have watched dogs' brains light up when shown photos of people and dogs they know, and watched the brains of sleeping rats as they dream. There is simply no question, and there is plenty of proof, that their minds are generally as similar to our own minds, as are their bodies. In light of so much new evidence, many scientists now agree that the scientific reality is: everything in the living world is on a continuous range, and this includes the similarities in the nervous systems of various kinds of creatures, and thus in their mental functions and emotional capacities.

When we lose a loved one, including a loved pet, we grieve. And some animals grieve, too. Any animal capable of emotional bonding shows grief when you'd expect it. Grief isn't solely about life or death; it's mostly about loss of companionship, loss of presence. Author Barbara J. King says that when two or more animals have shared a life, "Grief results from love lost."

We know that humans can enjoy life and love or miss companions. The remaining problem is that we tend to deny, or mistrust, the idea that any other creature can. This is a great gap in our appreciation and understanding of who we are and who we are here with on this only known living planet.

Albert Einstein said our task is to "widen our circle of compassion to embrace all living creatures and the whole of nature in its beauty." Unity of need becomes unity of purpose. To deflect disaster, this is where we must be headed next.

And if you'd like to know what's in it for you, Confucius is credited with saying, "He who wishes to secure the good of others, has already secured his own." Dr. Albert Schweitzer observed, "One thing I do know: the only ones among you who will be really happy are those who have sought and found how to serve."

Charles Darwin recognized that "The simplest reason would tell each individual that he ought to extend his social instincts and sympathies to the men of all nations and races . . . our sympathies becoming more tender and more widely diffused until they are extended to all sentient beings."

There is a spiritual component here, even for the non-religious. The ability to feel along with another is the minimum standard of religiosity, "because in compassion," says the former nun and author Karen Armstrong, "we de-throne ourselves from the center of our world."

The geometry of human progress is an expanding circle of compassion. Each time people like Copernicus, Darwin, and Einstein have widened the circle—moving us farther from the center of the universe, the center of time, the apex of creation, we got a better, more realistic view of who we are. We understood a little better that we are not alone, that we have company here. Each of us must learn this for ourselves, and so progress is slow.

Expanded views make us more civilized. But being civilized gets us only so far. The challenge now is to become more humanized. It may seem ironic but caring for other animals helps to humanize us. Humans have the capacity for compassion, so acting compassionately fulfills our human potential. The greatest realization is that all life is one. Over my lifetime, living with, studying, and working with many other animals in their world and ours has only broadened and deepened—and reaffirmed—my impression of our shared life and of the rich gifts offered by closeness and care for the other-than-humans among us.

In the pages that follow, Aysha Akhtar expands and expounds this great potential. She illuminates the above by sharing stories of caring, and yes of abuse, and of grieving. But above all, these stories are about recovery, renewal, and hope. Be soothed by these stories, and the shared destiny and healing that takes place within these pages. Then consider how you yourself might find a way to help heal another. This is how we will heal the world, one life at a time.

Prologue

I want to show you something."

Uncle Talup approached me as soon as I stepped out of the bathroom of our East London row house. I had just spent the afternoon watching a TV show about a girl with giant teddy bear companions while my two younger sisters napped and my older brother roamed the neighborhood with his Matchbox cars. Uncle Talup often babysat us until my parents came home from work. Although he was a close family friend, by Pakistani standards we called all adults *auntie* or *uncle* as a sign of respect.

I let Uncle Talup lead me by the hand up the dark, narrow stairs. Maybe he had a new game to show me. But we walked past the bedroom where I normally played with my brother and sisters and into my parents' bedroom. He closed the door and we sat on the edge of the double bed. I squinted my eyes at the sharp sunrays as they peeked around the edges of the yellow-and-brown-striped curtains and bounced off the floor-length mirror. Often, I stood in front of this mirror and asked the girl looking back at me if the world she lived in was different from mine. On this day, though, the mirror wasn't showing my imaginary friend. Something wasn't right.

"Here," Uncle Talup said. I followed his gaze downward to his baggy, white shalwar kameez pants.

I had just turned five years old the first time Uncle Talup molested me. His sexual abuse would continue for five more years and across two continents. He abused me weekly when he lived near my family's home in London. After my family moved to the United States, he visited us four, sometimes five times a year and continued the abuse, as though we had never been apart. Throughout those years, I remained silent, telling no one, not even my parents, what he was doing to me. That was one of his rules that he knew I would follow. I was an obedient girl. *Keep quiet.*

Uncle Talup's abuse launched a childhood marked by confusion. Although I was too young to articulate my thoughts at the time, I had so many questions, mostly about myself—my role as a good Pakistani girl who followed the rules, my duty to elders, my self-worth. And I sought answers to those questions feeling scared, embarrassed, and alone.

But one night, at only nine years old, clarity came.

This was one of those rare moments in life when insight doesn't seep in the usual trickles into our subconscious until the flow of information becomes too vast to ignore. No, the answer to my questions rushed to me in a torrent. And once I had the answer, it seemed so obvious.

My answer was a dog named Sylvester.

⚮

It's the only picture I have of him. It's a sunny, late November day. We had just returned from a romp in the woods, picking pinecones to spray with gold and silver sparkles as winter gifts. I kept tripping over him, as he braided his footsteps so close to mine, never leaving my side. In the photo, he's looking off to something beyond the garden gate that I can't see. Brown hair. Brown eyes. A red-and-white bandana is wrapped around his neck. He looks rugged, handsome, and adorable all at once.

Sylvester entered my life when I was nine years old. My grandparents and my Uncle Dave on my mother's side followed my parents from London to Virginia, where they adopted Sylvester from a litter of unwanted pups. He was part German shepherd, with a velvety face and a tuft of white fur on his chest. Like me, like each of us, Sylvester had his own story.

For much of my childhood, our lives became so intertwined that if you now tried to remove Sylvester from my story, it would unravel. I had never known an animal before, but I bonded instantly with Sylvester. In Virginia, my grandparents lived in the next building in our apartment duplex, fewer than fifty yards away from where I lived. I can't recall a single day when Sylvester and I were not together. We shared a friendship, a kinship, a love that was strong. We were *that girl and her dog*.

We also shared something else: abuse.

The first time I saw Sylvester being thrown against the wall—also by a man I knew well—was the moment that set me on a path to find the courage to end not only his abuse, but also my own.

Sylvester was the first in a long line of animals I would come to know. Through him, I became more aware of the worlds of other animals around me and developed a great sense of kinship with them.

As a child, I rescued orphaned birds and rehabilitated them. I read books on how to mash up hard-boiled eggs (it seems so wrong now) to feed baby birds with tweezers. I learned how to house birds in warm, shoebox nests, how to train them to look for worms under rocks, how to let them go when they were ready. I also rescued injured rabbits, squirrels, and mice and anxiously sat with them in my lap in the passenger seat of our green Buick station wagon as my mother rushed us to the local veterinarian.

Through animals, I developed a desire to heal. It was easy for me to take the skills I learned by caring for animals and apply them to humans. My mother was a nurse and she taught me that the general principles were the same, whether caring for humans or animals. To be a good healer, she told me, you need to understand how others are hurting and you need to want to help them. I was so frequently by my mother's side as her "little nurse's assistant" whenever one of my sisters or my brother was sick that everyone in my family knew what I would be when I grew up.

"Aysha will be a doctor."

As I pursued my studies in medicine, I continued to seek the company of animals. While doing rounds as a third-year medical student at the Eastern State psychiatric hospital in Williamsburg, Virginia, my cat Aslan suddenly turned ill. During medical school, Aslan (a name from one of my favorite childhood books) was my constant companion, draped over my shoulders as I pored over anatomy, physiology, and molecular biology books on long, cold nights. After four years with me, Aslan was succumbing to feline leukemia, an infectious disease he caught before I rescued him off the streets.

On a Thursday night, I drove three and a half hours to take Aslan to a specialty animal clinic. But nothing could be done to save him. His heart failed. Aslan's lungs filled with fluid, and he was struggling to breathe. I made the humane decision and ended Aslan's suffering. He died, purring, in my arms.

By the time I left the clinic, it was close to five A.M., Friday. I was to start my shift at the psychiatric hospital in three hours. Later that morning, I tearfully phoned the psychiatrist in charge of my rotation. I explained what had occurred and asked if I could have that day off to grieve. He said no.

I had no doubt that if my mother, brother, or friend had died or even been seriously ill, the psychiatrist would have allowed me at least a day off. My presence at the psychiatric hospital wasn't crucial by any means. My main job as a mere medical student was to do the scut work, running errands for staff. So I was astounded and dismayed by the psychiatrist's response. How could he not recognize the significance of a loss of a beloved animal companion? Or at the very least, how could he not recognize that this loss was significant for me? I could not understand how a doctor, one who studied the mind no less, could *not* see the importance of animals in our lives.

I was naïve. The psychiatrist was far from unique in his view of animals. There was a tendency among doctors to disregard the significance of our relationships with animals. The only time we had ever discussed our relationships with animals during my medical training was to emphasize how animals can injure us and be sources of infectious diseases. Both are relevant issues, but they offer a narrow view of the subject.

I felt that by not considering our relationships with animals, medicine was missing a vital component of our health. During my training, I was taught how health is more than just the absence of disease. In 1946, the World Health Organization defined *health* as "a state of complete physical, mental, and social well-being." While disease today largely relates to our experiences within the halls of our medical centers, health reflects our lives outside the hospital, outside the doctor's office. To truly heal and to keep someone healthy, we doctors have to lift our gazes from our checklists of diagnoses, medical procedures, and drugs. We have to consider the numerous influences that occur beyond the white walls of hospitals.

Each of us is like a connect-the-dot picture. In order to draw the right picture of health, we need to: (a) include the relevant dots that make up our lives, and (b) connect the dots in the correct way. Each dot in our lives influences our physical, mental, and social well-being. We now recognize that how we interact with and treat one another, how we share (or do not share) our resources, how we relate to our environment, how we shelter ourselves, how we govern ourselves, how we spend money, how we eat, how we work, how we play—in short, how we *live*—influence our health.

I learned firsthand how many factors influence my health. I did not escape Uncle Talup unscathed. I have struggled with depression my entire life. Although internal biology certainly plays a role, I have found that my tendency to fall into despair is often affected by the state of affairs around me. I am far from alone in this. Even as some physical illnesses have declined in the past few decades, a malady that affects us all grows. This disease slowly courses its way through our modern civilization and divides in number like a cancer cell every time we hear another story of violence, grief, and struggle.

We collectively suffer from a deep spiritual and emotional affliction. Even if we are less violent today as Steven Pinker argues in his book, *The Better Angels of Our Nature*, it certainly doesn't *feel* that way. Stories of not only violence, but also of pessimism and gloom constantly barrage us. Every time we grieve another mass shooting, every time we hear of another crime of hate, every time we see another child going hungry, we suffer a setback in our fight against this malaise. Almost one in three of us can't sleep and one in five takes at least one psychiatric drug. We pop pills to ease our sadness, our loneliness, our deepest fears. We may live longer, but we don't necessarily live better.

Health draws from every aspect of our lives—not just as individuals, but collectively. Our mental states are deeply impacted by those of others. We are a social species. Our relationships with one another matter because we are interdependent, perhaps more so now in our global world than ever before. As we are increasingly aware of others, our empathy and compassion also increase. With each generation, we extend our circle of empathy bit by bit to include those who were previously ignored—like battered women, the mentally disabled, and the transgender community. Our ever-widening empathy reflects our growing understanding that our well-being is tied to the well-being of others. I suffer when you suffer. We laugh when they laugh. The lives, struggles, and joys of far-flung strangers affect us all.

So, how do the lives of animals affect us? Although doctors are connecting more dots in our lives, we still largely overlook one crucial influence that has existed since our beginning: our relationships with animals. On those rare occasions when doctors turn their gaze toward animals, we rarely see beyond the surface. We focus only on a few types of animals and a few situations. But my experience with Sylvester and my abuse inspired me to seek more information about how animals affect our health—this dot that doctors too often fail to connect.

For much of my medical career, I downplayed my affection for animals when I was among my colleagues. I felt embarrassed. I know of many other doctors who were also reluctant to admit their kinship with animals as though, by admitting this, we were somehow lesser scientists and doctors. As though compassion for animals was a fault. But the truth is that I love animals with all my heart and soul, and would never wish for that to be any other way. Far from being a detriment to my work as a physician, it has made me a better healer.

No matter how slimy, how scaly, how smelly, or even how scary, animals matter to me. By denying this, I was denying an integral part of who I am. And that clouded my ability to understand my own suffering—which is deeply influenced not only by the lives of other humans, but also by animals. With this awareness, I can look upon my experience with Talup and with Sylvester with a sharper eye. Whatever possible paths my life could have taken, my bond with Sylvester and my empathy for him changed it for the better. Now, as a neurologist, I find myself asking one question again and again: Where does that empathy for animals come from?

In a groundbreaking book, biologist Edward O. Wilson introduced *biophilia* as ". . . the innately emotional affiliation of human beings to other living organisms." Biophilia is the hypothesis that humans naturally connect with nature and animals and that our affinity is rooted in our biology. It is a love of life in its simplest definition. It is part of who we are as fellow animals on this planet. Wilson was not just referring to animals, but also to plants and all other "living systems." We seek out nature. Our need to have green spaces in cities, our desire to hike in the woods, and our drive to preserve natural parks are all evidence of biophilia.

Wilson wasn't necessarily arguing that we all seek a bond with animals, but I believe that it is in our relationships with animals where our biophilia is especially evident. If you were to look at the migration of people in the Western world from rural areas into cities in the 19th and 20th centuries, you would find a steady increase in the number of animals kept as pets. Historians have traced the rise in pet keeping as it parallels our increasing urbanization. As we stepped away from rural living and lost daily contact with many animals, we sought them in other ways. We brought cats, dogs, birds, hamsters, and rabbits into our homes.

We choose to bring animals into our lives. They make the world a little less lonely. And a lot more fun. When we can't bring animals into our homes, we look for them elsewhere. We visit wildlife sanctuaries; we join bird watching clubs. We go to zoos and circuses, even as we increasingly feel uncomfortable seeing animals behind bars or performing for our entertainment. We take safaris in Africa. We seek a bond with animals. Our need to be with animals is so deep and instinctively strong that our biology is not just biophilia. It is *animalphilia.*

An episode of the television series *The X-Files* provides a humorous perspective on how animals provide us company and comfort. In a flip of the usual werewolf tale, where a monster bites a man and turns him into a werewolf by night, the main characters Mulder and Scully meet a were-monster, a reptilian-like creature who was bitten by a man. One day this peaceful and content insect-munching reptile wakes up and finds himself turned into a pudgy Australian. As a man, he begins thinking like a man and finds himself burdened by all the worries, fears, and self-doubts that only humans have. He realizes he needs a job, as he later complains to Mulder, so he gets one selling cell phones. But then he hates his job and wants to quit and do something else. But he can't, because how would he pay his bills? How can he get a loan for a mortgage on a house? How can he save enough for his retirement? "If I haven't written my novel by now," he laments to Mulder, "I'm never going to write it."

Burdened by these all-too-human worries, the were-monster visits a "witch doctor" (psychiatrist), who, rather than curing him, gives him drugs that only serve to muddle his thoughts. In a last effort to ditch his melancholia, the were-monster gets a puppy who he names Daggoo. As the camera lingers over the were-monster happily rolling on the floor playing with Daggoo, the monster tells Mulder, "I quickly realized that the only way to be happy as a human was to spend all your time in the company of non-humans."

Not all of us seek the company of animals or empathize with them, though. Nor does this companionship and empathy extend to all—or even most—animals. Humans now cause more suffering to animals than ever before in history. We have an extremely contradictory relationship with animals. Coinciding with our increasing affection for companion animals is our increasing distancing from those species we define as tools, pests, and food. But I believe the lives of these animals who are hidden from our view are also woven into ours. Most of us just don't know it yet.

This book is a journey to understand the very nature of health and how it is influenced by the lives of animals. Specifically, how does our empathy for animals—and lack of it—affect our health in the deepest sense of the word? In order to answer this question, I have tried to understand the many different ways we think about and relate with animals and how our empathy for them is evolving.

This journey has led me to a wide range of individuals including a Marine with post-traumatic stress disorder, a mobster whose life changed after one animal encounter, a convicted serial killer, a pediatrician with HIV, a former cattle rancher, and an industrial animal farmer. This is a story of ignorance, apathy, and cruelty, but ultimately, it is one of beauty, kindness, and healing.

Anthropologist Brian Fagan described in his book, *The Intimate Bond*, that, "our urge to make a connection with fellow creatures is so powerful that it takes a lot to override it." If indeed this urge is so strong, do we lose something when we ignore it? Do we lose something of ourselves? Perhaps most importantly, when we do recognize our kinship with animals, what do we gain?

I know what I gained from my kinship with Sylvester. And this knowledge changed the entire course of my life.

Our Symphony with Animals

PART ONE

Healing with Animals

CHAPTER ONE

What Is Home?

The alarm didn't go off this morning. I look over at the clock and realize I'm late for work, very late. I jump out of bed and step, barefoot, into a puddle of warm, slimy vomit. Silos! Where is that good-for-nothing feline?

Why do we do this? Why do we tolerate vomit congealing on the floor, poop rolling on the bed, fur clinging to our clothes, urine-soaked curtain hems, saliva-covered slippers, ripped-up furniture, acid breath, stinky food, litter boxes, rude sniffing (you know where), insolent hissing, defiant pissing, incessant barking, hairballs, scratches, bites, snarls, fleas, ticks, ear mites, hookworms, tapeworms, roundworms, and so on?

Animals inconvenience us. We rearrange our work and vacation schedules around them, spend our hard-earned dollars on medical bills for them, and do just about anything to indulge them. They are the perpetual teenagers that test our limits. They wolf food like undiscriminating gluttons, or they turn their precious noses from our offerings like fussy snobs. They tear up the house, scatter their messes, and leave all of it for us to clean up. The worst part is that they expect we will graciously bow down and accept it all. And they are right.

In our contract with animals—pets, specifically—we voluntarily agree to a certain amount of hard labor. Comedian Jerry Seinfeld once joked that if an alien race were to visit Earth and watch the hordes of humans scuttling after their dogs and scooping up their refuse, the aliens would think that dogs ran the place. In some ways, that idea is not so far-fetched—except that I would add cats and other companion animals to the list of lords and ladies of the manors.

No other species routinely adopts other animals. Yes, there are the anecdotes we all love to read about—a cow mothering a puppy, a goose befriending a lost owl. But animals don't go out in droves to bring members of other species into their lives and into their homes. What compels us to do this?

I think about this question as I sit in the waiting room of the American Society for the Prevention of Cruelty to Animals (ASPCA) adoption center in Manhattan's Upper East Side. On this Saturday afternoon, the adoption center bustles with visitors. Elderly men and women, couples, and parents with children come here to pet, adore, and sweet-talk demure dogs and coquettish cats. Visitors have one goal in mind: to add another member to their household. As I watch a young couple walk out with a terrier in tow, the sheer bliss in the dog's movements reflects theirs. Despite all the expenses, hassles, and nuisances, we seek animals simply because they bring us a joy that's irreplaceable and unique.

There is something so wondrous about animals. They experience the world in ways we cannot even begin to fathom, and they can see, smell, hear, and feel things that are beyond our capabilities. What is it like to be dog, a dolphin, or a mole? Although science has increasingly turned its collective head to the study of animal behavior, our ability to understand each animal's unique world is woefully limited. Too often, the most we can do is imagine what their experiences are like. When we do take the time to imagine the lives of other animals, we are often instilled with a childlike awe and a desire to emulate them. No wonder many superhero traits model the abilities of animals. Who among us has not fantasized about flying, breathing underwater, or having super hearing? Animals draw us out of our human-centric worldview. We may initially seek out animals because of their similarities to us, because of our shared evolutionary biology. But we derive pleasure from their differences. As a result, animals pull us in like nothing else can.

❦

I was sitting in the living room of our apartment with my sister Sahar when my brother burst through the front door and said, "Amagee and Abadgee got a dog!" I jumped up from the puzzle that I was completing with my sister. "A dog?" I asked, catching my brother's excitement. This was big news! No one we knew ever had a dog before and I never would have thought that our grandmother and grandfather would get one. Among Pakistanis, this was unheard of. Dogs—and, really, all animals—were considered dirty creatures who were meant to be separated from humans. Eager to learn more about our grandparents' break from tradition, Sahar and I grabbed our jackets from the shoe closet and raced with Kamran to the apartment building next door.

Since we moved to the United States from England, my family had been living in a twin apartment complex in Arlington, Virginia. We arrived in America in the late 1970's with high hopes. After three weeks of living in a motel near Washington, DC, my father was hired as a busboy at a hotel restaurant and he found us a cheap apartment. A year later, my grandparents, two of the four aunts, and their younger brother, Dave, followed us from London and moved into the building next door.

Eager to meet our grandparents' new dog, Sahar, Kamran, and I rushed into their garden apartment and found all of them clustered in one of the bedrooms. Our grandparents, aunts, and Dave were gathered around the bed. And there he was. A little brown puppy, wagging his tail a mile a minute. I shoved my way to the center of the bed and scooped the puppy onto my lap as though I had known dogs all my life. "What are you going to call him, Dave?" I asked as the dog nuzzled and licked my face. Dave wasn't his real, Pakistani name. He chose a Western name to fit in better. I never called Dave "Uncle Dave," since he was only ten years older than me and much more like an older brother.

"We're naming him Sylvester," he said.

That's perfect, I thought. Every Saturday morning, my sisters, brother, and I spent hours watching Loony Tunes cartoons. Of all the cartoon characters, cheeky Sylvester was one of my favorites. Never mind that it was "Sylvester the Cat." If cats have nine lives, well maybe giving our new puppy the name given to a cat would bring him good luck. And I did think of Sylvester as *our* puppy, not just my grandparents' or Dave's puppy. I knew that Sylvester and I were going to be buddies. I looked into his large, brown eyes and I thought of all the best spots to play and all of my secret places around the buildings that I was going to show him.

⌘

About ten years ago, I was driving to work when some part of my mind registered something in the middle of the lane in the opposite direction that should not have been there. During the morning traffic, I, like everyone else on the road, was in a hurry. I ignored what I saw and kept driving. A few miles later, though, the nagging doubt surfaced, and I realized that what I saw on the road was a turtle.

The turtle was still alive when I drove by but had frozen in the middle of the road. With the rush of cars, I knew the turtle didn't have a chance. I turned my car around and drove back to the spot. By that time, though, another car was already pulled over to the curb. Someone else had gotten there before me. I watched as a teenager walked out into the middle of the road, arms outstretched, to warn and halt the oncoming traffic. He gently lifted the turtle, who appeared unharmed, and carried him to the other side of the road to safety.

Anxious to get to work on time, I didn't approach the boy to thank him for his kindness. I've always regretted that and I often wondered what compelled him to take time from his busy schedule to help a little turtle when no one else did. I never found this out, but I did discover something else. Later at work, as I recalled how that boy helped an animal in danger, I smiled. The boy's empathy, even though it was not for me, made me happier.

Empathy derives from the German word *Einfühlung*, coined by philosopher Robert Vischer in 1873. *Einfühlung* means "feeling-in." At the time the word was introduced, *Einfühlung* related to how an observer can project his or her own feelings onto an object or subject to "enliven" it. An example is when one describes a willow tree as "weeping." It was not until the mid-1900s that empathy took on a different meaning. Psychologists shifted its definition as they turned their attention to the science of social relations. Over time, *empathy* came to mean the understanding and sharing of the feelings of another.

We often confuse empathy with sympathy and kindness. *Sympathy* is a concern for another who is distressed. But with sympathy there can be an emotional distancing that can sometimes tip into pity, causing a feeling of superiority and the belittling of another. Kindness is an extension of empathy, translated into action meant to help another, as I witnessed with the boy who rescued the turtle. In comparison to sympathy, empathy has more grip.

Primatologist Frans de Waal suggests that empathy has roots in our evolutionary history. Studies on animal behavior show that empathy is a trait we share with a variety of species. Perhaps it initially developed to help mothers of multiple species better care for their young, but the expression of empathy reaches well beyond maternal care. It even plays a role in how we react to other people's movements.

If you saw someone grimace after tasting something bitter, you would likely grimace as well. For years, researchers wondered why we often mimic the movements of others. In 1995, a team of neuroscientists recorded motor-evoked potentials—which signal that a muscle is about to move—when participants watched a person grasp for an object. The motor potentials matched those recorded when the participants actually grasped the objects themselves. Since that study, others have supported the idea that we possess mirror neuron systems that enable us to respond similarly when we perform an action and when we witness someone else perform the same action. We see examples of this empathetic mimicry every day. Yawn and watch the others around you also yawn. It's instinctive.

Emotional contagion is similar to mimicry, but rather than automatically emulating another's body movements, we instead pick up their emotions, including, sadness, joy, anger, and fear. Babies will cry when they hear other babies cry. If you are in a movie theater and the room breaks out in screams just as the crazy ax-wielding clown jumps out of the shadows—even if you knew it was coming—I dare you not to utter at least a whimpering yelp.

Mimicry and emotional contagion are considered to be the building blocks of more complex levels of empathy. Researchers today generally distinguish between two forms of empathy. Affective empathy refers to the sensations and emotions we experience in response to another's emotions. With affective empathy, we share the other's emotional state. When we experience cognitive empathy, on the other hand, we take in the mental perspective of another—and can better identify and understand what that person is thinking and feeling. Both components of empathy together help us understand another's experiences, intentions, and needs. The ability to empathize with others allows us to predict and understand their feelings, motivations, and actions.

Neuroscientist Tania Singer and her colleagues at the Max Planck Institute for Human Cognitive and Brain Sciences in Germany explored the neurological underpinning of affective empathy, specifically the shared experience of pain. We don't just feel pain physically; we experience it emotionally as well. When we are hit by a painful stimulus, such as an electric shock, signals travel from the site of the stimulus up to the brain, where there is overlap between the pain and emotion centers. As a result, our responses to pain can include unpleasant emotions such as anxiety, fear, or sorrow.

To understand how empathy affects the emotional experience of pain, Singer's team studied sixteen women who were accompanied by their romantic partners. In one situation, the women volunteered to receive painful shocks through electrodes attached to their hands. In another situation, the women were allowed to see when their partners received shocks. Using brain scans of the women, Singer found increased activity in many of the same parts of the brain (in parts of the cerebellum and brain stem) whether the women received shocks themselves or whether their partners received the shocks. When watching their partners get shocked, the women's brains lit up in the same emotional areas, but not in the painful sensory areas as when their own hands were shocked. "Empathy," Singer said, "works by tapping into a brain mechanism that already exists for our own pain. This makes us believe we are feeling pain emotionally even when we are not feeling it physically." Singer's study added further proof that empathy is wired into our brains.

How we experience empathy toward animals may not be so different from how we experience it toward other humans. Researchers from the Department of Psychology at Brandeis University and the Pennsylvania State University found that when we are shown pictures of either humans suffering or dogs suffering, there is a great deal of overlap in our neural responses to both.

Empathy is the glue that holds groups together. When we empathize with another, we are sharing their experiences, the good and the bad, the joy and the suffering. It is a crucial component in human development and it forms the foundation for kindness, compassion, morality, and altruism. In *The Empathic Civilization*, social theorist Jeremy Rifkin describes empathy as "the very means by which we create social life and advance civilization." Empathy enables us to care for one another, share our resources, and help others, including animals, in times of need.

But research has revealed something else: empathy is strengthened by similarity, proximity, and familiarity. We empathize more with those in the "in-group"—those who are like us, who are near us, and whom we personally know. In other words, we empathize more with the "here and now." As Kristin Dombek describes in *The Selfishness of Others*, empathetic accuracy evolved as a way of protecting one's in-group against outsiders. And the core in-groups are our families.

So let's start there.

Two dozen men and women of the Cy-Fair Volunteer Fire Department and other law enforcement personnel in Cypress, Texas, formed a traditional wall of honor. On this June day in 2016, they saluted one of their comrades for a final farewell as her body, draped with the Texas flag, was carried to its final burial site. The individual they were saluting was Bretagne, the last surviving 9/11 search-and-rescue dog.

In addition to rescuing humans trapped under the rubble of 9/11, Bretagne also searched for survivors during hurricanes Katrina and Rita. After her retirement at age nine, Bretagne continued to help others. She befriended first graders at Roberts Road Elementary School and helped them slowly gain confidence as they read to her. "She's part of Texas Task Force One," said Cy-Fair Volunteer Fire Department Chief Amy Ramon at Bretagne's funeral. "She's part of the Cy-Fair Fire Department. . . . It's very hard. Bretagne's part of our family . . . she's one of us."

Ramon's comment about Bretagne leads to an important question: What is family?

At the outset it seems like a simple question. According to Merriam-Webster's Dictionary, one definition of *family* is "a group of persons of common ancestry." Another is "the basic unit in society traditionally consisting of two parents rearing their children." But those definitions don't quite work anymore (if they ever did). Statistically, a family is no longer a mother, a father, and their biological children. Attitudes are changing and the traditional view of the family unit is eroding. We are opting for a more liberal view of family, which can include unmarried couples with children, gay or lesbian partners adopting children, single mothers or fathers with children, and couples who opt not to have children.

Family members are not restricted to our own species either. Since at least 2001, most US households have included companion animals. Today, it's about 70 percent. The trend to adopt animals is spreading throughout the world, even in places traditionally unaccustomed to considering animals as household companions. China is second and third behind the United States in cat and dog guardianship, respectively. Between 2006 and 2014, the number of companion animals in India grew from 7 million to 10 million. Our language is changing to reflect our emotional connection with animals. Since the 1990s, the terms *pet* and *owner* have been increasingly replaced with *companion*, *guardian*, and *mom* or *dad*. As our roles change, so do the roles of animals. Animals can take on any conventional human part in the family, even multiple roles. At different times in my life, Sylvester was to me a friend, brother, father, and child. Most of the time, though, he was uniquely Sylvester.

Though most US households with animals—and that's most US households—consider pets to be part of their family, US authorities didn't see it that way for a long time.

It took a major event to draw governmental attention to this.

⁓

Like so many others around the country, when Hurricane Katrina smashed against New Orleans, Louisiana, at the end of August 2005, I watched helplessly as the catastrophe unfolded before me on TV. More than 1,800 people, almost half of them elderly, died from the hurricane and its aftermath.

Disasters rarely create new situations. In most cases, they simply expose a city's underlying systemic vulnerabilities in infrastructure and in emergency planning. Katrina was no exception to this. But because its devastation was so marked and widespread in comparison to prior American disasters, Katrina really hit home for us just how unprepared we were.

Major catastrophes like Katrina can cause long-term, devastating effects. People who survive disasters consistently experience higher rates of depression, anxiety, acute stress, and post-traumatic stress disorder (PTSD). After Hurricane Mitch hit Honduras and Nicaragua in 1998, one in ten patients being seen for general health care and who lived in the most damaged areas suffered from PTSD. Six months after Hurricane Andrew struck Florida in 1992, anywhere from one in five to one in three survivors had PTSD. Katrina threw an especially hard blow. The Centers for Disease Control and Prevention (CDC) found that even seven weeks after Katrina, almost half of the survivors met the criteria to be diagnosed with PTSD. Young children are particularly vulnerable to mental trauma after major disasters. They have a harder time making sense of the event, expressing its emotional impact on them, and independently securing the emotional help they need.

Being separated from loved ones or being forced to leave them behind during emergencies is probably the single, hardest thing any of us can imagine doing and it can compound the mental stress disasters cause us. Mary Foster of the Associated Press captured one of the most iconic moments of Katrina that showed just how gut-wrenching being torn from a beloved animal can be. Amid the chaos, panic, and fear of the hurricane, a little boy and his family left their home to seek shelter at the Superdome in New Orleans. But the Superdome quickly became unsafe. Buses soon arrived to take desperate families elsewhere. When the little boy, clutching his dog, Snowball, and his parents were boarding a bus headed for Houston, a police officer took the dog away. The boy cried out hysterically, calling "Snowball, Snowball!" and then vomited.

Stories like this have been told again and again. When rescue workers from the local police and fire departments, the US Navy, the Coast Guard, and the National Guard were deployed to help, they did not include animals in their evacuation efforts. Rescue workers were overwhelmed helping human survivors, and evacuating animals poses additional and unique logistical hurdles. Unlike humans (at least most of them), you can't order animals to get on the boats and buses. Animals may be fearful and hide, and you might have to catch them. Some might threaten your safety or that of the people you are rescuing. You often need carriers for the smaller animals, crates for the middle-sized ones, and leashes for the larger ones. Rescuers were unprepared.

Rescuers forced many residents, in some cases by threat of arrest, to abandon their companion animals. Hundreds of thousands of animals perished because rescue workers refused to take animals on board boats, helicopters, and buses and into emergency shelters. According to Wayne Pacelle, former president of the Humane Society of the United States, considering that about 70 percent of American households include companion animals (and that New Orleans was not different from other US cities in this respect), it was likely that rescuers found animals in two out of every three homes—either huddled away with their humans or abandoned and alone.

Yet most animals were left to die. Images of emaciated and frightened animals struggling to stay afloat amid the toxic, rising waters, trembling on rooftops and clinging to floating boards symbolized how our state and federal agencies vastly underappreciated the role of animals in the American family. These agencies also didn't understand something else: by abandoning the animals, rescuers also endangered many of the very people they were trying to save.

⁓

It was hard enough to get help for man's best friend or even woman's best friend (if the cliché that women prefer cats is true). But how do you drum up enough empathy for help to rescue an animal who most people recognize only as a piece of meat on their dinner plate? How do you get help if your family includes a three-hundred-pound pig?

Retired schoolteacher Jim Parsons would soon learn the answer. If you were to walk about Louisiana's Garden District in the 2000s, you would expect to see Victorian, Greek revival, and Italianate antebellum mansions lavishly dressed with stained-glass windows, decorative brackets, Italianate columns, cupolas, and gabled roofs. A peek through the wrought-iron fences surrounding these matriarchal homes would reveal cool, lush, private gardens. You would likely have made your way to the almost two-hundred-year-old Lafayette Cemetery jam-packed with its eerie aboveground tombs. In the Garden District's fantastical and opulent setting, you would have been surprised to come across a humble pig casually strolling down the boulevard with her even more humble human dad.

Townsfolk knew Jim as the "pig guy." On mornings, he and Rooty, a potbellied pig, took one-and-a-half-hour walks about the town and Rooty attracted so much attention, she became a minor celebrity. "People would see us walking," Jim tells me, "and would stop and want to talk to me about her. They would want all these pictures with the pig—mom and dad with the pig, the kids with the pig, the whole family with the pig." Rooty loved to walk along St. Charles Avenue where courtly oak trees bestowed mounds of acorns. "Sometimes on our walks," Jim says, "Rooty would look at me, then go running up the street. There was this big brush near a restaurant, and she'd be rooting around for acorns. One person in the restaurant nearby would point Rooty out and all of a sudden, they'd have half of the restaurant out there looking at the pig." Although an ordinance prohibited traditionally farmed animals in the city, local police made an exception for the cheerful, pink pig. Instead of handing Jim a citation, police officers would instead ask for a photo.

Jim knew Rooty since she was a piglet. Ten years before Katrina hit, Jim's girlfriend Connie (now his wife) bamboozled him into adopting Rooty from a litter of piglets. Ever since she had read *Charlotte's Web* as a child, Connie wanted a pig. Reluctantly, Jim took the most timid of the litter back home, and it was love ever since.

In no time, the piglet took to her new life with Connie and Jim. And Jim took to Rooty. He easily housetrained her, and she quickly learned how to get what she wanted. Always curious, Rooty could force open refrigerators, unlatch cabinets, and rummage through closets. She followed Jim around like a dog, slept at his feet, and nuzzled him in the evenings. Jim loved her dearly. Never could he have predicted that one day, his love for Rooty would force him to make a terrible decision.

❧

When Katrina made landfall north of Miami on Thursday, August 25, 2005, it was classified as a Category 1 hurricane with 75 mph maximum sustained winds. The next day, it was reclassified as a Category 2 hurricane. By 7 A.M., Sunday, Katrina became a Category 5, with 160 mph maximum sustained winds. When the hurricane hit New Orleans on Monday, August 29, it knocked out the power in the city and punched a hole in the Superdome.

Like so many residents of New Orleans, Jim and Connie underestimated the impact Katrina was to make. They figured that their hundred-year-old home, which sat eight feet above the ground, was a safe place to ride out the storm. But by Monday evening, the house rattled and shook with increasing force, as if the toy of a giant. Jim worried. He wasn't so much concerned for himself, but for the other residents in his house, which included Connie, two friends, two cats, and Rooty. As the house swayed, Rooty became so anxious that Jim fed her a bowl of wine to help calm her and made a shelter of blankets in the closet for her to hide under for the night.

The next morning, Jim saw debris everywhere. Downed telephone poles and trees blocked the streets, and glass shards littered the front and backyard. But their house was intact. Jim and Connie thought the worse had come and gone. As Connie left to provide nursing care at the local hospital to those who were not so lucky, Jim stayed behind to clean up the debris and care for the animals. He cleared a small space free of glass in the backyard for Rooty; and as she was taking care of business, Jim walked to the front of the house to better check the damage. He looked over to a manhole in the middle of the street and gasped. Water was oozing out. Jim stood there, confused. Where was the water coming from? Without working landlines, cell phones, or electricity, Jim had no way of knowing that the nearby levy had just broken.

The water came fast. By the time Jim scurried to the backyard, the water had risen to Rooty's knees. Jim measured the rise of the water by the steps that led to his front door, twelve in all. Within two hours, the water reached the third step, and fish were swimming in their front yard. A few hours later, the water spilled over the fifth step. By nightfall, the ninth step.

Although Jim's house sat high in his neighborhood, he feared the water would soon creep in. By then, the water had flooded all the other houses around him. Over the next few days, helicopters flew in and evacuated most of the neighborhood, but not the animals. So Jim stayed put. He wasn't leaving unless he could take the animals with him.

The water kept rising. It reached a high point of five and a half feet, over the roof of a pickup truck parked next door. As the days passed, the water, reeking of an overturned sewage tank, swelled nastier and nastier. And the streets, empty of most life, turned quieter. One night, across the silence, Jim heard crying from a neighborhood house. "I went through that filthy water with an ax and broke down the door to that house and the ceiling had come off the roof and there was a cat. The people who owned the house had left food and water, thinking they would be back in a few days."

This was a common scenario. One of the most frequent reasons people give for leaving their animals behind during disasters is the belief that the calamities would be short-lived. Other reasons include underestimation of the severity of a disaster, poor emergency planning, inability to transport the animals, and difficulty finding animal-friendly shelters. Regardless of the explanation, the loss of an animal companion can take its toll. When the little boy was torn apart from Snowball, he not only lost the dog he loved, he also lost the support that Snowball provided for him.

In stressful times we cling to whatever sources of reassurance and stability we can. And for many of us, that includes animals.

Among primary school children from Slavonia, one of the Croatian regions heavily affected by war, children with companion animals coped better than children without animals. The former group had developed better capabilities in expressing their emotions, seeking social support, and problem solving. As a result, children with pets were less likely to suffer from emotional trauma compared to kids without them.

Similar results occur across demographics. It doesn't matter if you're young or old, rich or poor. Animals help soothe us during stressful times. And losing them can add to the trauma. In a study of 365 low-income African American women, the loss of an animal significantly predicted their post-disaster distress and bereavement, and this effect was above and beyond that of other losses and sources of stress. Likewise, the loss of animals during Katrina caused greater negative impact on mental health than the loss of homes. As compared with people who did not lose their animals during Katrina, those who did were more likely to suffer significantly from acute stress, peritraumatic dissociation (an emotional disconnection from the acute traumatic experience), depression, and PTSD. After 2008's Hurricane Ike, loss of animals among survivors in Galveston, Texas, was a significant predictor of lower mental health. Losing our animal companions causes us distress that is independent of other losses.

Animals provide steady comfort in the midst of chaos. As with human bonds, our love for animals can foster in us a sense of security and well-being. That love can shield us from stress, anxiety, and depression. We can become more resilient by the emotional safety, protection, and nonjudgmental support animals provide us. Studies find that the majority of people with companion animals feel that the animals are important to their well-being. Animals give us tactile comfort and recreational distraction from worries. Caress a purring cat or play ball with a dog and you will know what I mean. Perhaps most importantly, animals are reliable presences. We can count on them to be there for us. In return, we can promise to be there for them.

To his already crowded house, Jim added the abandoned cat. On the sixth day of flooding, Army soldiers in red berets from the 82nd Airborne Division came knocking at his door. The mayor of New Orleans had ordered a mandatory evacuation of the city, and the last of the holdouts in Jim's neighborhood had left. To the shock of the rescuers, though, Jim still hadn't left. "The soldiers came up in a boat," he says, "and they were carrying cameras and filming me and they cursed me out. They told me I was a crazy man and what the fuck am I doing here and why the fuck haven't I left? I told them I had a three-hundred-pound pig, two of my own cats, one of my neighbor's cats, and that I wasn't going anywhere and I went back in the house."

Although to the soldiers Jim's refusal to evacuate may have seemed absurd, he was far from alone in this regard. Disasters test us. They challenge us to recognize what truly matters. Universally, we make it clear that it is our loved ones who matter. Families come first. And catastrophes force us to quickly define who is family. During Katrina, thousands of people made it clear that their dogs, cats, pigs, and other animals were kin. Almost half of the people who rode out the storm did so because they refused to leave their animals behind. They had good reason not to evacuate. Later studies showed that people who fled were more likely to have lost a companion animal. Only 15 to 20 percent of lost animals were ever reunited with their human families. Most animals, including Snowball, were forever gone.

One-fifth to one-third of human evacuation failures during disasters are attributed to animal guardianship. After a mandatory evacuation was issued in Yuba County, California, following a major flood in 1997, the biggest reason why households without children refused to leave was fear of leaving their animals behind. And, with each additional dog or cat in the household, failure to evacuate doubled. Of those who did leave, many remained homeless, living in their cars or in campgrounds, to stay with their animals. Additionally, when investigators examined two separate disasters—a flood and a hazardous chemical spill—they found that 80 percent of those who returned prematurely to unsafe sites did so to rescue their animals. They risked their lives to save their pets.

Jim willingly risked his life. But, as day after day went by, he increasingly worried. Almost a week later, the stagnant water was down only to the hood of the truck. Jim realized that he and his housemates were going to be trapped for a long time. The oppressive heat and sewer bugs infesting the house weren't his biggest concerns. Fresh water was. And food. Jim and his two friends started rationing their water and they had just enough food for a few weeks more for themselves and for the cats. But they were rapidly running out of food for Rooty.

What was Jim to do? He had few options. Even if he could get the cats out, rescuers weren't taking Rooty. Would he have to watch her slowly starve? "I realized that if this lasted a whole month, then we were going to have to"—Jim sobs—"I was thinking that we may have to have the soldiers take her out. But then all the horrible stuff came to my mind. If they shot her, what would we do with the carcass?"

After twelve days, the floodwater was still five feet high. Jim made the hard decision to ask the National Guard to shoot Rooty.

≈

Imagine for a moment the grief Jim was going through at the time. Many people don't or can't understand. Although this is gradually changing, too often, instead of giving compassion and empathy, colleagues, friends, and even family members tell those who mourn an animal that they are being silly to care so much—after all, they are *just* animals. Get over it, they say. Buck up!

We laugh together and cry alone. Grief is even lonelier when an animal dies because it's less valued than grief over the death of another human. Sociologists, psychologists, and psychiatrists (as I found out when my cat Aslan died) have been slow to appreciate the impact of a loss of an animal. An animal's death can cause poor sleep, missed days from work, significant distress, and depression. Among those who lose animals they deeply love, the extent of their grief is similar to that of those mourning the death of a cherished person.

Jim may have felt even greater despair over potentially losing Rooty because of the unique situation he faced. Consider the heartbreak of being forced to leave an animal behind. A team of researchers found that people's distress after losing their animals during Hurricane Katrina was worse among those who'd abandoned them. Losing animals from forced abandonment not only heightened people's trauma, but it also slowed their recovery. If, as in Jim's case, a decision to euthanize an animal was involved in the loss, this could aggravate a sense of guilt, regret, or even failure. Interestingly, the investigators found that being forced to abandon an animal was more likely to cause symptoms of PTSD, whereas the actual death of an animal was more likely to cause severe depression. With Jim, add a walloping dose of guilt to the bereavement that comes with the death or probable death of a cherished animal and you have one sad man.

⤶

Just as Jim lost all hope to save Rooty, a miraculous thing happened. The phone rang. For the first time since Katrina hit, his landline worked. "When I answered the phone," Jim recalls, "it's this guy named Jeffrey Tam, the producer of *Canada AM*. He asked if I was the guy with the pig. He had seen the video footage from the 82nd Airborne. I said, 'Yes I am.' Then he said, 'We are going to come and rescue your pig.'"

After Tam's call to Jim, the Canadian TV crew contacted a search-and-rescue team from the International Fund for Animal Welfare (IFAW), which was already in the area looking for abandoned animals. For Stewart Cook, a photojournalist with IFAW, saving Rooty was one rescue that stood out. Stewart wrote:

> Approaching the home, we saw two people standing on the steps. "Do you have an animal to rescue?" someone

asked. "It's my pig," The man cried. "Can you take my pig?" We entered his home and were introduced to Rooty, a Vietnamese potbellied pig. "She's my baby," the man said with love. "I can't leave her." The day before mandatory evacuations had been ordered across New Orleans, the National Guard were patrolling in airboats and following through on those orders. "I asked them to shoot her," said the man, tears welling in his eyes, "but they wouldn't do it. I can't leave her to starve."

Rooty was rescued and taken to a sanctuary that housed an assortment of saved animals—cats, dogs, cows, horses, and billy goats, including one named Goliath who quickly befriended Rooty. When the water in his hometown receded, Jim reunited with Rooty. Upon seeing him at the sanctuary, Jim tells me, Rooty "came running out and rubbing against me."

Rooty died in 2015 at fifteen years old. Parsons can't talk about her death without tearing up. "You can imagine," he says today, "if you've had a pet for fifteen years. . . . She was such an important part of my life. Rooty became a family member and everyone knew that. They called her my daughter."

&c.

Ten days after Jim and I spoke, I receive a book in the mail. During our entire conversation he kept referring to a book, which he told me describes in great detail his experience during Katrina. "I'll send to you the book I wrote," he said. "All the information you are looking for is in the book. Everything we went through. It's all there."

Taking the book of out of its shipping package, I read the title, *Our Rooty: The True Tale of a New Orleans Pig.* The cover is a drawing of a pig's snout peeking out from a red-and-white-striped blanket. I flip through the pages, ready to read the harrowing details about Jim's experience that he promised he had documented. An illustrated children's book, it has about as many words as a page in the book you are now reading.

It isn't until many months later that I grasp the significance of this.

⬥

Though not the first disaster to strike animals, Hurricane Katrina called worldwide attention to the plight of animals—and the people who love them—like no prior disaster had. Stories like Jim's (though his had a happy ending) played out on TV screens, newspapers, and websites, prompting an outpouring of empathy. Americans donated more than $40 million to help animals impacted by the hurricane.

US authorities clearly underestimated the strength of the bond between people and their companion animals. Fortunately, the public outrage that followed led to landmark changes in disaster preparedness. Less than a year after Katrina, Congress passed the Pets Evacuation Transportation Standards (PETS) Act, which mandates that state and local governments include animal rescue as part of their emergency evacuation plans. It also authorized the use of funds for the "procurement, construction, leasing, or renovating of emergency shelter facilities and materials that will accommodate people with pets and service animals." In a political rarity, both Democrats and Republicans united in this effort. The act easily passed with bipartisan support.

It was a defining moment. For the first time, the federal government understood what the public already knew: helping humans and animals are not separate endeavors. If you want to save the former, you have to save the latter. The awareness brought about by Katrina and the PETS legislation has had a positive, measurable effect. By the time the next big hurricane, Irene, hit the East Coast in 2011, most residents safely evacuated with their animals.

Despite the progress in disaster preparation, however, the recognition of the human–animal bond in other situations has been sluggish.

❧

You would think we'd have learned. You would think that after Katrina, we would acknowledge the strength of the human bond with animals in all dimensions of life. But the human mind has a remarkable ability to apply new wisdom to only specific situations, ignoring its larger implications. And we are tugged and pulled into even those lessons like a dog being taken to the vet. We tuck in our chins, lower our eyes, and drag our feet—anything to avoid learning something new.

Victims of domestic violence are still fighting to have their animal companions recognized as family. Sherrilyn Grant learned just how hard that fight is after her boyfriend came home one day and tried to choke her.

I meet Sherrilyn at a brownstone apartment building in East DC. A pretty woman in her fifties with dyed honey-blonde hair, she lives temporarily at a friend's apartment. When I walk into the apartment, Chelsea, a Shih Tzu–Yorkshire terrier, and Blondie, a beagle-Labrador run up to meet me. As Sherrilyn tells me her story, Chelsea sits between us on the couch and Blondie rests her hefty head on Sherrilyn's feet. Things were working out great with her boyfriend, Sherrilyn tells me, until they moved in together. The previously attentive, soft-spoken man took to the bottle and became verbally abusive. He came home one evening, reeking of alcohol, and wrapped his hands around her neck. As she struggled to breathe she could hear Chelsea and Blondie barking furiously in the background. A neighbor heard the commotion and called the cops. Sherrilyn opted not to press charges against her boyfriend, but since the Washington, DC, house was his, he kicked her and the two dogs out. Suddenly the disabled veteran was homeless.

The local domestic violence service secured Sherrilyn a hotel room for ninety days—but Chelsea and Blondie weren't part of the deal. The service folks told Sherrilyn to turn her dogs over to an animal shelter. She wasn't having any of it. "These are not just dogs," she tells me as she angrily recalls their words. "They are my children. They're telling me to just give my dogs up?"

So Sherrilyn made a compromise. She used the hotel room to change and bathe and slept in her car with her dogs. After the ninety-day hotel arrangement ended, Sherrilyn shuffled from domestic violence shelters to family members and friends, looking for a place to stay. Very few allowed her dogs. For long stretches of the two years that followed, Sherrilyn, Chelsea, and Blondie lived out of her car.

Today, three years after her boyfriend assaulted her, Sherrilyn is still without a permanent place to live. "To suddenly be broke," she says, "to be hungry, to be destitute, to beg for a place to live." She shakes her head, pulls Chelsea onto her lap, caresses her furry face, and sobs. "These girls keep me from going over the edge. I feel empty without them. There's a space that they fill. They are my inspiration to keep going." She lifts up her head and looks at the two dogs. "I will always be there to make sure they have what they need. To make sure they have fresh water and food. While I still have breath, we will be together."

⌘

As troubling as Sherrilyn's situation is, it could be much worse. The 1917 story "A Jury of Her Peers" written by Pulitzer Prize–winning writer Susan Glaspell is one of the earliest to highlight a previously ignored truth about domestic violence. In the story, the protagonist, Mrs. Hale, is asked to accompany her husband along with the sheriff and his wife, Mrs. Peters, to the scene of a crime. The day before, Mr. Hale had discovered the body of his neighbor strangled in his bed with a rope. All the while the dead man's wife, Minnie, calmly sat downstairs.

As the sheriff and other men search around for evidence to convict Minnie, they joke about the unkempt house and the small domestic "trifles" women care about. But Mrs. Hale and Mrs. Peters notice something alarming about the trifles that ruled Minnie's life. Small things about the house add up to reveal a life of quiet desperation. The most telling is their discovery of an empty birdcage with a broken door, as though someone had been "rough with it." A few minutes later, they find the body of a canary with his neck broken.

With growing understanding, the women see what their husbands do not. Minnie's husband, after a lifetime of dominating and controlling her, killed her beloved bird. And that led Minnie to strangle her abusive husband. In an act of solidarity, the two women hide the bird's body—the only evidence that would lead to Minnie's conviction.

In the mid-1990s, Allie Phillips was a young attorney in Lansing, Michigan, prosecuting domestic violence cases when she noticed a disturbing pattern that supports the premise of Glaspell's story. On Phillips's normal court days, 90 percent of the victims wouldn't show up. She surmised that many of them were too scared to face their abusers or were not interested in taking legal action (often due to fear). However, a third reason never occurred to her until one of the victims showed up late and said, without looking her in the eyes, "I went back to my abuser last night. He killed one of my dogs and I still have two more dogs and a goat. I would rather go back and lose my life than to live with the guilt of having him kill my pets."

Phillips was dumbfounded. "No one in the mid-90s was really talking about the link between violence to animals and people," she tells me more than twenty years later. "I had never heard of such a thing." Revealing her naïveté, Phillips called a local domestic violence shelter and asked if they had room for this woman. The shelter said yes. "Then I said I'll have the police bring her over right now," Phillips tells me. "And she has two dogs and a goat, so we're going to bring them too. And the lady on the other end of the phone laughed at me and hung up."

Phillips got angry and determined. Over the next fifteen years, as she investigated the issue, she found only four family violence shelters out of more than two thousand in the United States that took animals. This was a major problem. "When I started researching how many pets are in the home," she says, "I realized that many of the victims weren't showing up at court because their animals were keeping them home."

Published studies have proven Phillips right. Research has repeatedly shown that family-violence victims—male, female, and transgender, throughout the United States, Europe, New Zealand, Australia, and elsewhere—often refuse to escape their abuse because they worry that the perpetrators will turn on their animals. In a survey of 107 battered women, 47 percent of those with companion animals reported that their abusers threatened or harmed the animals. More than half of them said their companion animals were important sources of emotional support. Another study showed that among women with companion animals, one of the most common reasons they delay seeking shelter is threats against the animals. And once in shelters, many of the women continue to worry about their animals' safety. Abusers had hurt the animals for revenge or to psychologically control their partners. In most cases, the animals were hurt in the victims' presence—and often in front of their children too.

If you are suffering at the hands of an intimate partner and have animal companions, what are you to do? Most shelters and safe houses (as they are frequently called) won't allow animals. Renting property, assuming you have the financial means, may also not be an option. Caroline Jones, the executive director of a safe house in Arlington, Virginia, tells me that many landlords won't rent to victims of abuse because they worry about violence on their property. So renting is largely out. You may be fortunate enough to have caring family and friends who will house you and the animals, but what if you don't?

In 2012, a woman without options confronted the managers of a shelter and caused them to overhaul their practice. The woman's boyfriend had tried to kill her with a hammer, but her Great Dane, Hank, jumped in between them, laid his body over hers, and took most of the blows. The man then threw Hank and the woman out of a second-story window. Although Hank suffered many broken bones, both he and the woman survived. When the woman and her dog arrived at Rose Brooks Center in Kansas City, Missouri, seeking sanctuary, they offered her a bed but refused to admit Hank. The woman was defiant. And for the first time in its history, the shelter opened its doors to a nonhuman.

Today, Rose Brooks has a state-of-the-art in-house animal shelter with kennels for dogs, cats, and other family animals. The center's chief executive officer, Susan Miller credits this needed change to Hank's fierce devotion and the unwavering love of the woman he saved. "She was not going to leave her pet alone [with the boyfriend]. He saved her life."

⁂

He saved my life. They comfort me. She gives me a reason to go on. These are the words you will commonly hear when sufferers of violence speak about their companion animals. They often provide abuse victims with their only source of comfort and companionship during violent times. In 2007, Dr. Ann Fitzgerald of Windsor University in Ontario, Canada, published a study titled "'They Gave Me a Reason to Live': The Protective Effects of Companion Animals on the Suicidality of Abused Women." From her study, Fitzgerald found that the presence of animals can both help battered women and heighten their risk of danger. Fitzgerald noticed that some women "stayed with their abusive partner longer than they otherwise would have because their 'pets kept them going' by providing them with the social support necessary to cope with the abuse."

Fortunately, with people like Allie Phillips taking up the cause, there is now a movement to provide shelter for all members of a family. Phillips has partnered with RedRover, an organization that was founded in 1987 to rescue and shelter animals during disasters. In 2008, RedRover started helping animals caught in the middle of domestic violence. This change was largely due to the efforts of Esperanza Zuniga. Having grown up with animal friends and witnessing her step-grandfather abuse animals, she fiercely advocated on their behalf. Zuniga implemented a needs-assessment study on the animal housing capabilities of domestic violence shelters. "We learned some very alarming statistics," Zuniga tells me. "One:

less than 5 percent of domestic violence shelters have the ability to have pets on-site, and two: over 70 percent of households in general that have children under the age of six have pets. So we realized if 70 percent of households have pets and yet less than 5 percent of domestic violence shelters are willing to house them, then obviously there is something happening to those pets or there is something happening to those families."

"And pets are often first in the line of fire because they are voiceless," Zuniga continues. "They can't talk back and say what happened. So we realized pets were often being used as pawns in these domestic violence situations and that the victims were being told, 'If you tell somebody what I'm doing, then I'm going to kill the dog.'"

As a result of Zuniga's findings, RedRover formed two programs to help domestic violence victims. First, the Domestic Violence Safe Escape grant program helps find foster care for animals if there are no family shelters that will take them. RedRover has a network of volunteers, boarding facilities, and veterinary clinics that will provide temporary housing for animals. Though many people will not part with their animals, foster care can be a viable alternative that allows both humans and animals to be in safer environments. Second, RedRover's Safe Housing grants provide financial assistance to domestic shelters to build on-site housing for animals.

As of the writing of this book, the combined efforts of Allie Phillips and RedRover helped increase the number of US shelters that house animals from 100 to 132. Only about 2,500 to go. But Phillips and RedRover are determined to keep going. Already those additional thirty-two shelters have made a tremendous impact on human and nonhuman lives.

The Sojourner Center in Phoenix, Arizona, is one of America's largest and longest-running domestic violence shelters. In 2015, with funding from RedRover, it built the first on-site animal housing shelter in Phoenix—and was able to bring together a mother and her son with their orange cat, Clark Kent. When Jennifer and Robert Pressler arrived at the Sojourner Center, they did not want to leave Clark behind. But the center had not yet finished building the animal shelter. RedRover found temporary housing elsewhere for Clark in the meantime. For twelve-year-old Robert, being separated from Clark was "devastating." Every day, Robert helped with the construction, doing whatever he could to speed up the process and bring Clark to the shelter. When the construction was completed, the shelter opened its doors to not only Clark but also to another cat and two dogs. "It feels good to know that I'm here right here next to my cat," Robert stated, "and he's here whenever I need someone to comfort me." Mother, son, and feline were reunited.

⁂

On a cold January afternoon in 1993, after completing my shift interning for an AIDS charity, I rushed across the Washington, DC, streets. It was almost five P.M., and I was hoping to get a few minutes inside my beloved National Air and Space Museum on the National Mall. On the way, as my stomach grumbled, I stopped to buy a pack of French fries from a street vendor. By the time I reached the museum, it was closed.

Although a handful of people milled about on the front steps, I noticed one person in particular. A woman dressed in ill-fitting layers of clothes was desperately searching through the trash cans outside the museum doors. She tore through food packages, inspected their contents, and tossed them aside. It seemed that this woman was in search of her dinner. I went up to her and offered my still-warm, untouched fries.

What she told me was the last thing I expected. She was not looking for food for herself, but for stray cats.

The woman explained that she had been rummaging through trash cans daily for about five years to feed a colony of cats. She never missed a day, even when she was sick. She was devoted to them. Before I could ask more questions, the woman quickly departed to search elsewhere. Since that day, I often wondered why this woman would spend so much of her time caring for homeless animals when she herself was homeless.

Most of us have seen them. Men and women, sometimes teenagers, sometimes couples with children, huddling on the cold streets wrapped in tattered blankets, begging for our pocket change.

The US Code of Federal Regulations defines *homelessness* as lacking "a fixed, regular and adequate nighttime residence"—and that includes shelters (which are temporary) and places not meant for regular sleeping accommodations. The homeless move from friend's place to friend's place (i.e., "couch surfing") or sleep in cars, shelters, junkyards, vacant buildings, or on the streets. On a single night in 2017, according to the US Department of Housing and Urban Development (HUD), 553,742 Americans were homeless. Due to the high turnover rate, though, about 3.5 million will be homeless at some point during any given year. But Genevieve Frederick thinks that number is much, much higher. "I disagree with HUD," she tells me. "Their methodology is so out of it. If I was a homeless person, especially if I was doing something that's not quite legal, and if I saw somebody that looked like a white, middle-aged, middle-class person walking towards me with a clipboard, I'm going to disappear." Since 2006, Frederick has dedicated her life to helping the homeless—but in a way that was almost unheard of before.

Frederick and her husband were visiting New York City from Nevada when she saw a homeless man with a "beautiful, healthy, mixed-breed dog at his side. It was hard for me to wrap my head around it," she tells me. "That this person had a dog and that he couldn't take care of himself. How was he taking care of the dog? And I kept thinking about it and thinking about it and I thought about how much my dogs mean to me."

Back in Nevada, Frederick came up with the idea that she could help feed the companion animals of the homeless in her hometown of Carson City. She contacted her veterinarian, Dr. Gary Ailes, and asked to put a collection bin in his reception area so that people could donate pet food. The food would then be distributed to local food banks where it could be directly handed out to the home-less. Ailes not only agreed to the collection bin, he sent out a press release to the local newspaper announcing the food drive. Before he and Frederick knew it, the drive took off. Hundreds of townsfolk donated food.

Frederick has since founded the nonprofit charity Feeding Pets of the Homeless. It's the only national organization with the single focus to help the homeless care for their companion animals. In addition to supplying pet food to food banks and homeless shelters, the organization sponsors wellness clinics throughout the nation by partnering with veterinarians who go out into the community to vaccinate and treat animals of the homeless. This effort helps the larger community by preventing rabies and other infectious dis-eases. Perhaps the most rewarding task for the organization's staff is to directly arrange for an animal's medical care. Using prepaid cell phones offered by state programs, homeless men and women across the country call the organization seeking assistance for animals who are injured or ill. Feeding Pets of the Homeless staff members then help find a local hospital that will treat the animal and pays the hospital directly for the animal's care.

Some people might find it unsettling that Feeding Pets of the Homeless focuses its efforts not on the homeless themselves but on their animals. For Frederick, helping the animals *is* helping the humans.

Up to one-fourth of the homeless have companion animals—mostly dogs, although Frederick has also seen cats, ferrets, dragon lizards, pigs, and rabbits as well. Sometimes the individuals already have animals when they become homeless. As we saw, this is common among victims of domestic violence and those displaced by natural disasters. Other times, the homeless come across stray dogs or cats. "And the animals start following them and they form a bond," Frederick says.

The bond that forms, Frederick tells me, is strong. "I've got tons of stories I could tell you about. We've seen where people have been on the verge of suicide. But if it weren't for that dog, they would have gone through with it. But that dog kept them in reality long enough so that they could get past that bad moment and move on. They often feel their last chance at being a responsible human is to take care of their animal. So they will do without food for themselves, they will forego medical treatment for themselves, they will sacrifice for their pets."

University of Colorado sociology professor Leslie Irvine conducted some of the most in-depth interviews with homeless people about their animals, and her findings confirm Frederick's observations. The dogs, one of the interviewees told Irvine, "eat before I do. They'll eat before I do, period." Many of the homeless echoed this theme. They also resented any suggestion that they cannot care for their animals (a common criticism) and should not have them. One respondent argued, "People think because you're homeless, you can't take care of a dog. . . . Even people that have houses abuse and mistreat and neglect their animals, so that has nothing to do with it, whether you have a house."

The interviewee has a point, and Frederick largely agrees with this sentiment. She points out that the animals are "out there all the time with their owners, which makes them the happiest animals on the planet. Because they're getting that attention from their owner 24/7. My own dogs are back home right now wondering where I am. And I can tell you that when I've talked to veterinarians and when I've attended these wellness clinics, most of these animals are very healthy." And on those occasions when a homeless person can't care for his or her animal, Feeding Pets of the Homeless may be able to assist.

Like the desperate man who called them on the phone one day, pleading for their help. Although he didn't have long to live, he wasn't worried about his health. It was his dog's well-being. He was, Frederick says, "a veteran living off the streets and he was terribly, terribly disfigured. His dog, Girley, had really severe pancreatitis and kidney failure. He had called a number of organizations, and no one would help. Our executive director took the phone call and said, 'We're going to get your dog to a hospital right away.'"

They saved the dog's life. The man was so grateful that he sent a letter to Feeding Pets of the Homeless, in which he wrote:

> When I finally had to ask for help for the one thing I hold dear to me, the only thing in the world I have left, not one agency, not one so called charity, not one vet that I contacted stepped forward to help. . . . I cannot express my gratitude to Pets of the Homeless as not only were they the only organization [that responded], their quick and decisive action saved my service animal who is more like my child, but also me, as I cannot tell anyone who has not experienced the feeling of isolated helplessness when your beloved friend is so sick and ill, you feel so disgusted that you do not have the resources to provide the lifesaving attention they need and you do everything you can possibly do and then you realize time is running out for them.

Despite success stories like these, Frederick is running uphill. Most homeless shelters do not allow animals (sound familiar?). Unlike the efforts to provide for companion animals at domestic violence shelters, there is no widespread appeal to build on-site animal housing in homeless shelters. Perhaps this is because the homeless are so marginalized by society, they receive little attention. Until a larger effort occurs, Feeding Pets of the Homeless will send pet crates to any homeless shelter in the country. The crates are brand new, collapsible, and become the property of the shelter so that they can be reused. Whether it is 20 degrees or 120 degrees outside, the homeless and their animals can be safe inside. It's vital, Frederick tells me, to help keep the people and animals together. "The animals give these people unconditional love, which they haven't received from society as a whole. They are invisible in society. The animals are their only companions. The people need them."

Frederick's words bring back to mind the woman I met outside the National Air and Space Museum. The cats, the woman told me, had come to know her and depend on her. What she didn't tell me, but what I now suspect, is that she had also come to depend on them.

Although I was fortunate enough to always have a roof over my head, Frederick's stories and the cat caretaker have me thinking about the concept of home. There's the place you keep your belongings, where you eat, sleep, shower, and watch television. But that is a house, a condo, an apartment—a physical structure. When we think of the word *home*, what is conjured is an image of tranquility, of safety and support, something that is less physical in nature and more emotional.

What makes a home then? Is it certain individuals and the emotional connection you have with them? Those who rely on you and upon whom you rely? Those who you run to when you are lonely, feeling low, or scared? Those who you think of first when you have some joy you want to share? For most of us, *home* means family.

For those who have no physical dwelling, or have one that is not safe due to an abusive situation, perhaps by keeping them together with their beloved animals, we can, at the very least, provide for them some level of home.

Home is someone who comforts you and helps you feel safe. When I was nine years old and Uncle Talup was waiting for me back at the apartment, home was Sylvester.

CHAPTER TWO

Finding Our Voices

I used to daydream about the tall, wide apartment building across the street from ours in Arlington, Virginia. Unlike our building, that one had a parking lot that wasn't full of weeds or broken and littered with jagged glass, beer cans, and cigarette butts. Its sloping lawns encouraged soft, cool naps under the beckoning arms of maple trees. Unscarred, shining cars would drive to the front door and deposit little ladies wearing tailored suits and fitted hats, fathers flashing Carrera sunglasses and mothers flaunting their Jordache-jeaned bottoms. I imagined the building's airy lobby with red, plush carpets, mirrored walls and chandeliers, and fresh-cut flowers and women's perfume scenting the air.

Our apartment building smelled of garlic and onions. Immigrants like us from Pakistan, India, China, the West Indies, Korea, Ghana, and the occasional white family mingled together, exhaling a stench that hit you before you entered the building. Villages of miscellaneous cousins, uncles, grandparents—and that one hanger-on whom no one ever quite knew how he fit into the family—packed into tight, sweaty two- and three-bedroom apartments. At early dinnertime, you could sometimes tell what country of origin the inhabitants were from just by inhaling the different cooking odors emanating underneath closed doors. Eventually, though, the smells combined so that all you came to recognize was fried garlic and onions. The walls breathed garlic and onions. Our clothes belched garlic and onions. My skin perspired garlic and onions. I hated the smell.

Some of my classmates trailed after me, calling me a "brownie," and made fun of the garlic-and-onion smell that followed me everywhere I went. Or they taunted me about the fact that I was so skinny, I wore pants underneath my pants to make my legs look fuller. If schoolmates weren't bothering me, the strange men who loitered about our parking lot were.

It wasn't all bad. We had a great hill for sledding and all the freedom we could want. But at our apartment building, we also had our terrorizing gang fights much like the territorial warfare over the playground. We had our chilling urban legends, like the one about the boys who fell to their doom when the elevator collapsed. We had our disheartening thefts, like when my prized secondhand boy's bike that my dad taught me to ride was stolen.

For all the problems we had, though, I would never have traded our apartment building for the one across the road. Ours allowed dogs.

As soon as Sylvester and I met, we took to each other like two pups from the same litter. There were the long walks when we explored the woods behind our apartment. To me, it was Narnia, a sweeping country that only Sylvester and I were allowed to enter. We visited Mr. and Mrs. Beaver's home near the tiny, trickling stream. We pranced with the centaurs. We drank tea with Mr. Tumnus. Oftentimes we disappeared into Narnia for hours and returned home for dinner scratched up, muddied up, and mucked up, wearing the evidence of our grand adventures.

There were the games, like "Vester in the Middle" in which Sylvester stood between my sisters and me, trying to grab the ball that we tossed back and forth. There was hide-and-seek in our grandparents' apartment where I always hid and Sylvester was always "it." A sister would hold Sylvester and count to one hundred as I found ever more ingenious places to hide in the small space. When released, Sylvester would race ahead, sniffing unseen trails until he found me, barking with excitement. We tried hiding one of my sisters instead of me, but Sylvester never cared to find her. He would just look up at me with his tongue hanging out, wagging his tail, content to be by my side.

And there were the secret times when I sat on a boulder in Narnia with Sylvester in my arms and shed the tears I hid from everyone else.

As we sat in the woods, nothing ever needed to be said between us. Sylvester waited with more patience than he ever showed at any other time and he would lick my hands and face as he whimpered. Girl and dog both crying. It was as though, somehow, he *knew*. And at the time, just believing that was enough.

Sylvester nurtured me in ways that no one else could. Animals remind us that the world is larger than us. They can teach us to look beyond the racism, poverty, and cruelty in our lives—to step out of our daily struggles and see the beauty that surrounds us.

Many of us carry within ourselves moments when an encounter with an animal exalted us and reminded us of our shared world. On a spring day not long ago, I walked a forest trail that parallels a stream. At the stream's widest point, I climbed atop a large tree trunk that had fallen and formed a natural bridge. As I walked the length of the log, my eyes remained on my feet, watching my steps. Halfway across the stream, I heard a noise ahead of me. I looked up and gasped. Not more than eight feet in front of me on the log stood a fox, tall and gangly with large, upright ears and black markings across her face. Her dense copper fur contrasted with the shimmering, translucent green of the newly awakened forest.

We surprised each other. We each stood preternaturally still. I was a little afraid, as I didn't know if foxes ever attacked humans.

Here I was blocking the fox's path across the stream, which she might have perceived as a threat. But she just stared at me for a few seconds, then turned with surefootedness on the log and sprinted in the opposite direction. My experience in the woods was transformed into something larger than me. As the fox and I beheld each other, I was not just the observer but also the observed.

When we encounter another animal, no matter how fleeting that moment may be, we know that we are not alone. And that is comforting. Sometimes at the most unexpected and even the most needed times, we are reminded of this. Nonhuman animals are like us and unlike us. I believe that ultimately it is their differences that can heal us when we most need it. When we empathize with and connect with animals, we expand our social circle beyond our species. This expansion can lead to remarkable, and often startling, benefits.

⊗

Walking about a cavernous, dimly lit room with a glass of white wine, I peer at stark photos of men and women. Straight, gay, lesbian, bisexual, transgender. The pictures aren't about the people though—at least not the people alone. Central to each story conveyed in the images is the love between dogs and their human parents, who happen to have HIV. It's December 1, 2015, World AIDS Day, and I am at the opening of a photographic art show at the FLATS Studio in Chicago titled, "When Dogs Heal."

This show is a joint effort between photographer Jesse Freidin, journalist Zach Stafford, and physician Robert Garofalo. Jesse had been photographing animal shelter volunteers across the country and exploring the healing relationships they develop with the animals when he, Rob, and Zach came up with an idea. How about launching a series of photos depicting the relationships between people with HIV and their dogs? "We were talking and we thought, Wouldn't it be interesting to try and retell the story of living with HIV?" Jesse tells me. "Especially since that story has been told over and over for so long, and unfortunately, I think people have gotten a little bit tired of hearing about it. I think that our society has heard about it too much and they have stopped caring about it. So we wanted to tell a story that hasn't been told before."

Rob Garofalo's personal narrative inspired the story the three wanted to tell. A national expert in adolescent medicine at Northwestern University's Lurie Children's Hospital in Chicago, Rob runs a clinical program for gay, lesbian, transgender, gender-non-conforming, and HIV-positive youth. As a doctor vigilant of the risk factors, Rob never would have expected that, one day, he too would be diagnosed with HIV. And that, for someone who talks with frankness every day with his HIV-positive patients, he would be so resistant to speak openly about his own illness.

Wiry with a bit of scruff on his otherwise clean-shaven face, Rob fidgets. He waves his arms, taps his fingers, and scratches his face as though he's physically trying to shed the ghosts that haunt him still. He tells me that when visiting Washington, DC, one day, a group of muggers attacked and raped him. Whether he got HIV from this group or not is unknown. Temporally it fits. But Rob doesn't want to give people a ready excuse for his HIV. "If I talk about the assault, then people think, 'Well, he didn't do anything wrong to get HIV,' [but] I could have just as easily gotten HIV like most people [do]. Who knows how I ultimately got HIV? It's unimportant."

Rob has been openly gay with his colleagues, friends, and family. But when he learned he had HIV, he was worried that the disapproval that wasn't there before would suddenly emerge. "I had renal cell carcinoma several years before, and that wasn't the same," he tells me. "It's different with cancer. As devastating and challenging as cancer was to my health and well-being, there was no question in my mind that my friends and family would be supportive. But when you have HIV those assumptions kind of go out the window. Whether it's reality based or not, you question whether your friends or family, or the people around you and your colleagues, are going to be supportive or whether there's going to be an element of judgment."

Rob was also judging himself. He hid his illness from those he most cared about. Tears roll down his face as he says to me, "There's a stigma that you impose on yourself, and I felt like I had disappointed my family and friends. I lived in this sort of self-imposed hell or isolation and I really struggled." The shame he felt caused him to shut down. "I wasn't eating," he says. "I wasn't sleeping. I was making all sorts of terrible decisions about my health and I was so self-destructive. I was engaging in all sorts of reckless behaviors—I don't need to explain to you what I mean here. I just didn't care."

During this time, Rob flew to New Jersey to visit his mom. "I remember going home one day, afterwards," he says. "And . . . this is going to make me cry. . . . My mom, she . . . my mom grabbed my face and she said, 'You can tell me that everything's okay, but I know it's not. And one day you're going to tell me.'" But Rob couldn't find his voice to tell her about his illness that day.

⬥

When I was five years old, I suddenly stopped talking. My parents spent sleepless nights worrying about me. They did everything they could to find out why I turned silent. They took me to audiologists to have my hearing checked, internists to make sure I had no physical illness, and behavioral specialists who could find nothing else wrong with me. Finally, school linguists told my parents that they found the cause. My parents would speak in both English and Urdu at home. By doing so, the linguists told my parents, they were confusing me. The linguists instructed my parents to speak only English in front of me.

It was bullshit. We know that now. Kids easily learn to speak two or more languages. Learning a second language does not cause language confusion, language delay, or cognitive deficit. In fact, according to studies at the Cornell Language Acquisition Lab, children who learn a second language can maintain greater attention and focus than children who know only one language.

I wasn't suffering from confusion about languages. I was suffering from something else. Something neither my parents nor the child behaviorists had any clue about. I stopped talking just after the first time Uncle Talup molested me.

When people get a blood clot in their brain, depending on the location of the stroke, language is often the first thing they lose. Language is also one of the last things they recover. The neural circuitry that constructs and coordinates our ability to speak and understand the nuances of human language aren't as interconnected as neural networks that support, for example, our emotional abilities. In contrast to the language centers, the areas that control our emotions run deep into the oldest, most primordial parts of the brain. Because it's one of the more recently developed traits in humans, language is one of the most fragile.

What my personal and, later, clinical experience taught me is that you don't have to suffer physical trauma to your brain to lose language. Psychological trauma can do it just as well. When we face harsh times, whether as children or adults, we often literally find ourselves at a loss for words. It's hard to describe to another our grief, anxiety, and fear during such times, in part because we realize that language fails us. Language simply can't fully convey the experiential. It's like trying to explain a nightmare to someone the next morning. The dream was frightening to you at the time, but when you describe it to someone, it sounds banal. Words can never describe the mood and atmosphere of your experience.

Even worse, words can't be trusted. They can be said carelessly. They can be used to mislead, pretend, lie, or hurt. So we retreat into a more basic and deeper part of our nature—one that does not so easily deceive. We hide inside our instincts and emotions.

Over a year's time, I began to speak again. Not because of any successful intervention on the part of my parents or psychologists, but because I gradually adapted to the new normal of my life, one that now included Uncle Talup. But I often wonder if my speech would have returned sooner had I known Sylvester back then.

⌘

At the 1961 annual meeting of the American Psychological Association (APA) held in New York City, child psychologist Boris Levinson stood up to speak. With his goatee and gaunt, tall body, Levinson looked "more like an evil sorcerer than a child psychologist." In front of a packed room, Levinson solemnly described a baffling case that was brought to him eight years prior by a desperate parent. When Levinson finished talking, the audience erupted into laughter and catcalls.

The case Levinson presented was that of a young boy who had become withdrawn. The child's mother had taken him to a number of psychologists and psychiatrists, but they were unable to communicate with him. After several attempts, they gave up on the boy. The frantic mother begged Levinson to take a look at her child. On the first session with the boy, Boris happened to have his golden retriever, Jingles, in the office with him. When the boy entered his office, Jingles did what Jingles often did. He ran to the boy and licked his face. To Levinson's surprise, rather than shirk from Jingles, the boy put his arms around the dog and spoke a few words of greeting to him.

Seeing this, Levinson questioned whether the child's problem was not as great as his mother had described or whether he'd just gotten the child on a good day. However, it later became apparent to Levinson that this behavior with Jingles was unusual for the child. Levinson considered whether or not it was Jingles that facilitated the boy's communication. His thoughts were confirmed as the child continued to improve in further sessions in Jingles's presence.

After describing this case to the audience at the APA meeting, Levinson then discussed two other cases in which disturbed children similarly improved in Jingles's company. Levinson suggested to the audience that animals might provide safe, accepting relationships for children that can help them open up about themselves. Dogs, he said, can act as co-therapists.

The audience, though, was not open to Levinson's idea. "They treated his work as a laughing matter," psychologist Stanley Coren recalls. "People started shouting, 'How much of your fee does the dog collect?' There were a lot of guffaws. It was quite clear that he was being thoroughly dismissed as being some kind of kook."

Fortunately, Levinson persevered. Other voices added to his, most notably Sigmund Freud's. Cherishing his own dogs, especially his Chow Chow Jofi, Freud let them have the run of his office. During therapy sessions, Jofi would lie alongside the couch while Freud petted her. Jofi was originally brought into the office to help *Freud* relax when he was talking with his patients. But Freud soon noticed how his patients were more likely to talk about themselves when Jofi was there.

Today, almost sixty years after Levinson's revelation with Jingles, child behaviorists widely acknowledge the calming presence animals can give us. Many libraries and schools bring in dogs and cats to help kids learn to read. The animals provide a mental safe space for children who have difficulty reading, have learning disabilities, or have anxiety disorders. In the company of friendly, charming felines and canines, children who struggle with reading slowly gain confidence.

In child-abuse cases, animals are recruited to help children candidly discuss their trauma. Jeeter, a golden retriever mix with a beige button nose, was the first dog given permission to appear in court to help with a sexual assault case. It started in 2003 when Ellen O'Neill-Stephens, a deputy prosecutor, brought her son's service dog to a juvenile court in Seattle, Washington, where she worked. Jeeter befriended children so easily that word of his charisma spread. One day, prosecutors asked for Jeeter's help on one of their cases. Eight-year-old twins, Erin and Jordan, had been sexually abused by their father. The prosecution's success in convicting the father depended on the girls' testimony, but the girls were scared.

How hard must it have been for those little girls to tell a room full of strangers what their father did to them! They may never have done so if it hadn't been for Jeeter, who they fondly remember even nine years after the trial.

"I remember seeing him drink out of a sink in the bathroom and thinking that was awesome," said Erin.

"I remember Jeeter slobbering on me," added Jordan.

The girls came to depend on Jeeter's comfort so much that they refused to testify without his presence. "It's hard to explain," said the twins' mother. "He just had a tenderness about him that helped them find the strength they needed to tell the story they couldn't." While the girls were waiting in the hall to testify, Jeeter approached them and put his head on their laps as though "he knew they needed him then." With Jeeter's help, the girls testified against their father.

Seeing how much solace Jeeter offered the girls, O'Neill-Stephens lobbied for his formal placement with the Prosecutor's Office to help other victims. Since then, prosecutors in New York, Arizona, Idaho, Indiana, and elsewhere have allowed trained dogs to appear in court to help abuse victims.

As I walk about the FLATS Studio in Chicago gazing at the photos of dogs and their human parents frolicking together, two things come to me. The first is that there is no master and no subservient in these images. The men and women aren't sitting above the animals with the dogs lying passively at their feet. In most of the photos, the people are down on the ground with the dogs or the dogs are lifted up and held. Humans and dogs side by side. They are partners in the truest sense of the word. The second thing that comes to mind also concerns the children's story that Jim Parsons sent me about his pig, Rooty, and their experiences during Hurricane Katrina. Through the numerous illustrations of Rooty, Jim conveys a shifting undercurrent of emotions—first fear, then grief, hope, and finally, bliss. These were all emotions that he was not able to wholly articulate to me, emotions that he was only able to openly express through a children's book.

During traumatic times, as adults, we don't just retreat into our emotional selves; we retreat into our *childhood* selves. Into our past selves when our vision of the world was in many ways much clearer. Yes, we gain intelligence and maturity—let's hope at least—into adulthood, but we also lose something in the process. As children, we weren't yet shackled by societal mores. We had few preconceptions and our perspective of the world had not yet narrowed. Acceptance had not yet been supplanted by judgment. Wonderment not yet hijacked by skepticism. Openness not threatened by suspicion.

Like Jim's children's book, the photos before me tell stories of previously broken people. Trauma comes in many forms and stigmatization is one of them. Although Americans are more accepting than ever of those with different sexual orientations, the dread of social condemnation still exists among LGBTQ communities. Many fear being marginalized and socially shunned due to their sexual orientation. The absence of social support is so painful to all of us that societies have frequently used solitary confinement, ostracism, and exile as methods of punishment against a variety of people.

Humans are not alone in suffering from isolation. To other mammals and many non-mammals, isolation is punishing. When my husband and I took a safari in Kenya several years ago, our tour guide, who knew the animals intimately, pointed out a wildebeest grazing by himself. Wildebeests are herd animals, but this solitary one, the guide told us, was defeated when he tried to supplant the leader of the pack. For his failure, his group had ostracized him.

African grey parrots experience detrimental physiological changes from social isolation when held in captivity in separate cages. When a caged parakeet dies, her cagemate often dies soon afterward and not from any recognizable physical cause. In her book *Animal Madness*, Laurel Braitman describes an early-20th-century zookeeper's observations of the animals at the San Diego Zoo: "Solitude brings melancholia to the majority of animals. They pine away and die from sheer loneliness, which explains many of their strange friendships." One such unusual friendship at the Berlin Zoo in 1924 involved a sad, lonely monkey. The monkey was cheered when the zookeepers gave him a porcupine for company.

Loneliness devastates. Ironically and sadly, to avoid judgment, many of the individuals in the photos at the FLATS Studio, like Rob Garafalo, had put themselves into a self-imposed exile.

No wonder, when the world lets us down, we escape back into our childhood selves. It's freeing. Perhaps that is why, at these times, we are more willing to embrace animals as confidantes united against the cruelties of this world. The cultural biases that taught us as adults that animals are lesser beings are forgotten. And the doors that may have kept us from readily accepting the friendship, love, and kindness animals offer us are suddenly wide open.

After the devastation of World War I, naturalist Henry Beston retreated for a year to the beach in Cape Cod on the Massachusetts coast, where the doors unlocked for him. In the mid-twenties, the Cape was wild, windswept, and isolated, except for the multitudes of animals who lived there. Among the animals, Beston felt a kinship that he had not felt before. In the second chapter of his 1928 book, *The Outermost House*, he introduces us to the flocks of birds he encountered on the beach. As Beston contemplated their nature, he took aim against the dominant view held by philosopher Rene Descartes and his followers that animals are merely unthinking, unfeeling machines:

> We need another and a wiser and perhaps a more mystical concept of animals. Remote from universal nature, and living by complicated artifice, man in civilization surveys the creature through the glass of his knowledge and sees thereby a feather magnified and the whole image in distortion. We patronize them for their incompleteness, for their tragic fate of having taken form so far below ourselves. And therein we err, and greatly err . . . they are not underlings; they are other nations, caught with ourselves in the net of life and time, fellow prisoners of the splendour and travail of the earth.

Children naturally get this. We are born with a curiosity about animals. Remember those days when we sought out animals and bonded with them so easily? It stemmed from an inherent belief that animals are like us in standing, no more, no less. Famous cartoonists like Walt Disney, Chuck Jones, and Charles M. Schulz intuitively knew this. The most memorable cartoon characters like Bugs Bunny, Scooby-Doo, Mickey Mouse, and Porky Pig are animals. In children's own stories, animals are written as characters with equally potent interior lives as humans. Kids fill their worlds with representations of animals on their clothes, in their bedrooms, and in books, television, and other forms of media. Nearly 90 percent of the characters in young children's books are drawn from the natural world, and the vast majority are animals. Animals in stories are used to teach children critical issues of maturation and identity and of love, conflict, abandonment, pain, sadness, loyalty, and challenge. Storytellers use dogs, mice, cats, chickens, and rabbits because children see animals as themselves.

When psychologist Boris Levinson was interviewing a seven-year-old boy named David, he used the boy's identification with a cat to heal him. David, who was adopted, had threatened to kill his younger sister, also an adopted child. He believed their separate biological parents surrendered them both because they deserved it. "He felt," Levinson wrote, "that it was not possible for his adoptive parents to love him since there must have been something inherently wicked about him which brought about his desertion." It took Levinson's cat to change David's mind. During sessions, David would caress the cat and feed her. When Levinson told David that he and his wife adopted the cat from an abandoned litter of kittens and that "we love this cat very much," David at first seemed skeptical. As he spent more time with the cat, though, he began to see something of himself in her. He came to understand that if an abandoned cat can be loved by his adoptive parents, then so can he. "I believe," Levinson wrote, "this was the turning point in David's recovery."

Pediatric psychologist Dr. Barbara Boat was working on a case in North Carolina in 1979 when she first saw just how much children identify with animals. She was caring for a brother and sister suspected of being sexually abused in a daycare home. "So this wonderful interviewer was trying to talk to the little boy," she tells me. "But he was literally scared speechless. But when the interviewer asked the boy if there were any animals at the daycare, the boy's eyes got huge and he asked her, How did she know?" The boy then described a man who did terrible sexual acts on a dog. Boat and the other clinician realized that the boy wasn't just describing what the man was doing to the dog, but also to him and his sister. "Animals," Dr. Boat says, "are a window into the world of children."

⁂

When we are at our most vulnerable—at a time when speech fails us—our friendships with animals prove to be so healing precisely because human language is not needed. An intrinsic, more intuitive way of knowing links us with other species. We communicate with other creatures by translating one another's body movements, eye expressions, postures, and sounds. Communicating this way requires in us the ability to imagine and understand what an animal is thinking and feeling. In other words, it requires empathy—the great connector. We may misinterpret each other from time to time, but we can't lie. We can't hide who we are from animals. They see right through us. Thankfully, they don't care if we are gay or straight, beautiful or scarred, or whether we live in the White House or in no house. They meet us where we are. All they ask from us is kindness and company.

As we bond with animals, the pain, loneliness, and fear that resulted from our traumas are replaced with companionship, consolation, and courage. And, when we have a hard time discussing ourselves with others, we often find that there is something incredibly connecting about talking about animals. It's safe.

When Rob Garofalo first travelled to other cities to find HIV-positive people who would be willing to pose with their dogs for the art show, he was doubtful. "We didn't know whether people would do it or not," he tells me. "I thought it was going to be really hard to find HIV-positive people that want to be this public about telling their stories. I thought, Well who we are going to find is white men, who of all people living with HIV are the least stigmatized. It's going to be really hard for us to find women or people of color or transgender people." To Rob's astonishment, many people of diverse backgrounds wanted to tell their stories. Or, more specifically, the stories of their dogs. "We would just go to a city and I would contact either case managers or HIV clinics, and it was amazing how many providers were, like, I have patients who always talk about their dogs."

For photographer Jesse Freidin, each photo reveals a never-before-told story of people living with HIV and how their dogs give them the courage to face their fears. He says to me, "It's just this incredibly beautiful, moving experience where we're in the studio for half an hour, and I'm talking to them while photographing them. There's a sense of joy and comfort and relief and complete honesty, because they know that I am really there to acknowledge one of the most important relationships in their entire life, and that is the relationship with their dog."

Rob credits his own dog for inspiring the art show. The day his mother held his face and told him she knew something was wrong, Rob flew back home to Chicago. "I think I cried the entire time," he tells me. "When I got home, I sat on my bed and I thought, I have to do something. I have to change this up." Rob decided to get a puppy.

The first night Rob brought Fred home, the little puppy howled in despair. Rob had never had a dog or any companion animal before, and friends advised him that he needed to thwart the potential development of separation anxiety. "They told me the very first night you should put Fred in a bathroom or in a crate," Rob says. "And he's going to cry, but let him cry. Just don't let him out." Rob tried, but Fred "screamed at the top of his lungs for hours." Finally Rob gave up. "I was like this is bullshit." Rob opened the door and Fred ran into his bed. They've been inseparable since.

Fred's energetic self brought peace and happiness back into Rob's life and helped him reengage with the world. With each new day, accompanied by Fred's unconditional love, Rob was able to leave behind the dark world of mistrust and isolation. "He saved my life. I don't say that with any hyperbole. I'm not sure where I would have been, but I was on such a destructive path that this little puppy, without even knowing it, righted that course. It's nothing short of a miracle." Rob's eyes water as he tells me about Fred. But this time, his tears are those of joy.

Before I end my conversation with Rob, I ask him if there is anything else he wants to discuss with me.

"No," he says. "But I'm going to show you pictures of my dog."

❧

Six months after Rob adopted Fred, he took Fred to New Jersey to meet his family. Rob was a changed man, spirited and optimistic. For the first time, he told his mother about his illness. That evening, after taking a shower, Rob spied his mother in the living room hugging Fred. She was telling Fred that he had given her her son back.

❧

We've known for a long time that compassion for and connection with animals can improve our well-being. For centuries, people with disabilities have been prescribed horseback riding for emotional as well as physical healing. In 1792, the Retreat in York, England, brought in animals to help treat mental patients as part of an enlightened approach to reduce the use of restraints and drugs. Even famed nurse Florence Nightingale recognized the beneficial role animals play in healing. Animals were very much a part of Nightingale's childhood and adult life. She was especially fond of cats and surrounded herself with them during her convalescence in her later years.

During her nursing years, Nightingale noted how animals helped her patients. In her seminal text, *Notes on Nursing* (1860), she gave nursing advice on the virtues of cleanliness, fresh air, sunlight, and noise control—things that are obvious today but weren't at the time—and wrote "a small pet animal is often an excellent companion for the sick, for long chronic cases especially."

Despite these and other historical anecdotes, such as the story of Boris Levinson, health professionals still considered them isolated examples. In science, if a tree falls in the forest and no one is around to measure and quantify it, it doesn't exist. Enter Erika Friedmann. In the late 1970s, while working on her biology dissertation, Friedmann made a startling discovery.

Friedmann and her partners conducted a study of ninety-two patients who were admitted to intensive care between 1975 and 1977 after having a heart attack or chest pain from heart disease. The researchers were studying how social support and isolation affect a patient's survival at one year after discharge. The researchers asked each patient a long inventory of questions that assessed their living situation, geographic mobility, social network, and socio-economic status.

"It was a burgeoning time when people really first started looking beyond the physical influences on health," Friedmann tells me. "They were looking at social and psychological influences, too. I was at Penn [University of Pennsylvania] and I was around people looking at social stability and social support. And we knew about the Roseto effect in Pennsylvania." The Roseto effect refers to the finding that residents of a close-knit community in Pennsylvania had lower heart attack risks than those from nearby towns, suggesting the positive effects of social support. In her study, Friedmann also asked patients about companion animals. "I had a dog, and I was looking at social support." she says. "Animals are social support, too."

It was the question about animals that gave the most exciting answers. Friedmann and her colleagues found that while 72 percent of patients without companion animals were still alive at the end of the year, 94 percent of those with animals had survived. It was a significant increase in survival. In their study, social support from humans didn't even have the large effect that animals did.

Why would the presence of companion animals prolong survival? Could it be that those patients with dogs simply got more exercise by walking their dogs, which improved heart health? No. Friedmann found that both dog and cat guardians lived longer. Perhaps those with animals were healthier in the first place? Again, the answer was no. The difference in survival occurred regardless of the severity of heart disease. Independent of all other factors that were studied, the mere presence of companion animals significantly improved survival after a cardiac event. That was a major finding.

When I ask Friedmann about the medical community's reaction to her findings, she smirks. "James Lynch was part of my dissertation team. And one day he was giving a presentation to a large audience. He's talking about my dissertation. Without giving anything away, he presented a study on an intervention that was found to be a significant factor in prolonging survival after heart attacks. There's this buzz in the room. And everyone was excited. They kept asking, What's the intervention, what's the intervention? When he finally told them the answer, pets, they were truly surprised. They were surprised that pets could cause such a result, but also surprised that we were even looking at this question. They were dismissive."

Scientists couldn't remain dismissive for long. Friedmann's pioneering study caught the attention of other researchers. Pretty soon, scientists began studying how our interactions with animals impact both our physical and emotional health. Studies have since indicated that contact with animals can reduce our risk of cardiovascular disease and increase longevity by lowering our blood pressure, baseline heart rate, and cholesterol. Animals can also reduce our cardiac reactivity to stress and promote faster recovery from stressors.

When you walk through your front door at the end of a stressful day and your critter greets you, can't you just feel your blood pressure lowering? Stroking an animal relaxes our autonomic systems, as measured by blood pressure, cortisol, and epinephrine levels, and by respiratory rates and skin temperature. Of course, if you are scared of certain animals, petting them won't relax you. And I can tell you, when my cat Silos jumps on my stomach and hollers at three A.M. demanding attention, my blood pressure is doing anything but going down. But in most situations, the presence of a friendly animal calms us. When my husband, Patrick, wants to take a nap, he seeks out Silos. His warm, purring body soothes better than any sedative.

Animal companionship also improves our mental health by decreasing loneliness, depression, and anxiety. And here's an important thing to note: Other species aren't just substitutes for humans. The social support animals provide is independent of human social support. Animals seem to affect us in ways that are unique. They don't judge us (at least we don't think they do). They are there for us no matter what. They offer us physical contact and compel us to strip away social inhibitions. "You can have twenty friends, but how many of them will hug you?" Friedmann asks me. "How many will look into your eyes and just be with you for a long time?" With animals, we learn to stop and be in the moment.

As I came to find with Sylvester, sometimes, when everything else fails, the support animals provide helps us overcome the hardest moments of our lives.

⬥

When Capt. Jason Haag returned to California, after a tour in Afghanistan, his wife, Elizabeth, immediately knew something was wrong. Jason had completed three tours of combat duty, leading Marine Corps troops in fighting across Iraq and Afghanistan. Elizabeth and her three children were excitedly awaiting Jason's arrival at the Marine Corps Base Camp Pendleton, north of San Diego, after ten months of separation. But as the bus carrying the returning soldiers unloaded eager men and women at the drop-off point, Jason was the last to get off. He gave his wife and kids a stiff hug and barely looked them in the eyes. Elizabeth tells me that she had a friend with her taking photos of what they thought would be a happy family reunion. But she doesn't share those photos with anyone. She tells me, "The look on his face was just empty."

When the Haag family arrived home at dinnertime, things got worse. The kids were all over Jason, excited to have their father back. Without a word, he brushed them off, took a shower, and retreated to his bedroom. By nine thirty P.M. he raged at his family and punched a hole in the wall.

Over the next several weeks, Jason's outbursts continued as he unraveled. He stayed out at night, drinking. He stayed in on Saturdays and Sundays, drinking. He was still on active duty and was supposed to check in daily for work at the base, which he was able to do without betraying his true emotions. It was his family that received the brunt of Jason's hostility. Jason was physically home, but he had left his personality behind on the battlefield.

Elizabeth was desperate. She tried talking with Jason, but that got her nowhere. When he wasn't yelling, he retreated into that secure world of silence. She discussed him with the wives of the commanding and executive officers. That backfired. "They made it a domestic issue," she tells me, "The commanding officer told me we both needed counseling. 'You two got married too young and this is just a midlife crisis Jason is having.' None of them want this stigma on their battalion that something is wrong." The executive officer sat down with Jason and said, "You need to find Jesus. Your wife needs to find Jesus." Elizabeth and Jason were referred to the chaplain.

Seven months later, Jason received orders to report to the Marine Corps base in Quantico. When the family packed up and moved to Virginia, Elizabeth had high hopes that the new environment would be good for Jason. She had no idea that his new job would deliver the hard blow that toppled him over the ledge.

Jason ran the officer candidate class, training new recruits. Their enthusiasm was hard enough for his seasoned heart to handle. But the worse parts were the field exercises he conducted that simulated real-life combat. Jason turned increasingly violent at home. He screamed at his kids. He threw things about the house. He shoved Elizabeth against walls.

A major working with Jason saw his struggle and stepped in. With his help, mental health specialists saw Jason, diagnosed him with post-traumatic stress disorder (PTSD), and deemed him unfit for work. With suddenly nothing to do, Jason's physical and emotional health deteriorated even further. He fought daily pain from bone spurs in his foot and leg, where he had been shot during a firefight in the middle of a dusty village near Baghdad, Iraq. In addition to suffering crushing migraines from a traumatic brain injury, Jason experienced crippling anxiety, depression, and fierce flashbacks. Many nights, he woke up drenched in sweat, screaming.

The first mention of symptoms correlating with PTSD dates back to 480 B.C.E. Greek historian Herodotus wrote of a Spartan soldier who was so shaken by battle that he was nicknamed "the Trembler." The soldier hanged himself in shame. During the mid- and late 19th century, the presence of anxiety symptoms, including shortness of breath, heart palpitations, and chest pains, were called Soldier's Heart and Da Costa Syndrome (named after a physician who noted these abnormalities during the American Civil War).

World War I brought more widespread recognition of these clusters of unusual behaviors and signs. Doctors noticed something strange among many of the soldiers arriving at casualty clearing stations after they were exposed to exploding shells. Though they showed no physical wounds, they were clearly damaged. The soldiers appeared to be suffering from a state of shock. They exhibited signs of trembling (described as "rather like a jelly shaking") headaches, ringing in the ears, dizziness, poor concentration, confusion, memory loss, and sleep disturbances. In 1915, Capt. Charles Myers of the Royal Army Medical Corps called this "shell shock."

In World War II, combat stress reaction, also known as "battle fatigue," replaced the term *shell shock*. However, influential American military leaders, such as Gen. George S. Patton, did not believe battle fatigue was real. Many doctors who came after Myers were forced to brave their own battles to call attention to the affliction soldiers lived with long after their time in war.

It wasn't until 1980 that the APA introduced PTSD as a psychological and mental disability. The evidence gathered from returning soldiers from the Vietnam War was too strong to ignore. PTSD was added to the third edition of the *Diagnostic and Statistical Manual of Mental Disorders* (DSM-III). At first, the DSM classified *trauma* as an event existing "outside the range of usual human experience," and sufferers of PTSD included soldiers returning from war, holocaust survivors, and victims of sexual violence. In 1994, the definition of *trauma* was expanded. Events counting as traumatic theoretically included minor car accidents, natural disasters, and learning about the death of a loved one. Many scholars argued that this definition was too broad and would lead to overdiagnosis of PTSD.

The most recent iteration of the DSM (DSM-5, issued in 2013) narrowed the defining borders somewhat by stipulating that the criteria for PTSD include those "exposed to actual or threatened death, serious injury, or sexual violence." This may include not only people who directly experience the traumatic event, but also those who witness it, such as first responders and those who may hear about it from a close friend or relative exposed to the trauma. In the way of all psychiatric and medical diagnoses, the definition of PTSD is an artificial construct, based on what we know and how we view the world at the time. It will likely continue to change in the future.

For now, symptoms and signs of PTSD include experiencing flashbacks, nightmares, decreased interest in activities, irritability or aggression, difficulty sleeping, feeling isolated, exaggerated blame of oneself or another, and hypervigilance (a state of increased alertness). Anywhere between 11–30 percent of American military veterans will have experienced PTSD in their lifetimes. Roughly twenty American veterans, many diagnosed with PTSD, commit suicide every day.

⬤

Out of work, Jason Haag spent the next year and half drugged up on thirty-two medications, twelve of them narcotics. Jason spent most of his time shut away from the world and his family, in the basement of their house. He locked the door and blacked out the windows. "It was the perfect setup for him," Elizabeth tells me. "There was a bathroom and shower down there. No door to the outside. Basically, it was a bomb shelter."

All day and night, Jason stayed in the basement, eating, drinking, playing video games, and abusing Vicodin and Percocet. Jason would wait for his wife and kids to go to sleep before he'd go upstairs to get food, so that he wouldn't have to see or interact with them. He communicated with his wife through text messages when he needed something. In the meantime, Elizabeth deliberately lost contact with other military spouses she'd once been close to. She didn't want people asking her what was wrong. She began seeing a therapist, who urged her to leave Jason before he did further harm to her and the children. But she couldn't leave. "I knew if I left him, he would be dead."

Jason wasn't suicidal. But he didn't care whether or not he woke up the next morning. Many times, he was just a pill away from overdosing. He simply checked out of life. Just making it out to a convenience store once in a week was a good week.

Elizabeth was determined to find a way to help him. She dragged him from doctor to doctor. He tried anti-anxiety meds, one-on-one therapy, group therapy, massage therapy, chronotherapy (to treat depression through deliberate shifts in sleep cycles and light exposure), acupuncture, yoga—nothing eased Jason's symptoms. Elizabeth was at the point of giving up. One day, she gave him an ultimatum. "I'll give you one more chance," she said. "Try one more thing and if it doesn't work—if you don't make it work—I'm taking the kids and I'm out of here."

That one more thing worked.

⬤

I first meet Jason outside a Panera Bread restaurant at a strip mall in Fredericksburg, Virginia. He reminds me of the head of a volunteer rescue group I joined in high school that I had a huge crush on. Same quiet voice. Same cool demeanor. Similar tattoos coloring their pale arms. They even spit tobacco the same—long and languid. Today, though, I'm crushing on the German shepherd by Jason's side. With his alert, upright ears and knowing, brown eyes, he is an adorable dog.

After greeting the pooch and Jason, we sit at one of the outside tables. "Looking back, I think I had PTSD as far back as 2003, after my first combat tour," Jason tells me. "I was having nightmares. The day we crossed the border from Kuwait into Iraq, you crossed into the world of the unknown. It was the most dangerous time in my life, and it changed me forever."

"What happened?" I ask him.

"March 22, 2003," he states without hesitation. "That was the most significant day in my life. Cause that was the day that I saw someone get blown up. I shot at someone for the first time. I got shot at for the first time. I saw people die for the first time. I lost friends."

"Did you see civilians killed? Did that affect you as well?"

"Yeah. A dead person is a dead person is a dead person."

In my experience with patients with PTSD, they generally display two predominant dispositions: easily excitable or detached, often swinging between the two. Jason is showing the latter behavior, a common defense against trauma. He never looks me directly in the eyes as we speak, and his voice is flat. His apparent apathy belies an unspeakable inner turmoil of emotions. What Jason does not tell me, but what I later learn from Elizabeth, is that during combat in 2003, Jason shot and killed an Iraqi teenage soldier. "It took years before Jason told me," she says. "He took the life of a teenage boy. He has children of his own and he lived in such a world of guilt. He cannot get over it."

Although the hurt started in 2003, Jason's breaking point occurred in 2010 after his last tour in Afghanistan.

"Why then?" I ask him.

He scratches his shaved head and shrugs. "I think it's all a cumulative effect. I think it's how it is with a lot of our troops as it just slowly builds and builds and builds and builds."

As a man walks by our table, the German shepherd stiffens and lifts his head off Jason's feet. The dog watches the man until he's a good distance away before relaxing again. Jason reaches down and caresses the dog. "I wasn't really a dog person growing up," he says. "I'd actually been bit by a dog a couple of different times. But, you know, the great thing about being blown up is that you don't remember a lot. So, it wasn't really seared in my mind." He nods at the dog. "Axel saved me."

Elizabeth's ultimatum was a wake-up call for Jason. The next day, he intercepted his usually reserved next-door neighbor as he was checking his mail. The neighbor was also a Marine veteran who had PTSD and who lived with a service dog. Jason mentioned the dog and asked his neighbor, "Does that work?"

The response was a grunt. Yes.

Jason googled the use of service dogs and found out about K9s for Warriors, a nonprofit organization that pairs dogs with military veterans who have PTSD. The dogs are rescued from high-kill shelters and undergo an evaluation period for their fitness and temperament as service dogs. If they fail this test, they are adopted out to loving homes. If they pass, they are matched with a vet during a three-week bonding and training session at the organization's Florida campus.

Because the demand for therapy dogs for PTSD sufferers is so high, Jason had to wait for seven months before he was paired with Axel. "I met Axel on a Sunday," Jason tells me. "On Monday morning we were out just everywhere. We went to a Chili's, a Home Depot, a Target, the beach, a park—and I mean I hadn't even been to the laundromat or dry cleaner in a year and a half. With Axel, I went to all those different places in one day." After graduating from the training, during which time Jason learned how to partner with Axel, they boarded a plane for home. Accompanied by Axel, Jason attended his son's lacrosse game, the first game he'd watched in over a year. With Axel by his side, the sharp sting of Jason's fears softened.

⸙

Studies have shown that we generally perceive scenarios containing animals as more friendly, relaxing, cooperative, constructive, safe, and humorous. People in these scenes are also viewed as being less tense, less dangerous, happier, healthier, and wiser than people in scenarios without animals. Stressful places like hospitals, offices, schools, and, lately, airports are taking advantage of the calming effects of animals. Just having an animal nearby makes the world a little less threatening, a little friendlier, even for those trained to fight.

One of the first documented therapeutic uses of animals among US soldiers took place during World War II. In 1944, Cpl. Bill Wynne came upon a stray dog while stationed in New Guinea. One of Wynne's tentmates found the little underfed and scrawny Yorkshire terrier in an abandoned foxhole on the side of the road. Wynne adopted the dog, named her Smoky, and for the next year and half they together survived air raids, typhoons, and twelve combat missions.

When Wynne caught dengue fever, he noticed how healing Smoky could be, not just for himself, but also for other soldiers. While he was recuperating at a hospital, Wynne's friends brought Smoky to visit him. Nurses were charmed by Smoky and asked to take her to visit other patients. Smoky spent nights sleeping with Wynne and days being carried by nurses from patient to patient to help cheer them. Patients were especially fond of the antics and tricks Smoky learned, like playing dead and riding a scooter. Pretty soon, word spread and Smoky and Wynne were invited to other hospitals.

Smoky was not the only animal who helped heal soldiers. Patients at the Army Air Corps Convalescent Hospital in Pawling, New York, were encouraged to work with animals as part of a program to help soldiers recover from the effects of "operational fatigue," an acute, short-term condition that is similar to PTSD. The soldiers benefitted from the "healing powers" of a range of animals, including horses, cows, pigs, chickens, turtles, snakes, and frogs.

Currently, only half of veterans with PTSD seek healthcare. This number is probably lower for active duty personnel, as many are concerned about the stigma of being labeled with PTSD. Among veterans who do seek help, a mere 40 percent substantially improve. That means only one-fifth of all veterans see significant reductions in the frequency, intensity, and duration of their PTSD symptoms.

Animals may provide the therapy these veterans lack. In addition to their calming effects, animals assist veterans by demanding care. Domesticated animals are dependent on someone for food, grooming, and, often, exercise. For former soldiers troubled by recurring thoughts of a traumatizing experience, it's helpful to have an animal nearby. The animals force the sufferers to shift their focus away from themselves and their demons and attend to the animals' needs.

Studies on those with PTSD find that a variety of animals, including pigs, sheep, chickens, opossums, horses, dogs, and cats, reduce depression and PTSD severity. In one study, psychologists noted an 82 percent reduction in symptoms. Many of the patients were able to cut back their need for medications. In one particular case, interacting with a dog for just one week enabled a patient to decrease the amount of anxiety and sleep medications by half. It's not clear if PTSD sufferers experience long-term benefits by being with animals, but there is now a concerted effort to answer this and other questions about animal assistance. The Veterans Administration is funding new studies to explore the effects animals have on a soldier's mental health.

◈

Axel and Jason have been together for more than three years now. Jason rarely leaves his house without Axel. Simply having him nearby helps Jason feel more secure. "You can see him right now," Jason tells me. "He watches the door and things like that for me all the time. He's gotten up a couple times to let me know people are going into that store so I don't get spooked."

Axel pulls Jason out of flashbacks, nightmares, and panic attacks by gently biting and licking his arms. "If I'm starting to get distressed, he'll come up to me and start pushing on me and he'll start acting like he's in distress." Jason chuckles. "I think it's a trick. He knows it will get me to pet him and comfort him. And that ends up calming me." With Axel's help, Jason is slowly reintegrating back into society.

I ask Jason how his wife felt when he brought Axel home from Florida.

He smiles. "She was jealous."

"I was jealous," Elizabeth confirms when I later ask her the same question. "Partly. I mean, I've known Jason since middle school and we've been best friends since high school. It's so frustrating to me that we've been together for so many years, and I couldn't take his illness away. And then a cute fluffy dog with big ears comes and makes it not all better, but a lot better."

"But mostly," she adds, "I was just so grateful. My husband is back. Axel is part of our family. My kids and I just love Axel. We just love him."

When Axel was adopted by K9s for Warriors, he was two days away from being euthanized at an animal shelter. "He was abused, badly," Jason tells me. "He was nine months old and only weighed 40 pounds. Every single one of his ribs was showing." On his cell phone, Jason shows me pictures of Axel at the time. "That's his face the day that he was brought back from the shelter." Despite his emaciated body, Axel's face doesn't look dejected. He looks hopeful.

"You can't tell me that he doesn't know that his life was just saved," Jason tells me as he expands his thoughts to all dogs and veterans. "And that bond between the dog and the vet is a little bit more because they're saving each other."

Axel clearly helps as an emotional guard dog by alerting Jason to potential threats and reducing his anxiety. But their relationship runs deeper. Animals provide support simply by the companionship they provide. Although, given our long history of domesticating dogs, they might seem the obvious choice when you need a healing boost, the mental benefits we experience through animals is not limited to dogs. Today, cats, horses, goats, pigs, rabbits, and even turkeys give emotional support not only to veterans but also to rape and child-abuse survivors, first responders, and people suffering from general anxiety and depression.

Psychologist Andrea Beetz proposes that oxytocin plays a key role in many of the beneficial effects we see through contact with animals. Produced as a hormone in the hypothalamus in our brains, oxytocin was classically associated with stimulating labor contractions and milk production in new mothers. Oxytocin promotes maternal care in animals and humans alike. In the past few decades, though, studies on oxytocin have suggested that it has more far-reaching effects.

Oxytocin circulates in both men and women. The list of what oxytocin has been found to do is long. It lowers heart rate and stress hormones and increases social interaction, generosity, bonding, and attachment. It also improves trust and decreases aggression, fear, and hyperarousal—countering the symptoms of PTSD. In an article for the APA, journalist Tori DeAngelis stated: "If hormones could win popularity contests, oxytocin might well be queen of the day." It facilitates our most positive and prosocial emotions and behaviors. Oxytocin helps us feel happy.

In a famous study led by neuroeconomist Paul Zak, half of the participants inhaled an oxytocin spray while the other half received a placebo. All the participants were then asked to decide how to split a sum of money with a stranger. Those who received the hormone offered the strangers 80 percent more money than those who received the placebo. The findings of this study confirmed previous findings by Zak and others that oxytocin fosters empathy and altruism.

In further studies, Zak and his colleagues found that oxytocin increases after people engage in social activities. The level of increase depends on the type of interaction and the closeness to the person you are interacting with. Zak wrote, "Studies showed that when humans engage in social activities with each other, oxytocin levels typically increase between 10 percent and 50 percent. The change in oxytocin, measured in blood, indexes the strength of the relationship between people. When your little daughter runs to hug you, your oxytocin could increase 100 percent. When a stranger shakes your hand, it might be 5 or 10 percent. If the stranger shaking your hand is attractive, oxytocin might increase 50 percent." Not only does oxytocin facilitate social behavior, it is also affected by such exchanges through a positive feedback loop. The more meaningful your social interaction with another, the more oxytocin is released.

Beetz and her colleagues found that many of the beneficial effects of oxytocin overlap with those produced by animal companionship. Two researchers from South Africa were among the first to test what biochemical changes occur after interactions with animals. They found increases in not only oxytocin but also other chemicals that make us feel good—endorphins, dopamine, and prolactin—in the bloodstream of both dogs and humans after five to twenty-four minutes of stroking a dog. The positive effect of this interaction, then, was mutual. Both dogs and humans benefited. This study also indicates that it's not likely that a single chemical like oxytocin can fully explain the human-animal bond.

Brain imaging reveals that the caudate, a section of the brain that lies between the cortex and the brainstem, activates in dogs similarly in response to hand signals indicating food and to the smells of familiar humans. The caudate is rich in receptors for dopamine. In humans, the caudate activates to pleasurable things. The comparable results in dogs suggest that they experience positive emotions around the people they know. And it's likely that other animals experience similar boosts in positive chemicals around the people with whom they bond.

Paul Zak jumped on the human-animal bond. He tested if oxytocin increases when humans engage with animals. In his larger study, neither dogs nor cats consistently increased oxytocin in humans. However, in a small-scale experiment, Zak found that oxytocin increases when different animals interact with one another, suggesting it facilitates interspecies friendships. Zak took blood samples from a dog and a goat, who regularly played with each other. He wrote, "Their play involved chasing each other, jumping towards each other, and engaging in simulated fighting (baring teeth and snarling)." Fifteen minutes after play, oxytocin increased 48 percent in the dog, suggesting that the dog was quite attached to the goat and viewed him as a friend. "More striking was the goat's reaction to the dog," Zak wrote. "It had a 210 percent increase in oxytocin. At that level of increase . . . we essentially found that the goat might have been in love with the dog. The only time I have seen such a surge in oxytocin in humans is when someone sees their loved one, is romantically attracted to someone, or is shown an enormous kindness."

Zak continues: "That animals of different species induce oxytocin release in each other suggests that they, like us, may be capable of love. It is quite possible that Fido and Boots may feel the same way about you as you do about them. You can even call it love."

And here is where we get to the important part of what the studies on the human-animal bond are pointing to. Not everyone who interacts with animals experiences the physical and mental boosts referred to earlier. It appears that, as with social relations among humans, the types of interactions between humans and other animals that will cause the most benefit are those that occur when we feel a sense of connection, empathy, and love for the animal—and, often, vice versa. People who are frightened of, indifferent to, or feel antipathy toward an animal will not experience that boost in oxytocin or any other beneficial effect. It is the mutual love and bonding between a human and an animal that fosters the most benefit. The stronger the bond, the greater the benefit.

Less than two months after my initial meeting with Jason Haag, I attend the K9s for Warriors annual gala at the Hamilton Live in downtown Washington, DC. In a room full of generals and colonels, TV personalities, military vets and families, Axel steals the show. On stage, he looks spiffy with a red-checkered tie around his neck. Jason is dressed in a navy suit and yellow bow tie. As I watch Jason and Axel together, I notice how strong their empathetic bond is for each other. When we experience empathy, we don't just feel it mentally. We process it with our bodies too. When two individuals share empathy, they not only subconsciously orient their emotions and moods to each other, but also their body movements. Axel's and Jason's bodies align. When Jason's head turns toward somewhere offstage, so does Axel's. They move almost in sync.

As Jason stands on the stage, looking a little nervous, he caresses Axel's ears. Then he announces to the room, "On Sunday, three new warriors will be going to K9 school. I served with them, and they are my friends." He goes silent and chokes up. The room hushes as the audience respectfully waits until he finds his voice.

"When they graduate . . . their lives will be changed forever."

THREE

Humanizing Ourselves

Two security guards woke up forty of Ohio's most dangerous men. On this cold morning in January 1977, the men were sleeping in the large, single dormitory of Ward 18 at the Lima State Hospital for the Criminally Insane. After the guards lined the inmates into a single file, they escorted them into the dining hall for breakfast. Thirty minutes later, the guards led the men back to their ward. That's when about ten of them jumped the guards and tied them up before they had a chance to reach a phone. The inmates then waited for the A.M. shift nurse who was expected to bring their anti-psychotic medications, Thorazine and Stelazine, within the hour. The men planned to take the nurse hostage and escape.

⌇

I walk past a security guard and greet twenty gentle souls. On this warm afternoon in October 2015, a chorus of meows, some deep and rumbling, some tinny and piercing, greets me. Cats! About ten cats rush up to say hello to me. Others sit or lie in different positions of repose, cautiously eyeing me. In this sunlit room, cats relax on the built-in floor-to-ceiling scratching posts, cat beds, climbing structures, and walkways. Orange cats, tabbies, calicos, black and white, long- and short-haired, big and small. Ironically, these cats have been brought to this maximum-security state prison to get a little freedom. They are just a few of the many critters living in prisons throughout the country helping inmates get a second chance.

The Pendleton Correctional Facility in Indiana opened its cat sanctuary in March 2015, thanks to Michelle Rains, an executive assistant and creator of FORWARD. The reformation part of the full name of the program—Felines and Offenders Rehabilitation With Affection, Reformation and Dedication—sounds a bit puritanical, yet Michelle is anything but. She's open and easy to chat with. The Animal Protection League brings in the cats from a shelter they run. There, the cats were caged. Here, they are free to roam about the sanctuary's two window-filled rooms and interact at will with people. Prison staff or the inmates' families can adopt the cats.

Before visiting the sanctuary, Michelle first takes me into a conference room to meet one of the inmates, Daniel, who works at the sanctuary. My initial thought upon seeing Daniel is that he's just a kid. He's twenty-three years old, though he looks sixteen. Pale skinned with ginger hair and eyebrows and wearing tan overalls, he's so soft spoken, I can barely hear him say hello when we are introduced.

The cats in the sanctuary are Daniel's pride and joy. "I love animals," he says almost immediately and goes into a long explanation. I have to lean in to hear him. "Growing up, we always had animals. You know, my mom and grandma and me all lived together under one roof for a while and we always had dogs and cats and one time we had a couple pigs. I don't know. My mom always worked a lot cause she's a single mom. And she married lots of times. And we moved around from house to house depending on who she was married to at the time. She wasn't very nice, and I had so many different stepdads. It didn't matter how bad things were, I'd always have the animals to hold and pet and take care of. They were a comfort, and I wasn't getting much affection anywhere else but from them. I'd always have affection as long as the animals were around."

When Daniel heard from another inmate that the cat sanctuary was being built, he put in a request to work there. "I talked to my old boss in the paint shop, cause she knows I love animals, because we talked about them," he says, "She told Miss Rains I'm a good worker." The inmates work at the prison for small change, which they use to buy snacks, books, magazines, soaps, shampoos, and toothpaste. Daniel was making twenty-five cents an hour at the paint shop. The pay for working at the sanctuary is fifteen cents per hour. But Daniel still jumped at the opportunity to care for the cats. "I would have done it for free."

Despite Daniel's eagerness, Michelle needed convincing to hire him. "I'm gonna be totally honest with you," she tells me. "I've told Daniel this before." She nods toward him. "I'm very selective on who I allow to go in there. This was going to have to be something where the guys that work in there have to put the cats before themselves. I don't like reading people's pasts, okay? Because they've been judged by somebody else. That's not my job." Michelle, however, needed to know about the inmates' pasts as part of a screening process to determine if she could trust them to take care of the cats and not harm them. "So I looked him up," Michelle continues. "I read the case and at first I was like, I can't do that."

I turn to Daniel, who sits silently with his head turned downward and his hands on his lap. "Can I ask what brought you here to prison?" I ask.

"I'm in here for the murder of my brother."

Oh. I try not to let the surprise show on my face. Given Daniel's demeanor, I assumed he was in here for something . . . less bad. "What happened?" I ask him. "Was there a fight?"

Not exactly. "It was like, we were just wrestling around and next thing you know it was like I was watching myself do it. I guess I was like . . . choking him."

Daniel was seventeen years old when he killed his ten-year-old stepbrother with seemingly no provocation. However, one of Daniel's many stepfathers allegedly raped him at the age of eight, and Daniel may have suffered from a mental illness. The ragged scars across his left wrist sketch a failed suicide attempt.

"Honestly I don't know why I killed him," Daniel says. "I don't know." He readily admitted to murdering his brother and asked for the death penalty, which was denied. Instead, he is serving a life sentence with no parole.

Michelle weighs in, "It sounded like everything was just so spontaneous, you know? So when I read his history, I'm thinking, How can I trust somebody like that?"

The following week, Daniel's boss pleaded with Michelle on the young inmate's behalf. "She said he is the best worker," Michelle tells me. "She said Daniel works hard. He is the most polite kid you will ever meet. She said just give him a try. So I talked to him and I told him you have once chance. And that was the best choice that I made for the whole sanctuary."

It might have also been the best choice Michelle could have made for Daniel. When Michelle, Daniel, and I enter the cat sanctuary, Daniel is transformed. No longer the nervous, shy boy, he now exudes excitement and confidence as he shows me around the rooms. As the cats get under our feet, Daniel lights up and smiles. He picks up a gray cat who rests comfortably on his shoulders, dainty feet dangling, as though they are old pals. Daniel tickles his belly. "This is Boomer," he says to me as Boomer purrs and licks Daniel's face. "He likes to climb on my shoulders as I walk around, and when he gets down, he likes to sit in my lap. And that little black-and-white one you're holding"—he nods to the kitten in my arms—"every time I'm trying to sweep or do something, she'll stand on her hind legs and wrap her paws around my leg and meow for me to pick her up or to pet her." I wince as the kitten kneads his tiny, sharp claws into my arms.

Except for the sight of furry rumps all around and the sounds of their meows, you would not know that so many cats live here. The place smells fresh. I can see why. Another inmate, Larry, meticulously cleans out the litter boxes and sweeps the floor. He's big and amiable. As he cleans, he periodically scoops up a different cat into his arms and hugs her without a hint of reserve.

"Daniel and Larry are the two best workers I have," Michelle says. "They are excellent with the cats. They learned their personalities; they know what they like, what they don't like. They put the cats before themselves. There is a security camera in here, and I pop it on every once in a while to make sure everything's going okay, and you'll see Daniel either working—he's picking up chairs, he's cleaning behind everything—or sitting down doing paperwork. There's always a cat on him."

I put down the kitten and pick up a large orange cat, who stretches his heavy paws on my legs, demanding my attention. The cat curls back his lips and smears his wet gums against my neck, leaving spittle. "And you know," Michelle continues, over the cat's loud purr, "he's just right there and loving on the cats and you don't see a prisoner. You see a kid."

Daniel takes me into a small adjoining room, which holds supplies and medicines. Three cats follow us. He picks up a notebook and flips the pages for me, showing me his neat and organized handwriting. Names of the cats run down one side and, on the other side of each page, notes are jotted down by date. "I write down how each cat is doing every day. If he throws up. If he has a rash. When they got their meds. It's my job to take care of them. They can't go out and get their own food and they can't do everything for themselves."

Daniel closes the logbook, places it on the table, and turns to me. "If anyone asks what I'm in here for, I'm not going to lie. I did it and I deserve what I get. It's just . . . I guess growing up . . . I don't trust too many people. Some days here are harder for me than others. But these cats are the reason I get up. I know I'm helping them. To come here every day and see the cats and they're happy to see you . . . they're my little babies."

Inmates like Daniel socialize the cats and, once one is adopted out, another is brought in. In return, the cats provide the only physical contact and affection many of the inmates receive. Other inmates, hearing about the sanctuary, flood Michelle with requests to work there.

It took Michelle almost ten years to get approval for the sanctuary. Besides concerns over the safety of the animals, a common argument made against allowing animals on prison grounds is that inmates, especially those who have committed the most violent crimes like Daniel, aren't worthy of the affection they would receive from animals. It's a privilege they don't deserve, administrators and prison staff often say. But slowly the tide is turning. In addition to acknowledging the improved level of care and attention the animals get here compared to overcrowded shelters, administrators can't deny the change that's occurring in prisoners across the country who have contact with animals. Researchers are now asking: Can animals help redeem people considered beyond repair?

To answer this question, it helps to go back in time to the first successful animal therapy program in a US prison and to the man who started it all.

⌘

An excerpt from a 1980 article in *Cats Magazine* titled "Tom: A Cat and His Patients" begins:

> *A male cat of questionable lineage was discovered on a Thursday evening almost two years ago in some shrubbery outside a shopping mall in Lima, Ohio. It was obvious to the finder that the cat had not eaten for several days, but after some degree of protest the derelict was successfully placed in a car and taken to the nearest grocery store, where a supply of cat food was purchased. The food was ravished by the semi-wild, emaciated cat. After being allowed to eat his fill, the cat was taken to the greenhouse of the Lima State Hospital for the Criminally Insane, which was known to be looking for a cat.*

The cat, named Tom, was one of a menagerie of animals who resided at the Lima State Hospital as part of an unprecedented animal therapy program, which began in 1975. Social worker David Lee's program was the first of its kind. Its success was so astounding that it transformed not only the lives of the inmates but also the image of the hospital which, I would soon learn, was one of the most scandal-plagued penal institutions in the country.

&

I knew I would like David Lee the instant I met him. So did my husband. A former Navy mechanic and ex-hunter, Patrick is tall and broad-shouldered and has a big head, literally. You wouldn't think that a West Virginia boy and a Pakistani girl would have much in common. But among the many things we share is our love for *Die Hard*, animals, and road trips. Hopping into Patrick's pickup truck, we cheerfully drove nine hours from Gaithersburg, Maryland, to Lima, Ohio.

David looks like a cross between an older hippie and Noah (or maybe that's the same look). His long, white locks just seem to flow all biblical like. At seventy-three years old, he is tall, lean, and spry. And no wonder. On his five-acre lot, David spends his days from morning till night feeding, watering, and caring for three dogs, four billy goats, five deer, five swans, seven peacocks, ten guinea hens, thirteen cats, twenty llamas, and so many chickens that even David can't keep track of them. Many of them are senior citizens, and David keeps adding more animals to his ark out of the goodness of his heart. Unwanted, injured, and retired animals find their way to his home. "It's like running an old folk's home here," he tells us as he leads Patrick and me around his property, introducing us to the various animals.

"Fatty!" David yells, "Fatty, here girl!" A rather rotund deer trots out from behind a wood shed and nudges her head against his hand. "This is Fatty. I just like petting this stupid, fat deer," he says with affection. "I just like the touch and I think that was the way with the guys on the ward."

"Do you name all the animals?" Patrick asks, as he pets a baby llama who looks like a cross between an Ewok and a Wookiee.

"I had better names at one time. But now with my macular degeneration, I just name them Fatty, Brownie, Skinny, Whitey . . . I can't see well. All I see when I look at you is a vague impression of a face."

"Well then," Patrick replies, "I must tell you I'm extremely handsome. Sort of a debonair look like Cary Grant or Gregory Peck."

David erupts into one of the heartiest laughs I have ever heard. That's the thing about David. He's so jolly and optimistic; you can't help but be the same around him. I can see how he would have made a great social worker.

David then introduces us to his flock of chickens. He hands us raisin bread to feed them, which apparently is a real treat. One by one they come out of various outhouses and sheds as they figure out what we are doing. One ridiculously cute chicken with a Muppet mop on her head darts out so fast and eagerly, I'm afraid she will crash into the nearby tree.

After we meet and feed the assembly of animals, David takes us into his garage. With vintage metal signs advertising Coke, Marlboro, and Captain Morgan and decorating the walls, it's a collector's dream. A four-stop traffic light stands in one corner and a still-working railway signal hoots its alarm bells every time a cat walks by. David sifts through stacks of dusty, cobweb-covered, cardboard boxes. "I have all my stuff here, somewhere. Now where is it? It has photos of my days at Lima." While he searches, I watch the chickens, peacocks, and cats who freely walk in and out of the garage. "Don't tell my wife, Kaye." I hear David's voice coming from behind a precariously high stack. "She doesn't like the animals coming in here and messing everything up. Aaah!" He grunts, then walks over to me and dumps in my lap a dubious-looking box. It smells of cat pee. Dried-up chicken droppings, some kind of animal pellets, and grime coat the top layer of photos, administrative reports, and scrapbooks from David's almost thirty years at Lima State Hospital. Among the paraphernalia is an impressive black-and-white aerial photo of the institution.

First known as the Lima State Hospital for the Criminally Insane, the institution was the stuff of horror movies. The second-largest poured-concrete building in the world (after the Pentagon), the hospital opened its doors in 1915 and was, at times during its ninety years of operation, the world's largest institution for the criminally insane. Any state prisoner, no matter his or her crime, who became violently, mentally ill or was deemed insane was sent to the hospital. Lima State Hospital also took patients from other hospitals who were too dangerous to handle. Over time, Lima State became known as the dumping ground for Ohio's most toxic patients. Townsfolk referred to the facility as the end of the line from which few ever returned.

⌘

David, Patrick, and I head out to the site of Lima State Hospital. In 1908, construction began for this $2.1 million state-of-the-art hospital. Situated on 628 acres, the massive institution consists of fourteen separate buildings grouped like a rectangle around a large, football field–size courtyard. An enclosed walkway, which provides access to the buildings, surrounds the courtyard. Ten smaller courtyards fit between the individual buildings.

The institution's doors closed in 2004. David has not been back here since he retired in 1991. He's amazed at the transformation. Broken windows mar the three-story brick buildings. Overgrown trees, bushes, and rank weeds block first-floor windows. Rampant vines have taken over the coiled, razor-wire fence that surrounds the institution. "Back in the day, there were no trees or plantings," David tells us. "Nothing. There was absolutely not a single tree on the premises. Just grass. Those vines there? They wouldn't have been allowed. A guy could easily climb up one, and up and over the fence he goes."

David shakes his head at the ruin before us. "There were twenty-four units or wards and each functioned like a miniprison. They each had their own sleeping areas, day halls, and bathrooms. You

see the second-story room there?" He points to the rounded section at the end of a building that is surrounded on all sides by large
windows. "Those were the day halls. Every ward has the same day
hall. A big corridor would connect it to the giant dormitory off to
the left and to the nurse's station to the right." A few lucky inmates
had their own cells; most slept in large sleeping rooms. "The dor-
mitories would sleep twenty, thirty, forty people."

It's hard to believe that this massive collection of sturdy, brick
buildings was simply abandoned after the institution closed down.
It was never refitted for any other purpose, as though the people of
Lima wanted to shut out any reminder of its haunted past. Now, the
buildings' only occupants are birds, mice, and raccoons—animals
who find shelter and bring life to an otherwise empty place. Perhaps, given the role animals played here in the past, that's fitting.

In an isolated place near the railroad tracks, Patrick, David, and I
count 502 graves. Deceased inmates who were unclaimed by family
are buried here. On each grave sits a squat, concrete marker, num-
bered by order of burial, and a small, white cross with a first initial
and last name. No epitaph. No date of death. Like the institution
itself, the cemetery is a forsaken place. The dead were deprived of
even their full names.

❧

The institution admitted its first patients on July 10, 1915. Transferred
from the Cleveland State Hospital, the prisoners arrived by train
and then marched the three miles from the train station to their
new facility in shackles and handcuffs. Within one year, the institution housed 1,166 patients, most of them male. Among the patients
were farmers and firemen, merchants and miners, blacksmiths
and butchers, peddlers and painters, cooks and clerks, waiters and
weavers, teachers and teamsters. Once admitted to the hospital,
a patient would be measured, weighed, photographed, given a
physical examination by a psychiatrist, ordered to give urine and
blood specimens, stripped, examined for "vermin," and bathed.

In its early years, the institution's inmates worked in the bakery, kitchen, laundry, ice plant, paint department, sewing room, tailor shop, plumbing shop, machine shop, mattress shop, carpentry shop, butcher shop, and dairy barn. On nearly 300 acres, inmates grew corn, wheat, hay, oats, and potatoes. Pastures were fenced, fields were sowed, barns were built. The institution generated and supplied its own electricity and heat. It maintained its own water treatment plant and sewage disposal. And the place boasted its own morgue.

The institution was a hulking concrete fortress meant to be a self-sufficient minicity. Citizens of Lima slept safely at night, knowing that dangerous criminals were securely tucked away. They snored soundly, believing that these poor, mentally ill men and women lived in "one of the most modern and best-equipped institutions of its kind" and received the best care the nation could offer. The truth turned out to be very different.

After it first opened, rumors about the institution's cruelty and experiments crept around dark corners, echoed down hollow halls, slithered under locked doors, and sought willing ears. Like David's. Because he had keys to most of the facility, David snuck into the medical records room and read old files. He also explored the cellar's marathon of tunnels, sometimes finding empty rooms, sometimes coming upon dead ends. The cellar's hospital morgue contained an ice-block drop to store bodies and the bomb shelter was complete with water drums and dried food. One of the rooms, David was told by an older employee, was the experimental dog lab. The Lima dog warden was said to have "donated" dogs to the hospital. In the windowless basement room, doctors transplanted organs from dog to dog after debarking them, a common procedure whereby experimenters remove sections of a dog's vocal cords to silence them. When word leaked out about the dog lab in the early 1960s, it was stopped. But other experiments continued on another vulnerable group—the patients themselves.

There was supposedly a hydro room deep underground. In older medical files, David read of hydrotherapy conducted on psychotic patients. "The files described strapping patients into a harness and lowering them into a vat of hot, hot water," he tells me. "Then they would be quickly hoisted up and then lowered into a vat of ice-cold water." The doctors' goal was to induce a convulsion, which they believed would help the patients become less psychotic and calmer.

Another experimental program was insulin shock therapy. In 1937, the institution's superintendent waxed poetic to reporters about the therapy's remarkable ability to "cure" patients. Psychiatrists injected patients with increasingly higher doses of insulin, which sharply dropped their blood sugar levels, to induce comas and convulsions. The medical staff put patients into daily comas over several weeks at a time, believing that a physiologic shock would control mental illness symptoms, especially among schizophrenics. (This was never proven and it later fell into disfavor by psychiatrists when antipsychotic drugs were developed.)

These experimental procedures occurred in part due to the fact that oversight of patients fell mostly to the ward's guards (also called attendants). David tells me the wards functioned independently and were essentially run by the guards. "They were in charge of the patients. All day. Every day. They took the patients to their meals. Took care of discipline. They had full control."

According to David, medications were used mostly to control the patients if they got out of hand. The attendants advised the doctors on how to treat the patients. "They loved suggesting shock treatment." Tuesdays were shock days. David often watched with dismay as doctors strapped down up to sixty patients for shock therapy on a single day. "The patients' convulsions during shock would lead to amnesia and they would be lethargic and docile for two days after."

Cruelty at the institution was routine. So were drudgery, humiliation, and degradation. Much of the staff believed these were just retributions against rapists, armed robbers, murderers, and child abusers. There was a profound lack of empathy for the very people staff members were supposed to help. They not only denied patients their rights and dignity but also their identities. As we'll see later in the book, stripping the identity of another, whether human or nonhuman, is a common psychological mechanism used to defend the indefensible.

"The doctors didn't get to know the patients," David says. "Other than the shock treatments, they saw the patients only once a year to evaluate whether they could be transferred out of the hospital. The psychology and social departments basically just wrote reports. They all stayed up front in the admin section. No one ever visited the patient wards."

David was an exception. Dressed in jeans and T-shirts, he spent most of his days in the patient wards, getting to know the inmates. By doing so, he saw things that were otherwise hidden. During one of his visits with a patient named Herman, David saw him take out a shoebox from under his bed, open the lid, and talk to what looked like an empty box. When David peered closely, he saw a cockroach looking up with his antennas twitching at him. "Herman was raising the cockroach," David says. "He told me that the roach was his best friend."

David didn't think much further about Herman's cockroach until months later, when three patients in a different ward got caught sneaking bread back from the dining hall. The bread wasn't for them, but for a hurt sparrow they found on a window ledge. They adopted the bird and hid him in a broom closet while they tried to nurse him back to health.

With these three men, David witnessed the innate, human desire to connect with other species. The pull was so strong that men broke the rules and risked punishment in an already brutal institution to care for another creature. David also noticed something else. This ward housed the facility's most depressed and noncommunicative patients. For the first time, the three patients caring for the bird acted like a group. They talked about the bird and worked together. "When I saw this, I thought, *Wow, they're actually getting along!*" David says. The men found companionship not only with the bird but also with one another.

David recalled how his own dogs were so important in his life and he wondered if animals could be a positive influence on more patients. But he didn't have a chance to test his theory, at least not for several more years.

❧

Back in Arlington, Virginia, classmates bullied me mercilessly. It might not have helped that at the beginning of the school year, I would smell the fresh, crisp pages of my textbooks, anticipating what new things I was going to learn. Or that I always wore a frown, told other kids that the free breakfasts the school gave me made me feel special, and dumpster dived for treasures in front of the frilly skirted girls, ribbons in their hair and with hands so soft. It probably didn't help that I let other kids hear me call to the sky and tell any aliens out there that if they wanted to come visit, well, they could just take me back with them, if they wouldn't mind.

It certainly didn't help that I preferred the company of a dog to all other people, even my sisters at times. It turns out that's not unusual. When faced with adversity, children often turn to their animals for support rather than to their own siblings, even when they know that the animals don't understand what they are saying. Sylvester ran with me when I fled the apartment. Sylvester put his right paw on my lap when I tattled to him. Sylvester never barked back at me to tell me I was lying.

Ironically, Sylvester was the catalyst that made school life a little easier for me. Sylvester followed me almost daily when I walked the mile and half to school. My grandparents (before they knew better) would let Sylvester out early in the mornings and he would wait for me by the entrance of my apartment building. When I trekked to school, Sylvester walked beside me as though it was the most natural thing to do. "Sylvester," I would yell. "Go back! Go home!" I would point in the direction back home and try to shoo him, as I feared he would get lost or hit by a car. But he just perked his ears and woofed at me as though I was kidding. He wasn't going to leave my side. When we reached school, Sylvester would turn back home, as though his duty with me was done for the morning.

One day, Sylvester followed me right through the school's double doors. As I waited for my first class to begin, Sylvester raced down the halls, touching his wet nose from kid to kid as though high-fiving them. And the other kids simply loved Sylvester! They ran with him and cheered him every time he dashed into a classroom. That was the most exciting thing to happen at the school in a long time.

The fun ended when class started. I left Sylvester wandering the halls, not knowing what to do, hoping he would make his way out before the teachers, or worse yet, the principal, saw him. But the principal did see him and traced him back to me. When the principal walked into my class and asked me in front of the other students to help him get Sylvester out, I expected him to be angry. Instead, he was smiling.

Although it was no magic bullet, this event helped change things for me bit by bit at school. Other kids became friendlier to me. I was the girl who brought her wonderful dog to school—and got away with it.

Harry Truman famously said, "If you want a friend in Washington, get a dog!" Actually, there is much dispute whether he ever uttered those words. But I bet when you just read his supposed quote, you instinctively agreed with it, didn't you? The quote has a double meaning. Animals might be the only friendly faces in the man-eat-man world of politics. Animals also connect us with one another. They make us more likeable. In the past 150 years, all the US presidents brought animal companions with them to the White House, with the exception of Donald Trump.

Recent studies have shed light on how animals act as social lubricants. Researchers found that strangers were more likely to approach and start friendly conversations with people in wheelchairs if they had animals with them. Animals are icebreakers. They can bring the most unlikely people together for a shared experience, much like David saw with the inmates taking care of the bird who, up until that point, had barely uttered a word to one another.

Animals melt the glaciers people build around themselves. A study of more than 2,500 people in the United States and in Australia found that those with companion animals were much more likely to get to know their neighbors and form friendships than people without animals. On our walks through our neighborhood, Patrick has to stop every time we come across a neighbor with a dog. This inevitably leads us to converse with the neighbors rather than just say a quick hello. A half-hour walk easily becomes an hour. Patrick will say to the dogs, "What a cute doggie! What a pretty boy! Are you having a good walk?" One investigator refers to this as "triangulation" in which a person addresses the animal instead of the human. We do this because animals are safe and won't quickly reject us. As a result, animals allow us to strip our social inhibitions. Patrick often gets down on the ground and rolls around with the dogs we meet. He's a friendly guy, but I can assure you this is not something he would do with a human neighbor, even if that neighbor was game.

Get on the ground, chat animals up, play with them—and you have some happy animals and more than a few happy spouses. Or if you are looking to get a date, take an animal with you. In 2008, a male researcher was able to get women's phone numbers 28 percent of the time when he had a dog with him as opposed to only 9 percent without a dog.

Animals connect us with one another. Part of the reason is that we like people who like animals. We often judge others by how they are with animals. Participants in a study were asked to rate people in drawings on different attributes such as intelligence, friendliness, and healthiness. They rated the cartoon people more positively if animals were in the drawings. Similarly, in a study of college students, participants rated psychotherapists as more trustworthy if they had a dog with them.

How people are with animals gives us insight into their moral character. As early as 1699, John Locke advised giving children animals to care for so that they would "be accustomed from their cradles to be tender to all sensible creatures." During the Victorian era, child advocates and educators encouraged households to teach children to be kind and responsible by caring for companion animals. Sarah Josepha Hale, magazine editor and author of *Mary's Lamb*, published an essay arguing that for boys in particular, animals are a "great preventative against the thoughtless cruelty and tyranny they are so apt to exercise toward all dependent beings." She believed that animals can teach people about kindness, love, loyalty, duty, and friendship.

However, these positive attributes can't be achieved without a healthy dose of empathy. It sparks prosocial behaviors that are intended to help or benefit others, like kindness and altruism. Such actions include giving emotional support, murmuring soothing words, or donating money to worthy causes. Kindness and altruism are the flames of our empathy. Empathy also kindles emotional intelligence. In his book *Emotional Intelligence*, Daniel Goleman describes emotional intelligence as the ability to recognize and manage the emotions in one's self and in others to guide behavior. It's strongly linked with improved social skills and relationships and with greater mental and physical health. Emotional intelligence is a measure of empathy and the ability to understand and connect with others. "Empathy is the fundamental people skill," Goleman writes. Empathy is so intrinsic to our relationships with one another that we label anyone who lacks it as dangerous and mentally ill.

We prefer empathetic and kind people. We even judge people's attractiveness based on these qualities. In a study published in 2014, researchers in China randomly assigned 120 male and female participants to one of three groups and asked them to rate sixty photos of women making neutral facial expressions. Two weeks later, the participants were asked again to rate the photos, but this time, one group of raters was given negative personality descriptors about the women in the photos, such as meanness. The second group was given positive personality descriptors such as kindness. A control group was shown the same photos without any descriptors. In the first experiment, all three groups similarly ranked the photos for attractiveness. However, in the next round, the group shown the photos with positive personality descriptors ranked the faces much higher in attractiveness than the other two groups. The group given negative descriptors ranked the photos the lowest in attractiveness. In other words, as the researchers wrote, "we find that 'what is good is beautiful.'"

Although this study has limitations (it only looked at a narrow demographic of Chinese women's faces between the ages of twenty and thirty), its findings support a growing series of studies that have revealed that we like people who are ethical. For example, researchers at the University of British Columbia suggest that, as early as five months of age, our attraction to kindness is evident. They found that infants preferred a puppet who showed kindness in a puppet show over a mean puppet. We gravitate toward empathetic people. In turn, those who show greater empathy tend to be more successful in life. In a study published in *PLoS ONE*, preadolescent children who extended kindness to others were generally happier, in better relationships with others, and more popular.

Fortunately, empathy isn't a scarce commodity. There's plenty to go around. Empathy is likely a mixture of nature and nurture, influenced by childhood experiences. Nevertheless, it can still be learned in those who developed little empathy early in life. We can strengthen our empathy like a muscle.

School programs, such as social-emotional learning programs, have proven successful in teaching empathy to children through lessons in kindness, relationship skills, and managing emotions. Teachers and therapists have also been using animals to promote empathy development in children—not only toward animals, but also toward other humans. In a yearlong school program in which children were randomly assigned to receive either lessons in kindness toward animals or to a control group, psychologist Frank Ascione found that children who learned empathy through animal companionship also showed greater empathy toward other humans. The stronger the bond a child has with an animal, the greater their empathy and social competence. Other school-based programs show that children learn empathy and become less aggressive and violent by being with animals. And there is growing evidence that for even the most violent adults among us, animals bring out their better human selves.

On our second day in Lima, Patrick, David, and I drive to the Fraternal Order of Eagles where up to twenty-five former employees of Lima State Hospital meet for lunch every month. Since today is free senior day at the county fair, David says, we are expecting about half of the regulars to join us.

The host leads us into a room that resembles a school cafeteria and seats us at a round table unaccountably draped with a fine, white cloth. As I peruse the menu, my mood deflates. I worried there would be no good vegan items, but I still clung to hope. Food is very important to me.

The rest of the group hasn't yet arrived. A few stragglers sit at the counter. Patrick asks David, "Do you talk a lot about your days at the hospital?"

"Ha! Mostly we just complain about our joints and what's breaking down now."

When the rest of the group arrives, that's exactly what they start doing. As we sip the drinks we ordered, Linda asks Dan how his heart is doing.

"I gotta get a heart monitor test," he says.

David jumps in. "I thought it was your knees that was the problem!"

"No, no. My heart," Dan says, shaking his head at the injustice of it. His hound-dog face, furred by a state-trooper style mustache, adds to his morose look.

Bill, who dragged in an oxygen tank with him and who breathes with a nasal cannula, turns to me and gets to the point: "I hear you have questions for us."

"Uh . . . yes," I say and take a sip of my iced tea. I don't know why, but Bill flusters me. "I am hoping you can tell me about your experience at the hospital."

"Well, I started as an attendant on Ward 20, but then they needed help on Ward 21. They needed large people on the super strong ward. Well," he points a finger at his abundant figure, "you can see."

Ward 21 was one of two Super Strong Wards, considered the most secure wards where the most violent or "troublesome" inmates were sent. "I worked the day shifts," Bill says. "Inmates had to sit in a chair all day. They couldn't talk. They couldn't talk when they went to their meals. They couldn't talk when they came back from their meals. They couldn't talk when—"

"Ha ha ha!" Dan interrupts. "It might be easier to say when they *could* talk!"

"They had to kneel at my desk and whisper to go to the bathroom." Bill pauses. "I guess they could talk in the shower. I don't know. We didn't go in there with them."

According to Bill, the inmates on the Super Strong Ward were ordered to literally sit in hard, wooden chairs all day and not utter a word unless requesting something of the attendant. Even then, they were only allowed to speak in a whisper. The inmates had to whisper to Bill to request the TV be turned on. There were no books. Nothing else to pass the day. "I didn't find any of inmates very interesting," Bill says. Who would be interesting given nothing to do?

Our meals arrive and we dig in. I look over my plain baked potato and steamed broccoli and eye David's plate of French fries with envy. He looks gloriously satisfied munching the hot, salty fries. After a few minutes, Bill turns to me. "Have you gone out to see David's animals?"

"Yes, Patrick and I were there all day yesterday. Have you been?"

"Nope. Llamas spit."

Unlike the others at the table, Bill shows no interest in David's animals; and as the conversation proceeds, it becomes clear he views animals with contempt. Is that why he makes me uncomfortable?

Dan returns the discussion to the inmates on Ward 21. "Part of the reason why the inmates just sat there was because of all the medications they had to take."

Ah yes, the meds that put the men to sleep. The Super Strong Wards were considered by many to be the cruelest places in the institution. Punishment was swift and severe and guards forced inmates into total seclusion if they didn't follow orders, including, allegedly, trivial ones. I'm surprised to learn that some of the others at the table, particularly Bill, defend these practices even today as necessary to prevent fights and riots among the inmates. Maybe I shouldn't be surprised. His disdain toward the inmates is not dissimilar from his feelings about animals. He equally denies them his compassion.

Bill tells me that only a few employees "might have gone a little too far." The alleged abuses, he says, were exceptions. Certainly not the norm.

But some social workers, nurses, psychiatrists, and occasionally attendants, spoke out about the wrongful treatments of patients. When they did, they were ignored, punished, or pressured to remain silent. Lima State Hospital continued its practices as normal for decades, until two diligent reporters and a photographer from Ohio's largest newspaper, *The Plain Dealer*, conducted an undercover investigation in 1971.

During their six-week investigation, reporters Richard Widman and Theodore Whelan and photographer William Wynne interviewed patients and former patients and their families and sifted through thousands of death certificates and coroner's reports. They interviewed hospital attendants, security guards, doctors, and social workers who were previously silenced. The reporters found that many of the rumors were indeed reality. They detailed accounts of widespread brutality at the institution, including:

- Attendants forcing inmates to perform sexual acts.
- Attendants beating patients for "infractions" such as pantomiming a song.

- Attendants stripping patients naked, including a pregnant woman, and locking them in cold, barren solitary cells.
- Nurses strapping a young woman's hands overhead to a mesh, wire screen in the window of a solitary cell as an attendant beat her to unconsciousness with a chamber pot.
- Staff labeling the suspicious hangings of twenty-six patients as suicides.

Following these and other findings, a grand jury indicted twenty-six male and five female Lima State Hospital employees. A subsequent federal court order led to a litany of reforms at the hospital, beginning with the hiring of a new superintendent, William Balson. One of the first things Balson did was close down the strong wards.

"Then Balson calls six of us into his office," David says to me as he chews a fry with gusto. "Balson must have heard good things about us. He said that if we had any ideas to help him make changes, he would sure like to hear them."

David sent Balson a memo requesting that three parakeets with cages and two aquariums be allowed on two wards for a period of sixty days to test if they could brighten up the lives of the patients. One day later, he found his memo in his mailbox with a note from Balson. It simply said, "Go for it."

⟨⟩

Back at David's house, David shows Patrick and me photos of former Lima State Hospital patients with different animals. "This is Frank," he says of the man in a photo with a black-and-white cat draped over his shoulders. "He was the 'FBI man.' He would talk into his wrist, calling into FBI headquarters. We had a lot of guys who said they were undercover for the FBI or CIA!" He laughs and we all jump as the train whistle blows an alarm when a hen passes by. "Anyway," David continues, "Frank took care of that cat. He used to sneak food back to him. Oh, how he loved that cat!"

That cat was a much later addition to the institution. For his sixty-day trial period, David started with birds and fish in two male wards: one that housed the most depressed and suicidal patients, and another that housed the geriatrics. Immediately upon seeing the animals, patients asked to take care of them. So David gave some patients the responsibility of feeding the fish, cleaning the aquariums, or tending the birds. David monitored each patient's progress and mental health and kept careful notes. He also tracked the progress of two wards almost identical in patient makeup, staffing, and care—but with no animals—as a control group.

Within just three weeks, David saw amazing results. As soon as any guest would enter the test wards, patients would take them to see "my fish" or "my birds." By four weeks, the parakeets were all named, spent more time out of the cages, and perched the days away on the patients' shoulders. David's trial was working.

David tells us, "I couldn't believe it. To understand this place—it's the loneliest place you can imagine. First of all you're all by yourself. Second of all you're doing mostly a life sentence without any hope. Typically they had no family. And loneliness is probably equally as dangerous as the mental illness itself. Patients who normally just spent all day pacing the wards were now still pacing the wards, but with birds on their shoulders. And they were talking to the fish and birds and talking *about* them. It was like that movie, what was it? When the people in a coma all wake up?"

"Awakenings?" I suggest.

"Oh, yeah. Depressed, almost catatonic people at Lima suddenly were awake."

In a place where everyone and everything else was hostile and cold, the inmates found the birds and fish to be friendly and warm. Animals stirred deep within them a sense of connectedness that was missing in their lives. After all, animals are living beings with individual personalities, eccentricities, and quirks, who adapt to our behaviors and customs just as we adapt to theirs. Men who were previously silent were cooing to the birds. Fish were swimming up the tanks to the hands that greeted them. Birds were alighting on patients' arms and sitting with them in the TV room. And through their shared relationships with animals, the inmates found common ground. Suddenly, the inmates were responding not only to the animals but also to one another. The animals lifted the gloom and eased the despair of some of the most desolate of men.

The men and women at Lima State Hospital weren't just mentally ill. They weren't just criminals. They weren't even just dangerous criminals. They were individuals who, from the moment they entered the institution, were told and shown in one form or another, that they were society's castoffs. At best they were left to rot. At worst, they were degraded, subjugated, and beaten as if staff saw only demons left within them. With that kind of systematic campaign against you, combined with the awareness of your violent past deeds, it's hard not to believe that you are indeed less than human.

I stated before that animals don't judge us. Well, that's not entirely true. They don't judge us in the way we judge one another. They care nothing about our past lives, our possessions, or our outward appearances—they cut through all of that and get to the heart of the matter. Animals in our care assess us mainly by one criterion: Are we kind?

A juvenile inmate who worked with dogs in a recent prison program called Project POOCH, aptly said that "how much a dog can love you depends on you." Animals aren't merely mirrors of who we are. They don't just reflect our emotions—they have emotions of their own that respond to ours. How they respond can tell us a lot about ourselves.

When the birds and fish responded to the inmates by feeding off their hands and landing on their arms, they were sending the inmates a message they were desperate to hear: *I trust you.* They were telling men and women who had been judged as being beyond redemption that there was still something good in them. Coming from creatures who assess us solely by the gentleness of our voices and the softness of our touch, that is a powerful message.

After sixty days, David's trial was a success. Balson gave him permission to continue the program and within one year, the results were irrefutable. Compared with patients in the control wards, patients on the wards with animals required half the amount of medicines, had fewer violent incidents, and made no suicide attempts. The other wards had eight suicide attempts.

"The difference was so significant," David says to Patrick and me as he shuffles through piles of photos in his garage. "It was just hard to believe. Men who would spend eighteen hours a day in bed were up and social. They were bragging about their birds and fish! Oh man, it was so cool! And this was back in the seventies when nobody was even thinking that stuff."

One patient who David tells us about was a man named Lichen, who was in for robbery. "And maybe he was a pedophile," David says. "I can't remember. But he was very mentally ill. There was an aquarium on his ward with angelfish, and he would put his hand in the water and they would come up to him. Only to him. It never worked with anyone else. When he was finally going to be transferred to another hospital, he said he would not go unless he could take his angelfish with him." He laughs. "Oh man! I had never before heard of anyone refusing to go home or at least someplace better! Because let me tell you, we were the worst!"

This man considered the fish so much a part of his family that he would not even leave a mental institution without them. Fortunately, David convinced the receiving hospital to take the aquarium, under Lichen's promise that he would be the one to care for the fish.

After Lichen, other patients refused to leave the institution without their cherished animals, including one man who had been at the hospital for a year without uttering a single word. Medications and psychotherapy had no impact. "One day, after making sure he would not be a danger to the animal," David says, "I gave him a cockatiel to keep in his room." Within days, the man had the female bird, curiously named Gilbert, trained on his shoulder and was encouraging her to whistle. David says, "About a week later, as I was passing his room, he said, to my surprise, 'Birdseed.' That was the first word he ever said there." Slowly, the man began talking more, at first mostly to Gilbert, who was his constant companion. Then within two months, the inmate was interacting with others. By the time of his release, he was dramatically improved. His only request to the hospital was granted: that Gilbert be allowed to go home with him.

Over the next several years, David expanded the animal program into fifteen of the nineteen remaining wards. "All of a sudden it caught fire and every ward was asking for animals," David says. Eventually, besides the fish, more than two hundred animals—chinchillas, rabbits, guinea pigs, birds of various kinds, and cats roamed the halls of the institution, sunned in the greenhouse, or slept in the sheds and small barns the inmates built. David shows us photos of laughing men feeding, caressing, and playing with the llamas, deer, goats, sheep, ducks, chickens, and a very talkative goose. The once-sterile halls and yards were full of life—and hope.

"It made my job easier," David says, "and it seemed like the guards started to see that their jobs were easier because they didn't have to fight all the time. Because these guys were pretty satisfied just hanging around with their animals."

Studies now show that animal prison programs increase self-control, patience, and self-esteem in inmates. Additionally, the presence of animals increases not only the morale of the inmates, but also the staff, reducing violence and improving interactions between the two groups. With animals present, tensions between the two groups who are often pitted against each other melt away.

In one prison program, researchers assessed the inmates' social skills and social sensitivity, their ability to interpret communication from others, and their sensitivity to norms governing appropriate social behavior. The investigators divided the inmates into an experimental and a control group. Members of the former group participated in an intensive program to train shelter dogs to improve their chances for adoption. The results of the study showed substantially improved social skills and social sensitivity among the inmates who spent time with the dogs.

Animal programs may also reduce crime by reducing recidivism or re-offense rate. One such program in Washington State reported that the state's average three-year recidivism rate is 28 percent, but only 5 percent for inmates who participated in an animal program. Other programs have shown similar findings. These studies are few and the reduced recidivism is probably not due to just one cause. But what the Washington and other studies suggest is that the benefits animal companionship provide us is not just seen on an individual level, but also for society at large.

Animal therapy programs like those at Pendleton and Lima State Hospital may work simply by boosting inmates' confidence, improving their vocational skills (and thus helping them get jobs after release from prison), teaching them responsibility, and reducing depression. Empathy isn't necessarily the cause behind these improvements. The question remains then: Can animals strengthen empathy in the unempathetic and the violent?

David shows Patrick and me a photo of a man, a deer, and a goose, all three jumping together. They look like they were thoroughly enjoying one another's company. David says, "I would often start the inmates like this guy first caring for the animals out in the barn before I allowed them to have any in their cells—a lot of men were asking to have their own pet live with them in their cells." David was careful to gradually place the animals into the care of only those patients who proved responsible and had no history of animal abuse. "That was my cardinal rule. Pet safety came first. We had two cannibals"—he chuckles—"I wouldn't let them anywhere near the animals."

Cannibals aside, the institution's image dramatically changed after animals entered. Instead of writing news articles depicting atrocities, reporters from the *Smithsonian Magazine*, *60 Minutes*, the *National Enquirer*, *Reader's Digest*, and *ABC World News Tonight* flocked to the hospital to tell inspiring stories of animals reaching their human companions in ways that no one else could. In turn, the inmates showed remarkable tenderness and patience with the animals.

"We had some mean parakeets," David says. "I mean *mean*! And within a week and a half, the guys had the birds on their shoulders and I would wonder, Man, how did they do that?" Another had trained a gerbil to ring a bell when she wanted food—a feat, to be sure. Yet another inmate who stroked a gerbil cupped protectively in his hands as he spoke to reporters told them, "In the past, I never had that really deep-down compassion-type feeling for any kind of animal. As a boy, I used to go hunting quite a lot and shoot rabbits. I never even thought they were animals. . . . Now, after seeing the birds and the guinea pigs and the hamsters and the gerbils and the rabbits on the ward and coming close to them, you really understand the necessity of feeling for these animals and not harming them."

A young patient who had become suicidal while serving time for armed robbery credits a parrot named Christy for teaching him kindness. "I had never felt compassion," he said. When he was finally released, he got a job with the Atlanta Humane Society establishing a federal program recruiting the help of animals in mental health institutions.

In the last chapter, we saw how animals help calm us by lowering our blood pressure, heart rate, and stress hormones. We relax with animals. They don't compete with us like other humans and they offer us emotional and psychological release. As a result, animals defuse a lot of the human-generated pressure in our lives. Take Ron Kirkpatrick, who was in Lima for abduction and rape. He was known as "Killer" because he had killed another inmate at a North Carolina prison years ago. But to a yellow cockatoo named Babe, he was the gentle man who adopted him and took care of him in his small cell. To Kirkpatrick, Babe was the antidote to his pent-up rage toward himself and the other inmates and staff. Gesturing to Babe, who was perched on a tree limb, Kirkpatrick told reporters, "I used to argue with the attendants. . . . Now I just come in and talk to the bird, and I just don't yell at anyone anymore."

David tells me that Kirkpatrick just loved Babe. "All he talked about was Babe. How Babe was doing today. What new treat Babe discovered." What science had not yet revealed at the time was that while Kirkpatrick was with Babe, his oxytocin levels likely increased. Similarly, levels of mesotocin, an oxytocin-like neurochemical in birds, may have increased in Babe. As mentioned earlier, oxytocin puts us in a better mood, which enables us to feel more empathetic toward others. When you are tense, hurt, or angry, empathy can be as hard to hold on to as a wet bar of soap. Animals can diffuse those negative emotions. Another inmate told reporters, "I'll tell you, if somebody came to my room and started arguing, I'd push him out the door. . . . All I gotta do is go in my room and watch my fish. If those fish can live in peace with each other, I can." Animals, by increasing our oxytocin levels, make it easier for us to grasp onto empathy.

Recent studies indicate that oxytocin sharpens our understanding of one another. Higher levels can help us better decode the emotional meaning of nonverbal cues. For example, researchers had thirty adults inhale oxytocin and then examine photos of people's eyes. Compared to the placebo group, the oxytocin group was better at interpreting the emotions of the people in the photos. In the words of the researchers, oxytocin improves "mind reading."

I now realize another reason why Bill, the former attendant on Ward 21, unnerved me. His face and body showed little emotion, which made it hard to read him. Many times, I couldn't tell if he was joking with me or being dead serious. Two-thirds of human communication is nonverbal and we need nonverbal cues to decipher what others mean. Through words alone, we have a hard time telling if someone is being sarcastic, making a joke, intentionally being hurtful, or even means what they say. We need to see if he is smiling or frowning, if he looks directly into our eyes or avoids them, if he closes his arms or rests them comfortably by his side. That's why the use of emoticons has proven popular for many forms of written communication now—words don't fully convey our meanings. And people can use words to mislead or intentionally lie. But it's very hard to lie nonverbally. Your boss may tell you the company is not going to lay people off, but if you can read his body and face well, you might figure out that it's time to look for a new job.

The more we practice deciphering nonverbal cues, the better our empathetic skills will be. Animals are perfect for this. When we are with animals, we return to that deeper language, one that better conveys our true emotions than the spoken word. To form a true reciprocal relationship with other animals, you have to interpret the animals' sounds and the meanings behind their body movements. And you have to hone your skills in helping them understand you.

Empathy for another requires self-awareness. We can't fully read another's feelings and take in their perspective unless we can decipher our own. Otherwise we would just be projecting our own emotions onto another. With animals, you have to be cognizant of the stance of your body, the tone of your voice, and the position of your hands. You have to be aware of your emotions. Are you giving off threatening vibes? Do you sound calm? Or is there a bite in your voice? Animals demand attention to our own verbal and nonverbal cues and perspectives. What messages are we sending them?

A complex synergy of emotional and cognitive empathy helps us best to understand not only ourselves but also what another sees, feels, hears, thinks, and what they might need or want. It's a continual process. We use both types of empathy back and forth, and the combination of information we gather helps motivate us to act with compassion and ethics. With animals, we are trying to decipher the perspectives of seemingly very different beings. Through their companionship, animals teach us to "read minds"—not just theirs but ours as well.

I was glad to hear that as time passed, David started bringing to the hospital only animals who had been injured, neglected, or homeless like Tom the cat, mentioned in *Cats Magazine*. Other injured and homeless critters included a disabled goose, a one-footed finch, and a fawn whose mother was killed when developers knocked down an old home. "It just made sense to me," David says. "The inmates were broken. The animals were broken. I figured the patients could feel that they were also helping to save the animals. I think the inmates also identified with the disabled and unwanted animals."

David's words remind me of Daniel at Pendleton. Socializing the cats to find them good homes gives him a purpose in life, but his link with these animals goes deeper. In a sense—and by no means am I justifying Daniel's murder of his stepbrother—Daniel was just as unwanted as the cats. Maybe that was a factor in his sudden, and still-inexplicable, act of murder. Before his life at the penitentiary, he was yanked from home to home every time his mother remarried. Perhaps in part because he identifies with the sanctuary cats, helping them is especially rewarding.

Patients on Ward 4 at Lima State Hospital were exceedingly fond of Roscoe. A big, green one-eyed Amazonian parrot, Roscoe sparkled with animal magnetism. David tells me that it was as if Roscoe could spot a sad, depressed person pacing the halls and would land on his shoulder. Then later, you would find the same person bringing him a treat from the dining room or letting Roscoe sit with him while he watched TV. "I was told lots of times that Roscoe was the best therapist of the entire staff," David says.

There's another thing about animals that might explain how and why we can learn empathy through them. It's something that science can't yet measure. When we are in relationships with animals, we are making emotional connections with creatures who don't share human goals and aspirations. They draw us out of our self-absorptions. They enable us to gain an external perspective on those values we think are important. They motivate us to become less driven and obsessed with goals and more accepting of our own shortcomings and weaknesses. Animals bring us down to earth.

Soulful interactions with animals restore within us a sense of balance and harmony. They help us feel connectedness and unity with all life. With that bond comes true empathy—the ability to recognize that even with our distinctions, we are not so different in the ways that count. Animals, like Roscoe, remind us that we too are fragile beings. And that's okay.

⊸⊷

Over the many years at Lima State Hospital, there were a few problems concerning the animals. On one ward, patients plugged the water fountain drain and flooded the floor so that two cockatiels could take a bath. Bonehead, the adored black-and-white goat, kept setting off the security alarms and annoying the guards. Billy the goat got into the ceramics room and knocked over the pottery that inmates had spent hours creating. The "dueling Jesuses"—two schizophrenics who believed they were Jesus reborn—fought, viciously at times, over who got to care for a particular rabbit. But for all the small and often funny bothers, the inmates who bonded with animals felt a love that was unique and sincere. And for many of them, their inner angels unfolded their wings.

On that frigid January morning of the riot of 1977, passions heated on Ward 18 like electrons bouncing off the insides of a particle accelerator. With the guards tied up, the ten rioters, mostly murderers, paced the halls in anticipation of the arrival of the nurse. This nurse was a holdout from the days before the reforms and was particularly severe with the inmates. Nevertheless, the majority of the ward's inmates refused to join the riot.

The ward was in a lock-down area, meaning that, other than being escorted out for meals three times a day, the patients lived their entire lives within its walls. The ward consisted of two main areas, the day hall and the dormitory, where forty beds circled the room. Kidnapping the nurse would be the rioters' ticket out of the confines of those walls, their pass to freedom. But where was she? They grew impatient. Unable to control their pent-up energy, the rioters smashed the TV, tipped over the water fountain, split the chairs, ripped the couches, and shattered the windows.

It was this last action that caused the rioters' undoing. Police in a patrol car roving the exterior saw the broken windows and glass and notified security. Fifteen minutes later, instead of seeing the morning nurse when the entrance door lock was turned, the agitators were met by a team of twenty very angry guards carrying sticks. When the guards entered, they found almost everything in the day hall destroyed, broken, and flooded. The only things left untouched were an aquarium and a birdcage. The nonrioting patients had surrounded their beloved fish and two cockatiels to protect them from the mob.

PART TWO

Breaking with Animals

FOUR

The Making of a Murderer

After doing my chores after school one day, I walked into my grandparents' apartment seeking Sylvester. Immediately upon entering, I heard Dave yelling and Sylvester yelping. My heart raced. What was going on? I found the two of them in one of the bedrooms, and what I saw would be seared into my memory for the rest of my life.

Dave was slamming Sylvester against a wall. Again and again. Sylvester wasn't big, and it was easy for Dave to throw him far and hard. Sylvester cried out each time his small body hit the wall. Rather than try to run away in between throws, Sylvester tucked his tail between his legs, lowered his head, and whimpered back to Dave as though trying to placate him.

"Dave!" I cried out. "What are you doing to Sylvester?"

"I'm training him," Dave replied.

"He's hurt. That's hurting him!"

"Look what he did over there!" Dave pointed behind the bed where there was a puddle of pee. "He needs to learn. This is how I train him. This is normal to train a dog this way."

I stayed until Dave finished to make sure Sylvester was okay and to comfort him. But Dave's words lingered as I left the apartment. I felt a jumble of emotions I was too young to know how to process. I loved Sylvester, and watching him get hurt grieved me like I never thought possible. I was also angry with Dave for hurting Sylvester. But Dave was older than me; he was practically an adult. I was only a child. It was the same rationalization I was using to keep silent about my own abuse. Maybe training dogs this way *was* normal.

Over the next five months, as Dave continued to abuse Sylvester, I put aside my empathy. I loved Sylvester, and hated knowing that he was getting hurt, and yet I acceded to Dave's reasoning for hurting him. My natural empathy for Sylvester was overridden by Dave's rationalization. How did this happen?

How do any of us comply with cruelty to animals? Collectively, we do this every day. When Ringling Brothers and Barnum & Bailey Circus announced long before its closing that it was phasing out elephant acts, decades after being condemned by animal protection groups for using bullhooks, isolation, starvation, and electric prods to break elephants into submission, circus defenders mourned the "end of an era." When stories emerge about the number of animals struck by cars, people joke about roadkill. When we are confronted with the brutish lives of animals who end up on our dinner plates, we tell ourselves, "These animals are here for us to eat." Each time we brush off the intentional harming of an animal, are we not tacitly condoning violence? Despite the innate human capacity to connect with other animals, we can just as easily suppress any empathy for them. How?

In the last section we saw how empathy for animals can help our well-being by improving our emotional, physical, and social health. Is there a flip side to this? Does lack of empathy for animals harm us—as individuals and as a society? Additionally, how is empathy for animals lost or suppressed in the first place? To explore these and other questions, this next section looks at the causes and effects of breaking our empathy with animals.

To begin, perhaps I can gain some answers by probing extreme forms of violence. Empathy can play a compelling role in restraining aggressive behaviors like murder. A strong link exists between violence toward animals and violence toward humans. Published studies suggest that many serial and mass murderers (those who kill many people in a single spree) abused animals as children and that their failure to develop empathy for both animals and humans may stem from a shared root. These killers are outliers on the spectrum of human violence and their extreme attitudes and behaviors toward animals (and humans) may bring to focus the more nebulous attitudes of the average person. Can such a killer's experience with animals illuminate how any of us can override our empathy for animals? Moreover, just as empathy can be learned, can it be unlearned?

Unfortunately, studies on animal abuse among serial and mass murderers are not wholly informative. One major limitation of examinations of human-animal violence is that they are rather superficial—they are more like a checklist: Did the person hurt animals? If yes, at what age and what was the circumstance? I had already reviewed the litany of published studies, but they didn't provide full insight as to *why* violent people abuse animals and how that abuse starts. Throughout the writing of this book, I have met people who lived through intense situations. I would not have gained the understanding that I did about their circumstances if I had not spoken with them myself. That's certainly true when trying to understand a patient's ailments and needs. Published studies, while important, are not enough. Nothing replaces the value of speaking with someone one-on-one.

I made a resolution. I was neither sure that my idea would work nor that I would gain anything of value. But my gut told me that it would. Rather than only relying on published data for answers to my questions, I decided to go one step further.

I decided to meet a serial killer and ask myself.

Of course, I have no idea where to start. How does one go about meeting a serial killer? It's not something they taught me in medical school. So I start my journey where anyone else would: I google it.

In my search, I read about former Supervisory Special Agent Alan Brantley of the FBI's Investigative Support Unit (also known as the Behavioral Science Unit). Brantley joined the FBI in 1983 after working his way through college at the Dorothea Dix Hospital and serving as a psychologist for the North Carolina Central Prison. Once with the FBI, Brantley built upon his pioneering predecessors' work in criminal profiling and interviewed numerous violent men and women over more than two decades. He is frequently cited for confirming the connection between animal abuse and human violence. If you are looking for clues on serial murders and animals, Brantley is the right guy to talk to. He gives me helpful advice on how to best use my background in psychiatry—a critical component of neurology—to contact and interview violent killers.

I then research convicted serial murderers who have a reported history of abusing animals and who acknowledged their crimes. This last criterion is critical as it increases the chance that the person will speak truthfully with me. Among the names at the top of my search results is Keith Jesperson, who currently is serving a life sentence without parole in the Oregon State Penitentiary. His few prior interviews about his murders suggest to me that he might speak openly about his behaviors toward animals.

Between 1990 and 1995, Jesperson murdered eight women by strangulation, after raping most of them. Previously married and a father of three, Jesperson met most of his victims while driving across country for a long-haul trucking company. He targeted easy prey—vulnerable women such as prostitutes or transients—gambling that they could disappear for a long time before anyone noticed them missing.

Craving attention, Jesperson left an anonymous note on the bathroom wall of a truck stop and sent a letter to reporters bragging about his murders. Because he signed the letter with a smiley face, reporters dubbed him "the Happy Face Killer." Jesperson's five-year killing spree ended only when he murdered a woman whom the police could tie him to directly: his girlfriend, Julie Ann Winningham.

I write to Jesperson explaining that I am a doctor exploring empathy for humans and animals and asking if I could meet with him to discuss his history. Based on Brantley's advice, I make it clear to Jesperson that he will be in control over what is discussed. Also, after much deliberation and hesitation, I do something I had not discussed with Brantley. Along with the letter, I slip into the envelope a headshot photo that I use for professional purposes. I am running the risk that Jesperson might speak with me solely because I am a woman (many people can't determine my gender based on my name alone). But I am willing to take the chance if it might open the door for me. As Brantley suggested, I need to gain Jesperson's trust. Perhaps he will be more willing to write back to me if he sees that I put all my cards on the table, so to speak, and can put a face to my name.

Less than a week after I mail my letter, I find one from Keith Jesperson in the post office box I set up. Amazed that he replied so quickly, I tear open the envelope, which includes a visitor form for me to complete. His six-page, handwritten letter includes:

> Dear Aysha,
>
> You say you want to talk to me here. I guess so. Been a long time since someone so pretty sat across from me with such a pretty smile and long hair. Aren't you afraid you'll fall madly in love with me and want to sweep me off my feet . . .
>
> I'll be in charge? What kind of crap is that? Seriously, Aysha, it isn't about control at all. If we do this, we need to put that kind of thought behind us. We move ahead with a mutual task at hand. All I ask is that you be honest with me and yourself. Come with an open mind. I've been lied to before.
>
> At beginning of each visit and at end, we can embrace, hug, kiss, shake hands, stare into each other's eyes—get excited OR NOT.

You can set up a phone account with Telmate. We should not get ahead of ourselves. I don't want to waste your time or mine in all of this. Have a job in here and between doing art and answering mail and exercising, little time is left to write at a life's story.

Take care,
Keith

Jesperson first wants to chat by phone to gauge me before meeting in person. Fair enough. That will give me a chance to assess him, too. A few days after receiving his letter, I start a series of weekly phone calls with Jesperson. These conversations end up being some of the most horrifying, disturbing, annoying—and surprising—that I have ever had.

⟨≈⟩

"All killers are serial killers," Jesperson tells me during one of our phone calls. We have been conversing over the phone and through letters for about three weeks. "It's just that most of them get caught the first time."

"Why do you say that?" I ask.

"I believe that with everyone that has ever killed anyone, they want to kill again. It's in their blood."

Keith Jesperson got his first taste of killing before the age of nine. Born in 1955 in Chilliwack, British Columbia, Jesperson was the middle child with two brothers and two sisters. Growing up in the country, surrounded by apple orchards and farmland, his family kept many animals, including dogs, horses, ducks, and sheep. According to Jesperson, any animal that was not a dog or a farm animal was considered a nuisance. His father provided BB guns for him and his brothers and encouraged them to hunt unwanted animals. Jesperson learned how to use many weapons, including rifles and bows, at an early age. "I could shoot fifty yards at a gopher," he boasts.

Jesperson killed lots of animals. His most frequent animal victims were gophers or "sage rats," as he often calls them. Local farmers paid small change to Jesperson and his brothers to kill gophers and other animals. "We have all these rats, and the farmers wanted to get rid of the gophers and the coyotes and the rabbits. They asked people to bounty-hunt them. We didn't see it as hurting animals. We were destroying them because it's of little value to the community. . . . Everyone was doing it."

He goes on: "Farmers would provide us with these traps, and we'd snare [the gophers]. We'd pull this trap out of the hole with this trapped gopher, and my brother Brad or Bruce, or myself, would have a club and we'd beat him to death."

Sometimes Jesperson "dispatched" the gophers and other animals without much thought, as a matter of routine. Other times, he took great pleasure in hurting them. Jesperson says that his father recorded the bloodbath on one occasion using thirty-five-millimeter film. "My dad is video-recording this and narrating the show. He's laughing about it as we're clubbing them to death. We were all laughing. As my dad narrates, he said, 'Here's some natural-born killers dispatching a gopher.'"

Over the phone, I wince. "How many gophers do you think you killed overall?" I ask.

"Thousands."

I wasn't expecting this. "Thousands?"

"Thousands of gophers," he confirms. "Weekends we'd go out and I'd shoot five hundred rounds and whether I hit all the gophers—let's say I hit half of them—so I killed two hundred and fifty gophers on a weekend."

"Did you ever take pause about shooting gophers? Did you ever consider the suffering you were causing them?"

"Shooting gophers was like shooting targets. Kill and move on."

Jesperson tells me about a cat he killed when he was older at a mobile park owned by his father. A tenant had called Jesperson to fix the leaky plumbing in her house. "So I was in there fixing the sink underneath the cupboard," Jesperson says, "and this cat was in the cupboard. I laid my hand down, and he clamped onto my hand . . . clawing the hell out of my hand. So I came out from underneath of the sink with this cat on my hand and I tried to get it off. I ran outside and I threw it onto the pavement. I threw my hand down as hard as I could and threw this cat into this pavement. And then I reached down, grabbed the cat, and strangled it."

"Why did you kill the cat?" I ask him. "You shook the cat off. You could have ended it there and let him go, right?"

Jesperson agrees. "The cat could have run away, but then I just killed it. I grabbed it and strangled it. I was mad at it. I was angry. . . . I have issues."

"Did you feel any remorse after killing the cat?"

"Not at the time. I'm sure there was some kind of thrill that I was killing this cat because this cat clawed me and I was getting even with it."

Jesperson tells me that, from prison, he wrote a letter about this cat to the *Statesman Journal*, an Oregon newspaper, "sometime in '96 or '97." The letter was in response to another cat killing, committed by two local football players. Intrigued, I make a mental note to track down the letter.

Jesperson was twenty-one years old when he killed the cat. Later in life, he poisoned a flock of seagulls for soiling his truck. He fed them potato chips laced with strychnine. "I killed about fifty seagulls. I never gave it another thought." He also recalls killing a dog at the mobile park with a bow and arrow. "It was getting in the trash, and I chased it home. I actually went back, found the owner's house, and I told him to take the dog in his house and he pretty much told me to go screw myself . . . and so I just nocked an arrow, drove it into the side of the dog. Stuck it right to the telephone pole."

❦

In 1963, psychiatrist John M. Macdonald published the first study to suggest that certain behaviors in childhood could indicate later violence. While at the Colorado Psychopathic Hospital, Macdonald looked at the early behaviors of forty-eight psychotic patients and compared them to nonpsychotic patients, all of whom had threatened to kill someone. Among the cruelest patients, some "boasted of their sadistic exploits and took pleasure in describing their hunting triumphs and their skill in karate or judo." One man took satisfaction in repeatedly describing to his wife how he eviscerated a cow by tying him to his tractor. Macdonald identified three characteristics that were repeatedly found among the most violent patients: bed-wetting beyond the age of five, fire-setting, and childhood cruelty toward animals. These traits became known as the Macdonald Triad.

At the time of Macdonald's study, cruelty to animals was not considered significant by criminologists and was certainly not viewed as a psychiatric issue. The APA did not recognize animal cruelty as a sign of a psychiatric disorder until 1987, when it published the revised DSM-III. In this edition, animal cruelty was added as a criterion for antisocial personality disorder (APD) in adults (commonly referred to as sociopathy) and conduct disorder (often considered a precursor to APD) in children and teens.

It wasn't until Robert K. Ressler expanded on Macdonald's study two decades later that criminologists more readily identified animal abuse with other forms of violent behavior. Ressler joined the FBI in 1970, after having served as a criminal investigation officer in the Military Police Corps for the US Army. Credited with coining the term *serial killer* and interviewing some of the country's most notorious murderers, Ressler was among the first FBI investigators to report the strong connection between violent murder and animal abuse.

With the help of his FBI colleagues and Ann Burgess, an expert in forensic nursing, Ressler originated and developed the FBI's first research program of violent offenders. Between 1979 and 1983, he and fellow profiler John E. Douglas visited prisons around the country and interviewed offenders such as Richard Trenton Chase (aka the Vampire Killer), Edmund Kemper, Ted Bundy, and David Berkowitz (aka the Son of Sam). In total, they interviewed thirty-six convicted serial and sexual murderers (those who appeared to gain sexual satisfaction from the torture and/or murder, or have an otherwise sexual component to their crimes). Ressler and his colleagues then looked at how often these murderers displayed certain behaviors, including fire-setting, bed-wetting, and animal cruelty during their childhood, adolescence, and adulthood. More than one out of three killers revealed that they had been cruel to animals in both childhood and adulthood. Almost half were cruel to animals while they were teenagers.

Although Ressler's study found patterns of behavior among the murderers interviewed that corroborated some of Macdonald's findings, later studies on the Triad found inconsistent results. There is now general agreement among psychologists that the presence of bed-wetting and fire-starting in a child does not predict future violent behavior. However, abuse of animals could not be so readily dismissed. Unlike the other two behaviors, animal abuse is an act of violence against a living being. The psychological ramification of harming a creature who can suffer can't simply be lumped together with other forms of atypical behavior, like bed-wetting in later childhood. In 2001, psychologist Frank Ascione, a leading authority on the connection between animal abuse and other forms of violence, reviewed the existing data and concluded: "Taken together, these studies suggest that animal abuse may be characteristic of the developmental histories of between one in four and nearly two in three violent adult offenders."

The range of findings in Ascione's review reflects inherent obstacles in studying cruelty to animals. The first obstacle is defining animal abuse. We can all reasonably define what bed-wetting is, for example, but what is animal abuse? Ascione defined it as a "socially unacceptable behavior that intentionally causes unnecessary pain, suffering or distress to, and/or death of, an animal." Although his definition is one of the most frequently used, it has been criticized as being too narrow. Under this definition, strangling a cat would be considered animal abuse. Shooting a dog or cat for the pleasure of it would also fit. But what about shooting gophers or coyotes? Is that animal abuse? If Jesperson shot a coyote because the animal was considered a nuisance, then that would likely be considered "socially acceptable" behavior. Do we include Jesperson's hunting of wild animals for pleasure under the definition of animal abuse? If we do, how does that affect our acceptance of sport hunting? If we don't, why do we only accept the harming of certain animals, such as dogs and cats, as abuse, but not other animals?

How we define cruelty to animals is very dependent on our fickle views about them. What our society accepts today may very well change tomorrow.

A second obstacle is the difficulty in determining if a person abused animals in the past. Will people tell the truth or will they even be able to accurately recall the events? Questioning friends, former teachers, or family about a person's past faces similar issues. Parents tend to significantly underestimate their children's involvement in cruelty toward animals, instead passing it off as "kids being kids." Or they simply don't recognize cruelty when it exists.

In reviewing court or medical records, what is revealed is based on who originally asked the questions about animal abuse, how those questions were asked, and how the answers were described in the records. Most importantly, information depends on whether someone asked the question about animal abuse in the first place. Despite the increased awareness about the link between animal violence and human violence, many in law enforcement, medicine, and the social sciences still do not ask sufficient questions to closely examine this link.

Because of these and other reasons, it's likely that studies underestimate the frequency of animal abuse. Responding to Ressler's FBI study that found about half of the killers abused animals, Alan Brantley stated, "We believe that the real figure was much higher." Regardless of the limitations of studies on this topic, however, a history of animal abuse remains one of the most consistent findings among violent adults. Childhood animal cruelty, especially repeated acts of animal cruelty, is a harbinger of adult violence.

⤶

"Goddamn it!"

Sitting in my living room, I hold Keith Jesperson's latest letter in my hand. He and I have been communicating for a little over two months now. I had made myself a strong cup of Irish breakfast tea, then settled in a comfortable chair. I need the tea for fortification to read Jesperson's letter. During my prior conversations with him, I worked hard to remain impassive when he described his killings in his trademark unemotional way, but his descriptions of his violence were taking an emotional toll on me. After every communication, I needed to step away from the horrors and cleanse my emotional palate. I would hug my husband and my cat or zone out watching *Seinfeld* reruns.

And though Jesperson was always polite, he continued to say sexually evocative things to me, both on the phone and in his letters. On several occasions, I asked him to stop, and he would do so for a short while, but his restraint never lasted long.

So I was expecting more of the same from Jesperson when I opened his latest letter, but instead of ranting against the media and writing things like "when you show up [for your visit], you can give me a tongue," he writes that he no longer wants to speak with me.

I'm stunned. I don't understand why he suddenly decided to cut me off. We had just talked on the phone the day before he wrote this letter. Our conversation went fine. He seemed interested in communicating with me. What went wrong?

I'm not ready to end my conversations with him. I'm fully aware that Jesperson may not always be truthful with me, and I cross-reference everything he tells me and ask the same questions in different ways to check for consistency in his responses. I suspect that he exaggerates some things, like how many gophers he killed. Even so, our discussions are proving to be insightful—as much by what he doesn't tell me as by what he does. We have barely scratched the surface, though. I mentioned earlier that most research on the human-animal violence link is rather superficial. With Jesperson,

I have the opportunity to dig more deeply and examine not only why and how he became cruel to animals, but also the more subtle nuances of his relationships with animals. I don't expect to conclusively understand how empathy is suppressed based on examining one man alone, but at least my conversations with Jesperson can reveal if I'm asking the right questions.

In the evening, I leave Jesperson a voice message.

"Hi, Mr. Jesperson. Uh . . . Keith. This is Dr. Akhtar. I received your letter saying you don't want to talk with me anymore and that you had concerns. Will you give me a call so that I can address your concerns?"

I should have stopped here.

"I don't understand what went wrong," I blurt out. "Will you call me so that we can talk about this? I think we can continue our conversations if you just call me so that I can understand what your concerns are. You know how to call me. Just call me back this Saturday at our usual time or any Saturday. Actually, you can just call me whenever and I will pick up the phone. So. Just call me whenever it's most convenient for you. I hope you can call me so I can have a chance to uuuhhhh—"

I hang up. Mid-sentence. Patrick is listening and laughs. "Aysha, you started out strong, but then you got desperate. You sounded like he's a boyfriend who just broke up with you, and you're trying to get him back!"

Patrick is right. What the hell is wrong with me? During prior conversations with Jesperson, I always spoke confidently and professionally. If he tried to rile me up, as he occasionally did with his lewd comments, I brushed them aside and continued with my questions. But I am now nervous. I thought I had gained Jesperson's trust. I feel rejected. By a serial killer! Could there be anything more ludicrous?

"What an idiot I am." I murmur to Patrick. "What am I going to do?"

I do what every rejected person wishes she could do after leaving an embarrassing voice mail. I call the phone service company, confirm that Jesperson has not yet heard my message, and ask them if they can delete it. They do.

I leave another voice message. But not before I write it out—with Patrick's help.

Will Jesperson call me back?

⌘

Overnight, I consider why Jesperson suddenly refused to speak with me. The explanation that comes to mind is that *he* fears rejection from *me*. During our last call, Jesperson asked if I was going to visit him, meet him face-to-face. I told him I was traveling a lot and that it might be several months before I could get to Oregon. My response obviously bothered him. His last letter reflected anger. He wrote, "Your [first] letter suggested urgency to set up visiting. Yet, you are now not in a hurry to get in here."

I am traveling a lot, but he does have a point. I have not yet filled out the form to request visitation rights at the prison. I have been divided. I know, intellectually, that I might gain important insight by sitting across from Jesperson and watching his nonverbal cues. Emotionally, though, I have no desire to meet him. I'm not sure that I even need to anymore. We've been progressing just fine with our phone calls. Jesperson previously mentioned the possibility of Skyping but quickly dismissed the idea. He said to me, "I'd rather have you here in person so I can look at your pretty little eyeballs." This doesn't exactly entice me.

Jesperson obviously has trouble relating to women. He is directly revealing to me his distrust of women, his difficulty accepting rejection by them, and his need to exert control over them. When I later discuss this with Dr. Eric Hickey, one of the foremost experts on criminal psychology, he affirms my thoughts. "He doesn't have the issues with men that he has with women," Dr. Hickey postulates. "With you, he has to dominate; he has to control the relationship. And if he feels in any way a sense that he's losing control, he's going to say goodbye. At least to play the game with you to get that control back. He doesn't want you to go away, but he wants you to know he's in control of the interviews."

If that is what Jesperson is trying to do, his attempt is so amateurish, I almost feel sorry for him. Even worse, I fell for it! Before I first reached out to Jesperson and even after, I armed myself with the right tools. I had exhaustively researched Jesperson. I talked to multiple experts in the field. I went into this situation prepared. Or so I thought.

He got to me. Jesperson got to me. Is he hoping that I will call him back and ask for a second chance, which as it turns out, is exactly what I did?

I didn't have to wait long for the answer. He calls the next morning. I don't promise to visit him, but my asking for "an opportunity to address [his] concerns" is enough to put me in his good graces again, and we are back to our scheduled conversations.

❧

"Manipulation. Domination. Control," wrote FBI profiler John E. Douglas. "These are the three watchwords of violent serial offenders." Through shows like *Criminal Minds* and movies like *The Silence of the Lambs*, it's now common knowledge that killers like Jesperson often feel a need to dominate and control others. But what is not often known is how someone like Jesperson comes to feel that need.

What astonishes me most about Jesperson is that he wasn't always cruel to animals, and I suspect that his fears of rejection and need to exert control over others started, in part, through his early attempts to connect with animals. Sigmund Freud noted that children identify strongly with animals: "The child does not yet show any trace of the pride which afterwards moves the adult civilized man to set up a sharp dividing line between his own nature and that of all other animals." However, just as childhood identification with animals can be rewarding if animals are treated kindly, it can equally be demoralizing if animals are abused.

When Jesperson was six years old, he tried to help a crow with a broken wing. "When I picked it up, I saw it was hurt and I just thought it would be the good thing to do," he tells me. "I thought I'd nurse it back to health. I was trying to make it all better, feeding it. I thought it might be my pet."

Jesperson kept the crow in a box in his bedroom as he tried to nurse her. One day, his brother ended Jesperson's hope of healing the crow. "My brother, he ran around with the neighbors who were into animal abuse and so forth, and I just got home. And they kind of told me I wasn't doing it any good by keeping it alive. So they killed it." They killed the crow by throwing the box she was in out of the bedroom window, smashing it against the driveway. Jesperson retaliated by throwing his brother's model airplanes out the window. "And of course I was being punished," he says. "My dad came home and punished me for breaking my brother's airplanes. His idea was it was just a dumb crow anyway."

One of the closest relationships Jesperson had was with his dog, Duke. Jesperson was five years old when his family adopted Duke. "Duke wound up being my dog," Jesperson tells me. "I guess he claimed me. Duke and I were like inseparable; everywhere I went, there was my dog. If my mother saw Duke around, she knew I was around. He was my buddy. I didn't have many friends growing up."

When I ask what was so special about his relationship with Duke, he replies, "There was no hugging, no kissing, no companionship in the family. The social comforts of a dog is really . . . there's no-holds-barred kind of thing. They give it unconditionally. And we were friends—the dog and I were friends. Duke slept on my bed every night. That's where he slept. He was on my bed."

I think back to Sylvester. How many of us as children sought the company of animals when human companionship either wasn't there for us or wasn't enough? According to a *New York Times* article, seven-to-ten-year-old children named on average two companion animals each when listing the ten most important individuals in their lives. In another report, when children were asked, "Whom do you turn to when you are feeling sad, angry, happy or wanting to share a secret?" nearly half of them mentioned their companion animals.

Both Jesperson and I developed loving relationships with animals and, like me, Jesperson tried to nurse animals back to health. We also share something else: both of us witnessed animal abuse. Yes, Jesperson took part in animal cruelty, but, like me, he also witnessed it by others, especially by authority figures like his older brother and father. He saw them abusing animals before he did so himself. According to psychologist Dr. Randall Lockwood, children who witness animal abuse "are often driven to suppress their own feelings of kindness and tenderness toward a pet because they can't bear the pain caused by their own empathy for the abused animal."

Jesperson the adult is incapable of expressing to me the pain he felt when his brother killed the crow, but Jesperson the child must have felt it deeply. The incident remains a vivid memory for him. Every time Jesperson's family members severed his connection with an animal, did they amputate a part of his empathy?

Although this does not offer a full explanation—human behavior is too complex—Lockwood's theory may partly explain Daniel's sudden turn to murder. When I met Daniel at the Pendleton Correctional cat sanctuary in Indiana, I was appalled to learn about his terrible murder of his stepbrother while witnessing how kind he was with animals. Like many victims of domestic violence (as his story suggests), Daniel found solace in animals. But even their company wasn't secure. He told me that his stepfathers forced him to leave the animals with his grandmother, including one cat with whom he strongly bonded. "Aidan was just for me," Daniel told me. "He would sit on my shoulders as I walked around the house. I'd go and visit him at my grandmother's after my stepdad made me leave him there. But one time I didn't make it to my grandmother's for about a week, and when I did, she told me Aidan was dead. He was hit by a car." Could the repeated, forced loss of animals have unraveled some of the threads that held Daniel's sanity together and provoked his impulsive murder?

Although Daniel had violently killed another human being, his empathy for animals remains strong. Jesperson has killed

humans and animals without remorse. As a child, I tried to suppress my empathy for Sylvester in order to align my view with
Dave's. But I never abused an animal or a human. My empathy
toward all life remained, and remains still. Why did Daniel, Jesperson, and I veer into different directions? It can't be explained
by gender alone. Both girls and boys abuse animals. One theory
is that witnessing infrequent or milder forms of animal abuse
may lead to greater empathy, while frequent exposure of animal
abuse desensitizes an individual to suffering. Additionally, evidence suggests that the younger children are when they witness
animal abuse, whether male or female, the more likely they are
to abuse animals themselves. Jesperson witnessed animal cruelty
at a younger age and far more frequently than I did, and Daniel
never saw an animal physically abused. This could explain some
of our eventual differences.

I think there is another reason too. Those around me, even
Dave for the most part, validated my relationships with animals.
They never mocked my love for Sylvester and allowed me generous
freedom to play with and care for him. The same cannot be said
for Daniel's parents. And Jesperson's family, neighbors, and friends
went even further. Not only did they not support his kindness
toward animals but they mutilated it. Either through their example
or through punishment (like killing the crow and punishing Jesperson for his retaliation), they actively encouraged Jesperson to
switch off his empathy.

Jesperson tells me his friends and neighbors thought nothing of
hurting and killing animals. "I've known neighbors that put cats
in gunnysacks, put rocks in it, and then threw them in the river."
Some, he says, killed baby pigeons by stepping on them. Even if
this claim is not true, Jesperson saw plenty of animal abuse in
other ways. Children who grow up witnessing animals abused or
neglected are more likely to view such treatment as acceptable and
to emulate those patterns of abuse.

Of all the influencing factors, it was probably Jesperson's father
who most squashed his empathy for and nurtured his cruelty

toward animals. Jesperson tells me, "I watched my father take a two-by-four to a horse and beat him because he bit him. He always thought he owned animals and could do whatever he wanted."

Jesperson's father was present when he, as an adult, strangled the cat at the mobile park. I ask him how his father reacted.

"Let me explain my father for you. My father would say he saw the whole incident, and I think it set him back a little bit. But from that point on, he would brag or tell it almost like a joke. He'd tell people, if you have a cat to kill, just hand it to Keith."

Jesperson is extremely ambivalent toward his father, who died years ago. Sometimes Jesperson describes his father as his mentor, other times as someone so controlling he "took up all the air in the room." He describes his father as going into alcoholic rages at times. When Jesperson did something that upset his father, his punishments were sometimes severe. "He didn't beat me often," Jesperson says. "But when he did, he took it seriously. He beat me with a belt scientifically. He would start from my butt and serially whip me down to my knees and then back up. I couldn't walk. My clothes would cling to me because of all the blood and fluid seeping through."

Violence begets violence. Those who abuse animals or other humans are frequently from troubled families where they have witnessed violence or are themselves victims of physical, emotional, or sexual abuse. Violence over another is a powerful means to exert control, especially when one's control over other parts of his life is tenuous. For Daniel, this need for control may have manifested by the murder of his stepbrother. For Jesperson, it was through the killing of countless animals and eight women.

When Jesperson was young, his father tried to dominate the one relationship that Jesperson could depend on. "One day, my dad and I were out hunting with Duke," Jesperson tells me, "but Duke wouldn't hunt. He wouldn't go after the animals. I watched my father take Duke and throw him into the ravine. I said to him, 'Duke isn't a hunting dog. He's never been trained. You can't expect him to hunt all of a sudden.' When he threw Duke into the ravine,

I thought he killed him. But Duke came crawling out of the ravine and he never went near my dad again. And I wouldn't let my dad near him."

Eventually, though, Jesperson's father won ultimate control over Duke. When Jesperson was sixteen, his father told him that Duke got into poison and that he had to "put the dog down." He said he had buried Duke in the nearby park. Jesperson was suspicious. "Dad wouldn't give me a straight answer. I went back to the park a couple of weeks later and I tried to find the burial site where he put the dog. I made it up there, and there was no burial site. I actually smelled the decaying flesh. I went over, and I crossed this creek, and there was Duke laying dead against this hill."

⌘

About four months after our first phone call, Jesperson informs me that the paperwork I went ahead and submitted for visitation was cleared. He writes:

> *Aysha,*
>   *Today I'm 61 years old. My brother Bruce is 63 today. . . .*
> *You have been approved!! Yahoooo! Female company!!!*

I am approved for a "privileged visit," meaning that I would be in a visiting room with no barrier between Jesperson and I.

> *We can embrace,* Jesperson writes. *And I'll hold you close to me, or maybe not. We'll play it by ear . . . .*

On the last page of the letter, he outlined his hand.

But then Jesperson cuts off ties with me a second time. Less than two weeks after he wrote the letter, he again writes to me: *I've taken you off my visitor's list. Don't bother writing any more. We are done.*

Even though I was approved for visitation, I had still not made any commitment with Jesperson. Okay, if making that commitment is what it will take to continue conversations with him, then so be it. I leave a voice mail, again asking "to address his concerns" and say that I would like to arrange a time to visit him. He takes a little longer to get back to me this time. When he calls after three days, I tell him I am now ready to visit him.

"We can get married when you get here," he says.

"You know I'm married, Keith."

"Will you wear traditional garb from Pakistan? I like those long, flowing clothes on women. They're so feminine."

"I'm not going to do that, Keith."

After a ten-minute call, I'm back in again. Three weeks later I'm in a rental car heading about an hour south of Portland to the Oregon State Penitentiary.

⁓

Salem is the seat of Oregon's state government. Locals also refer to the town as Oregon's prison capital. It houses five prisons. Of these, Oregon State Penitentiary is the oldest and largest. Situated on 194 acres in the heart of the city, this maximum-security, all-male prison is the site of Oregon's death row, where executions are carried out by lethal injection.

On a Thursday afternoon, I gaze at the twenty-five-foot, reinforced concrete wall, which encircles the prison. I enter the main building and join a small group of other penitentiary visitors—wives, girl-friends, fathers, and grandparents. Once we go through security, a staff member escorts us down a ramp through two sets of locked steel doors into the visiting room. The room is not what I expected. Large, brightly lit, and divided into two main sections, the room is inviting with comfortable couches, chairs, and coffee tables. Vending machines line up against one wall. A row of shelves holding books and board games stands against another wall. As I enter, I see inmates already seated in the couches and chairs in anticipation of their visitors.

Jesperson is sitting in a chair underneath a window. When I approach him, he stands up. Good God, the man is large. You could fit three of me into him like Russian dolls.

"Keith?" I ask, extending my right hand.

"Aysha?"

We shake hands. "I recognized you immediately from your photos online," I say. "Thank you for meeting with me." I sit down on the other side of the small coffee table in the chair opposite him.

We sit in silence for some seconds, each sizing up the other. With grayed hair buzzed close to his scalp, he is dressed in white sneakers, blue denim pants, and a blue button-down, long-sleeved shirt, stamped with the words "Oregon State Penitentiary Inmate." I wear dark slacks, a gray shirt, and a cardigan. Jesperson's face remains wooden as he stares at me.

"You look darker than your photo," he says.

"Yeah, well, that photo was taken in the winter. I'm darker in the summer."

I'm a little nervous. I flew all the way across the country and suddenly don't know what I am going to say to him. I jump up and ask, "Would you like a drink from the vending machine?"

"Do they have Mountain Dew? I can't get up and walk around. I'm supposed to stay here during the visit."

I look around at the two guards seated in opposite corners of the room. I walk to the vending machines and purchase a Mountain Dew.

"Thank you," he says when I hand it to him.

"You're welcome." I start walking back toward the vending machines. There are snacks, too.

"Would you like something to eat?" I ask him.

"I would like to eat you."

I pause and look back at him. "What do you mean by that, Keith?"

"Nothing. I'm just messing with you."

"Uh-huh." I get a cranberry juice for myself, then return and sit down.

"As you can see, I'm a cheap date," he says, holding up his Mountain Dew. He watches me as I take a sip of my drink. "How was your flight?"

"It was uneventful."

"What hotel are you staying at?"

"The Howard Johnson."

"You must travel cheap. What's your room like?"

I laugh softly. I am *not* going to describe to him what is essentially a bedroom. "It's not a place you want to spend time in," I say.

He looks at me a moment. It seems he understands I'm not going to say more about my room.

"I haven't had a female visitor in a long time. I'm so excited you're here."

He doesn't look excited. He doesn't look . . . anything. His face doesn't betray any emotion.

"Does anyone in your family visit you?" I ask.

"Not for a long time. I rarely get a visitor. Is your husband upset that you're here visiting me?"

I don't tell Jesperson that, in fact, Patrick *is* upset. He's uneasy about Jesperson's behavior toward me and concerned about how meeting him would affect me, given my past with Talup and how badly I handled that one voice mail I left for Jesperson. But in my typical cavalier fashion, I brush aside Patrick's concerns. I reason with him, and myself, that I have built up a strong armor now.

Ignoring Jesperson's question, I listen to the many conversations in the room as they ping off the walls and fuse into a low buzz. One inmate sitting near us is talking intently with a woman in a business suit who shows him documents. His lawyer? In a corner, a young woman holds hands with and nuzzles an inmate. A male visitor plays cards with another inmate.

Over my silence, Jesperson urges, "Is your husband worried you are going to marry me?"

I smirk at this. "That's not a concern, Keith."

He startles me by smiling back. Throughout our discussions over the phone, I never once heard a smile in his voice. Tiny lines crinkle around his gray-blue eyes. His upper and lower rows of teeth each have a middle tooth missing. I am thoroughly comfortable now. I allow our conversation to flow naturally as it did whenever we spoke by phone. I ask him about Felix, a dog who was brought in to chase the geese away from the lawns, but has since become the unofficial prison mascot.

"Felix brings a lot of life here," Jesperson says. "He allows us to feel more human. He doesn't judge you. He just takes you away from here. . . . Sometimes he gains a lot of weight because all the guys are slipping him food."

"Keith, you have liked and even loved some dogs and also killed other dogs. Why the difference?"

"It's all a matter of context. I didn't just go around killing every animal out there. I killed some animals. Not every animal. I killed animals because it was the thing to do at the time, like with the sage rats—I'm killing these animals, and I think nothing. Or it was for a reason."

"What kind of reason?"

"In the mobile park, my dad provided guns for me to chase the cats and dogs away. The dogs and cats kept coming back because the tenants who lived there owned them. But they weren't on a leash, and my dad felt they needed to be on a leash. One day I'm driving by the mobile park, and I see a stray dog, and I shoot him. It yelps and jumps two feet into the arms of its owner. I didn't notice the owner before. I didn't care about the killing. But when the owner saw me hurt the animal in front of him, I felt this small." He holds up his thumb and index finger.

Hurting animals didn't weigh on Jesperson's moral consciousness at the time, but being caught did. I turn the conversation back to Felix. Jesperson lives in the A-block, or honor block, and gets to see Felix often. It's a funny thing. Serial murderers are often considered model prisoners. They tend to keep to themselves and not cause trouble. "The I-5 killer [Randall Woodfield] lives in A-block too," Jesperson tells me. "I've met him and talked with him. He's arrogant."

"Why do you say that?" I'm curious to hear one serial murderer's take on another.

"Because he says he didn't do it." He shakes his head. "Give me a break. They all say they didn't do it."

"You think you're a good judge of people?"

"There isn't much to judge. . . . I can tell what kind of person you are." Before I realize what he's doing, he reaches out and grabs my hands. His hands swallow mine. I notice a green bandage and splint on his left pinkie. He says, "I know that you're a good person."

I pull my hands back and nod at his bandage. "What happened to your finger?"

"I jammed it in the laundry cart and broke it."

I picture his large hands and the hurt they have caused. I'm now ready to move past the chitchat.

"Why women?" I ask.

"What's that?"

"Why did you kill women?"

He sits back in his chair and thinks for a moment. "There's a sort of arrogance. They feel they can say and do anything and nothing will happen to them. Men see me, see how big I am, and don't mess with me." He leans forward. "Also, I'm vulnerable to women. I love women—the way they look, taste, feel, smell. I'm a romantic. So when I feel something could be romantic and then that's not what's going to happen, I get angry."

Rain drizzles against the open windows above us and a chill breeze blows through. I wrap my sweater tightly around me.

Since we started conversing over the phone, Keith has refused to discuss his murders of the women. I think he dangled that information in front of me as a reward only if I visited him in person. Even now, I sense that he is not ready to disclose his murders to me. I change the subject.

"Keith, let me ask you again. Why did you write that letter to the newspaper about killing the cat?" I have still not found his letter about the cat he strangled at the mobile park. The newspaper archives prior to 2000 are not so well organized.

"The cat was someone's pet."

"What if the cat wasn't someone's pet? Would you see that differently?"

"It's still someone's pet. The animals are still part of the community. All animals belong to someone or they belong to society on the whole."

Society on the whole. I consider these words. When my sister traveled to Costa Rica, the attendant at the rental car office handed her the car keys and said, "Please don't hurt our animals." Throughout her trip, my sister encountered a sense of shared responsibility among Costa Ricans in caring for animals. If we followed Costa Rica's lead and viewed all animals as society's animals, as *our* animals under *our* care, would we be much less accepting of violence toward them?

I ask Jesperson, "Out of all the animals you killed, why write about that one cat?"

"It's not just one cat. It's *the* cat. It was the fulcrum point, which changed my life. There isn't much difference in killing a cat or a human. I think it had some effect on me later on when I became a murderer. Strangling worked before so I figured it would work again. The cat killing desensitized me."

I don't agree with Jesperson. He was desensitized long before he killed the cat. But strangling the cat and the eight women might have given him greater satisfaction than killing by other means. A study looked at the most sadistic serial killers—those who had tortured their victims prior to killing them. Of these, almost two-thirds were reported to have previously injured or killed animals and half had tortured the animals before killing them. These killers took pleasure in causing their victims to suffer and they often used the same techniques of torture and killing against both animal and human victims. The FBI's Alan Brantley told me that murderers like Jesperson "like to engage all of their senses. Sight, sound, smell, touch, taste. And they get right up close and very personal. I mean when you strangle somebody, you literally see the life going out of their eyes and their face, and you see them struggle. You see the fear and the panic and the just sheer terror. For a lot of these guys with that very sadistic feature, it really enhances the experience. It is very arousing for them."

Jesperson continues. "People have a tendency to separate the two, animals and humans. One life is the same as another. They both struggle to stay alive."

❧

"Murder isn't cheap," Jesperson tells me with complete seriousness the next morning. I had counted on him talking about his murders. If he didn't, my understanding of his behaviors would be incomplete. I arrived as soon as the visitor doors opened to get as much face time as possible with Jesperson. This seems to have pleased him. He's willing to talk about the women now.

Jesperson describes how he rented a machine to clean up all the blood in his living room after he killed Taunja Bennett, his first human victim. "I met her at a bar and took her back to my place. Thought she was interested. But I was getting mixed signals. When she showed she wasn't interested in sex, I got angry. I punched her in the face."

I look up at the wall behind Jesperson. The animated movie *Despicable Me* is playing on the mounted, large flat-screen TV. I look back at Jesperson. I had read everything out there about Jesperson's murders. But it is a very different experience to be sitting across from the man and hearing him describe the murders to me. And one of the hardest things I have ever had to do is sit and listen.

Without emotion, he tells me how he repeatedly punched Bennett. He bloodied her face and broke her nose. Blood was flying all over the walls and ceiling.

Oh God.

"When I did stop [punching her]," he says, apparently not noticing the loathing on my face, "I saw what I had done and I thought, 'I don't want to go to jail.' So I killed her. It took about four minutes to strangle her. My hands were as white as this." He points to the fake marble tabletop between us.

I'm nauseated. I get up and excuse myself, knowing his eyes follow me. I walk into the restroom and try to throw up, but I just have dry heaves. As a trained neurologist, I had taken care of patients with severe psychiatric diseases and personality disorders, including sociopaths. Some were violent. But I always maintained a dispassionate and clinical demeanor. I had a clear role to play, which was to help heal them. This is different. I am not Jesperson's doctor. There is no white coat or clipboard between us. Throughout our visit, Jesperson sits with an uncanny stillness. His gaze rarely leaves my face and he closely watches my expressions. If Jesperson wants a reaction out of me, I am not going to give him that. Not this time. I wash my face and hands under cold tap water and walk back out.

I make no comment as I sit down, my face impassive. He continues right back where he left off, describing in detail how he raped and killed the other women. As he describes his murders, I muse at how his life so eerily matches the story of Tom Nero, the protagonist in William Hogarth's The Four Stages of Cruelty. A social critic and artist, Hogarth released a series of four prints in 1751. Each print furthers the narrative of fictional character Nero—perhaps named after the tyrannical Roman emperor—to depict how mistreatment of animals is part of a larger, social pattern of violence.

The *First Stage of Cruelty* shows a group of boys, most of them participating in or encouraging some form of animal abuse. Nero is pushing an arrow into the rectum of a terrified dog while another boy pleads with him to stop. In the *Second Stage of Cruelty*, animal abuse is more widespread and institutionalized. Nero has progressed from a schoolboy inflicting cruelty on animals for recreation to a man who does so as a routine part of his job. The second print shows Nero beating his horse, who has collapsed under the strain of the cart he his pulling. Another man bludgeons a lamb to death. An angered bull tosses his tormenter. Also depicted is violence against humans. A driver naps while a child is crushed under the weight of his cart and posters in the background advertise cockfighting and boxing matches. In *Cruelty in Perfection*, Nero is a highway robber and has murdered his pregnant lover. Her body lays prostrate on the floor, with her throat slit and her wrist and index finger almost severed. In the final print, *The Reward of Cruelty*, Nero is convicted of and hanged for murder, his body publicly dissected, and, in ironic justice, a dog feeds on his heart.

At the end of the morning visiting hours, Jesperson asks me if am going to return in the afternoon. I look at him. *What am I doing here?* I want to leave Jesperson far behind and forget all about him. But I just say, "I don't know."

❧

I do return in the afternoon. I know I will be kicking myself later if I do not use the available time to learn as much from Jesperson as possible. When I enter the visiting room, he has the game of cribbage set up on the table. Yesterday, we discussed having him teach me how to play. Mentally drained from our conversation this morning, I don't feel like talking right now, anyway. Perhaps I could just observe him for a while as we play the game.

We don't get far into cribbage, though, before Jesperson says that he doesn't think he can teach the game properly during the time we have. We then play the game *Sorry* for about twenty minutes before we give that up. It is a newer, jacked-up version with the rules missing from the box. We make up our own rules, but neither of us is really into it. Jesperson wants to talk.

Okay. We will talk. First, I need a cup of tea. I get up and purchase a hot, black tea from a vending machine. I take a sip and grimace. The tea tastes like hot water flavored with eight granules of instant decaf coffee.

"I want to tell you a secret," he tells me as I sit back down.

"Okay." I gulp a desperate sip of my "tea." What is he going to tell me now?

"When I was thirteen, my brothers and I are sitting around a campfire and my dad tells us of a night when he had a premonition. He was traveling down a road and had a premonition that something bad just happened there. He pulled over, and there was a cop there who told him it wasn't a safe place to pull over—a man was run over and killed there the night before. We all thought, 'Oh that's scary,' when Dad told us this. He told us this same story when I was fourteen, then fifteen. One night, when I'm eighteen, Dad is drunk and he tells me that he was driving down that road at that same spot the night the man was killed. Dad thought he hit something but kept going. The next day he drove out there, and that's when he heard that a man was killed the night before."

"You think your dad ran over that man?"

"When I asked Dad about this the next day after he was all sober, I asked him why didn't he go to the police and tell them what happened and that it was an accident. He said, 'Listen, you forget about what you heard; it never happened.' My dad taught me that as long as we did things behind closed doors and no one knew about it, it was okay."

Yeah, I know how that is. Sylvester was abused behind closed doors. I was abused behind closed doors.

"Did you ever hear a deer cry?" Jesperson asks, suddenly switching topics.

"No. I didn't know they could."

"Deer will actually cry and bawl. . . . You ever hear a rabbit cry?"

"No."

"A rabbit will scream, will actually cry or scream. That's what draws the coyotes in to kill the rabbit. They'll actually start bawling. We're so used to animals saying nothing. Did you watch that movie *Powder*, where this kid has extra powers and he puts his hands on the animal and he actually can see and feel the animal's fear?"

"You mentioned this movie before. I've never seen it."

"He grabs onto this person that shot the deer, and he puts his hand on the deer, and the guy's actually able to feel what the deer is going through, and from that point on the guy doesn't want to hunt deer anymore."

"Tell me about the deer you heard cry."

"When I shot the deer, I shot too high and too forward. I had to hunt that deer down for hours before I could get another shot and kill him. It was bawling. It was crying. That's how I tracked it, because it was crying over the fact that the arrow had gone into the shoulder blade and didn't go through any vitals. It was limping around on one leg. Sooner or later a coyote would have gotten it or something, but I had to track that deer for hours before I could finally get a good shot at it to put the deer down. I refused to go hunting for deer after that, I just refused to. I refused to go hunting for elk and deer after that happened in Canada in the fall of '82."

"Why do you think this affected you?"

"Because I actually heard him cry. I went out there thinking they don't make sounds, so it's okay. Hearing the deer bawl was sickening. That moment I heard him and heard that they actually have a voice."

Over the loudspeaker, an announcer informs us that visiting hours are over for the day. I fly back home the next morning and will not see Jesperson again. We stand up, shake hands, and say our goodbyes. He heads in the direction where inmates line up to return to their cells, and I go the other way. Something compels me to turn around and I watch Jesperson as he walks with a slight limp from an old leg injury and from arthritic knees. For the briefest of moments, I see him not as the brutal killer that he most certainly is, but as an aging, lonely man.

"Bye, Keith," I say again.

He stops and turns to me. He looks surprised. "Bye," he says quietly.

❧

Patrick is right, again. Two nights later, for the first time in twenty years, I dream about Uncle Talup.

❧

Why did I do this? Did I get what I wanted? Back at home, I reflect on my rather cavalier attitude about meeting Jesperson. I come to the conclusion that despite the emotional turmoil he caused me, it was worth it. I learned far more than I expected, not only about him but also myself.

I must admit that when I first wrote to Jesperon, I had preconceived notions of what I would hear from him. I expected that Jesperson's only relationships with animals were those that revolved around cruelty. However, even though Jesperson showed immense cruelty and apathy toward those he killed, he also showed moments of unexpected humanity. Although these two sides were evident with many of the men I read about at Lima State Hospital, I still did not anticipate this dichotomy in a serial killer. I fell prey to my own bias.

Jesperson had natural empathy for animals as a child and even, occasionally, as an adult. It comes through when he talks about the deer he shot who cried. But he learned early on that kindness toward animals leads to painful results—punishment for his retaliatory action after his brother killed his crow, deceit by his father who killed Duke. And Jesperson's neighbors and family, and most importantly, his father, taught him that violence toward animals was acceptable. Every time Jesperson cruelly treated an animal and got away with it or was rewarded by attention from his father, his behavior was reinforced. Ultimately, his nascent empathy was largely crushed by the weight of his many years of practiced cruelty.

A psychiatrist has never formally examined Jesperson and diagnosed him as having a personality disorder like APD. Commonly thought of as sociopathy or psychopathy—two distinct personality disorders with some overlap—APD is characterized by, among other things, lack of empathy for others and little to no remorse. But even if Jesperson was diagnosed with APD, it would be far too easy to stick a label on him as an explanation for his violence. Does APD cause the violence? Or does the violence cause APD? Which comes first?

We must look at the totality of Jesperson's life, including his relationships with animals. In 1964, Margaret Mead noted: "One of the most dangerous things that can happen to a child is to kill or torture an animal and not be held responsible." There is no one-to-one direct correlation between harming animals and harming humans. After all, Dave did not go on to abuse humans after hurting Sylvester. There are many complicating factors that have to be accounted for, including family dynamics, mental conditions, and genetics. However, there is a rising tide of evidence verifying that people who inflict violence on animals, and are actively or even passively encouraged to do so, are more likely to do the same toward humans.

Empathy is an essential component in our moral development. Without it, we are unable to imagine the lives of others and their suffering and a have a desire to relieve it. In this sense, criminology professor Piers Beirne argues, empathy for animals and humans is probably strongly linked. For Jesperson, women and animals share a vulnerability that he exploited. The women he killed, mostly sex workers and homeless, were on the margins of society. Easily overlooked. Not unlike most animals. If someone had intervened early in Jesperson's life and nurtured his inherent kindness toward animals, he might have learned to view women with empathy rather than as targets for his venom.

Jesperson reawakened an emotional reaction to my own abuse—something I arrogantly thought was far behind me. Naturally, his descriptions of his raping and killing women played a role in this. But it is more than that. I did not anticipate just how much I would come to know about myself through a serial murderer.

Violence is not just a product of an individual's psychology, but also of social and cultural influences. Through his surrounding culture, Jesperson was habituated to accept violence. So was I. I was taught to be a good Pakistani girl and to respect my elders, authority, and traditions. If an elder tells you to do something, you do it. If an adult leads you by your hand to the bedroom, you go with him. Even though I was disturbed by Uncle Talup's behavior toward me, I also, over time, came to see it as nothing out of the ordinary. It was just my life. It was routine.

I now also understand why I didn't question Dave too deeply when he hurt Sylvester.

"This is normal," Dave said to me.

Throughout history, these three words championed willful ignorance. These three words excused discrimination. These three words fueled dominion over the powerless. And these three words tricked me into accepting Sylvester's abuse and mine.

It's hard to recognize violence when it is seen as ordinary. Just as I, as a child, did not fully recognize the violence in my life either toward me or toward Sylvester, neither did Jesperson. But I can look at *his* life and see the warning signs that led to his murders. Jesperson knows right from wrong and he has a ready rationale for each murder. How much does his ability to justify his killing of women stem from learning to justify each act of cruelty toward animals? As with his murders, he has in his mind a reasonable answer for why he killed each animal. Additionally, he defends many of his actions toward animals by deferring to cultural attitudes (including those of his neighbors and family). "Everyone was doing it," or "It was part of the job." When cultural norms overlook or justify one kind of cruelty, do we open the doors for all forms of cruelty? Are we, as a society, culpable in the making of Jesperson?

"Violent killers like Jesperson are the tip of the iceberg," Dr. Hickey later tells me. "They are the harbinger of things to come. They are telling us what's going on with our society."

One month after my visit with Jesperson, I finally track down his letter to the *Statesman Journal*.

On November 23, 1996, in Salem, Oregon, police arrested two McNary High School students for bludgeoning a tabby cat to death. According to the police, eighteen-year-olds Thomas Shepard and Darle Dudley used wooden clubs to kill the cat after he wandered into Shepard's home. The cat was one of many strays that Shepard's stepmother had been feeding. When the stepmother found the cat's body in a trash can, she called the police.

It wasn't so much the arrest of the two students that caused a raging debate in the town's newspaper; rather, it was a remark by McNary football coach Tom Smythe. After learning of the arrest of Shepard, one of his prized football players, Smythe told reporters: "Let's put this in perspective. [Shepard] didn't rape, maim or pillage anyone. He committed a foolish act that cost a dumb animal its life."

For nearly two weeks, the *Statesman Journal* received more letters about the killing of the cat and Smythe's remarks than on any other subject. Among the letters was Jesperson's:

> *It's in the crime journals of all major law enforcement agencies. Abusive behavior toward animals is one of the symptoms on the road to being a murderer.*
>
> *It was in my early adulthood that my aggression toward animals increased.*
>
> *My father witnessed me throwing a cat against the pavement and then strangling it to death. We owned the rental in which the cat was found.*
>
> *Instead of telling me it was wrong, he was kind of proud of the way I took care of it. He even bragged about the way I took care of the stray cats and dogs in our mobile home park.*
>
> *All this did was to spawn in me the urge to kill again. I began to think of what it would be like to kill a human being. The thought stayed with me for years, until one night it happened.*
>
> *I killed a woman by beating her almost to death and finished her off by strangulation. No longer did I search for animals to mistreat. I now looked for people to kill. And I did.*
>
> *I killed over and over until I was caught. Now I'm paying for it with the rest of my life behind bars.*
>
> *We should stop the cruelty to anything before it develops into a bigger problem, like me. Violence and aggression may cause bigger problems than just the senseless beating of a cat.*
>
> *Keith Jesperson*

FIVE

It's Just an Animal

D ave continued to hurt Sylvester. He blamed Sylvester's rambunctiousness for his broken bones and injuries. Every time he slammed Sylvester against a wall, punched him in the face, or kicked his little body, I shed secret tears. But I remained silent.

After four months, I thought about calling the police. I looked up the number for the local police station, then hesitated. What would I say to the police? I loved Dave and, despite what he was doing to Sylvester, I didn't want to get him into trouble. And what if the police didn't care about what was happening to Sylvester? What if they saw nothing wrong with what Dave was doing and agreed that he was just training a dog? I had seen police come by our buildings many times to talk to the people living there or make arrests. Possessing and selling drugs and guns was a common activity. In my neighborhood, cops were our enemies. Even if we weren't doing anything illegal, we always dreaded that the police would find *something* against us.

Yet in full view of the police, neighbors chained dogs cruelly for hours in the extreme cold or heat and collared cats with gaping wounds wandered about. A lot of people hurt animals openly without fear of the police.

I never did make that call. I was nervous about calling the police and I convinced myself that they wouldn't care anyway. "It's just an animal," they would say. And I was probably right.

But attitudes have evolved since then.

Somewhat.

⚬

Outside an expansive seventh-floor auditorium, I gaze at the sweeping Manhattan skyline. The Police Academy in Queens, New York, is holding a training session today on animal cruelty for its police force. I first reached out to the New York Police Department (NYPD) to learn how police today would handle a call about animal abuse. It turns out that New York is ahead of its time. Headed by Sergeant Mike Murphy, the NYPD's Animal Cruelty Investigation Squad is the nation's first-ever unit of detectives who work full-time investigating animal cruelty.

Murphy invited me to attend this training session, which is jointly taught by the NYPD and the ASPCA. The police were always required by law to investigate animal cruelty if they saw it or received a tip-off. But up until a few years ago, the bulk of that policing role fell to the ASPCA. Whenever a 911 call of animal abuse came into the police system, it was usually routed to the ASPCA. Now, through a new collaboration, the NYPD takes the primary role in investigating animal cruelty and enforcing animal cruelty laws in New York. This change has led to rippling effects. Suddenly, the number of men and women inspecting animal abuse went from about eighteen ASPCA employees to the thirty-four thousand police men and women throughout all five of New York's boroughs. Additionally, the NYPD formed a new unit of detectives to solely investigate animal cruelty cases. Now the ASPCA can focus its energies and expertise on providing instrumental support, such as training the entire police force in identifying animal abuse, understanding animal protection laws, and knowing what to do if a 911 call comes in pleading for someone to help a dog, cat, or other animal in need.

On this Saturday morning, three hundred men and women—rookie cops to senior sergeants and detectives—pack into the auditorium. I sit near the front row with a cup of hot, black coffee in hand. First up to the podium is Sergeant Murphy. His soft voice, tinged with a Brooklyn accent, doesn't quite match his body type. I keep expecting a deep roar to emanate from his thick neck and body.

"Ted Bundy. Jeffrey Dahmer. Dennis Rader," he announces to the audience. "They all had histories of hurting animals before killing, eating, and mutilating people. When they do bad things to animals, they do bad things to people. When investigating these crimes, be nosy. When investigating people, look at the animals. When investigating animals, look at the people."

After Murphy's brief introduction, a young woman from the ASPCA takes over. "If you have an animal case, call us at the ASPCA. We'll help you. We have a hotline. We'll walk you through it." The ASPCA's helpline operates twenty-four hours a day to support the NYPD and instruct the officers on how to handle and transport animals. The ASPCA directs the police to take animals to their animal hospital on Ninety-Second Street in Manhattan or to one of many partner veterinary hospitals in the area. At the hospitals, veterinarians will provide medical care for free, if needed, and initiate forensic examinations and documentation. This last action has proven to be instrumental in successfully prosecuting animal abusers.

"Be prepared; there may be media," the ASPCA representative says. "There was [footage] of a man who kicked a cat twenty-five feet in the air. That video went viral."

An attorney with the ASPCA gets up next and asks the audience, "Who here has investigated an animal case?" I look around. Only a smattering of hands is raised. "The most common forms of animal cruelty you will see are inadequate shelter, abandonment, confinement in vehicles, an animal in extreme temperature, and animal fighting. Animal cruelty can be an overt act or an act of omission, and it applies to any animal." She next shows photos. Audience members, whose eyes were glazed, are suddenly alert. One photo is of a cat drowned in bleach, another of a squirrel riddled with gunshots. "Overt acts," she says. Then she shows photos of emaciated animals and animals with open, painful-looking sores. "Cruelty by neglect. Owners have an obligation to provide veterinary care. 'I can't afford it' is not an excuse."

One by one throughout the morning, miserable images and videos are displayed on the screen. Images of bloodied, beaten cats. Poisoned raccoons. Burned rabbits. Then a speaker projects a series of photos of animal fighting rings and equipment: a concrete dog-fighting pit covered in feces and blood; treadmills where dogs are forced to run up to three hours at a time to prepare for a dogfight; rape stands used to breed dogs; weight-pulling machines, heavy chains, and spurs. All equipment made for the sole purpose of watching animals maim and kill one another. This is big business.

Some of the largest cases the NYPD investigates involve animal-fighting rings. These operations run deep underground with extensive networks throughout the country and even the world. Murphy described to me how one of the men they are investigating for running a cockfighting network in New York frequently travels back and forth to Mexico. He is suspected of overseeing further animal-fighting rings there and possibly other crimes. "Crime doesn't happen in a vacuum," John Goodwin of the Humane Society of the United States once said. "When you have violent people betting large sums of money, you're going to have problems."

Dogfighting, cockfighting, and other similar activities partner with money laundering, drug cartels, human trafficking, prostitution, gambling, and gangs. Murphy frequently sends members of his team undercover to penetrate the heavy defenses surrounding animal-fighting networks. These investigations take months, sometimes years, and they usually include detectives outside of his squad, each focusing on different connecting crimes. "Where there's animal fighting," one of the presenters say, "there's gangs, guns, drugs, and lots of money involved."

The room erupts into laughter, and I look up from my coffee cup. The large screen shows an image of cockfighting paraphernalia, including a blue, passport-looking book embossed with gold lettering on the cover that says in large print: EL COCK OFFICIAL RECORD BOOK.

I laugh along with the audience, but then we all quickly sober as a video of a cockfight runs. I've never seen a cockfight before and am shocked at how violent and swift they are. In the video, men strap two cocks with spurs, place them into a concrete pit, and stand back and watch. In barely a minute, the two birds attack and practically annihilate each other. Feathers, skin, bone bits, and blood fly everywhere. I hear someone in the audience gasp, "Holy cow!"

The presenter says, "Whoever loses the most blood is the loser in the cockfight."

As I look upon the image of the bloodied fighting pit and imagine the mind-set that enables people to cause such suffering, I think, no, the presenter is wrong. Everyone loses in this fight.

⸎

Over the lunch break, I sit with the other detectives of Murphy's squad in a private room reserved for the presenters and hosts. Eight detectives are assigned to the squad, formed in 2015. All had been working for the NYPD for years—some worked on homicides, some on gang violence, others on drug crimes. All highly experienced. The detectives are so eager to share their animal investigation experiences with me that I get the sense that many other cops dismiss them for not working on "serious issues" anymore.

One of the detectives, Lisa Bergen, shows me a photo on her cell phone of her dogs, Paco and Pebbles. The two dogs lounge in a kiddie swimming pool in their backyard as Paco holds a water-spouting garden hose in his mouth, looking extremely satisfied. "I had been in the force for almost seven years," Lisa tells me, "but when I heard of this new unit, I put in a request to join."

When I ask her why, she shows me a photo on another phone. I wince. The photo shows a dog's body, burned and charred.

Someone had wrapped the dog in a blanket, then set him on fire. "For reasons like this," Lisa says. "They're innocent. You're being the voice for the voiceless. Look, I did a lot of DV [domestic violence]. You get a victim calling for help. We go out, then they drop the charges. They call for help again another time and then drop the charges again. They don't want to press charges. With animals, you don't need them to press charges. You help on their behalf and they're always so grateful to be helped. Doesn't matter how abused they are, they still show love when helped."

This last point is reiterated almost word for word when I speak to another detective on the squad. Tara Cuccias tells me, "In our unit, we have hardened street cops, and this is the most rewarding thing we've ever done. Animals are so thankful. No matter how abused, they are always so grateful."

After our lunch break, we head back to the auditorium to look at images of x-rays of bone fractures, broken ribs, and skull trauma. I don't want to look at any more sad photos so I spend more time watching the audience members, curious about their reactions. Some cops appear bored. A few others lean forward in their chairs, eyes glued to the screen, scribbling down notes. Most look somewhere in between. Howard Lawrence, who worked for the NYPD for twenty-five years before joining the ASPCA to serve as their NYPD liaison, later tells me that the feedback he has received about the class ranges from cops demanding that they "show less pictures, they're disgusting" to "this is one of the best classes I've ever taken." He tells me, "We got a lot of kickback in the beginning. People saying we already have enough to do. I worked in the police force since 1983 and back then DWIs [driving while influenced], domestic violence—they weren't taken seriously. Now they are. It's routine. I expect the same to happen with animal cruelty. More cops now are getting it."

What more cops are now getting is that animal cruelty is part of a much larger social picture of violence. And not just the most extreme forms of violence. The Keith Jespersons of the world are the exceptions, at the end of the spectrum of behavior. Most animal abuse links with "everyday" crimes.

People who abuse animals are more likely to commit other violent acts. A study of 261 incarcerated male inmates at medium- and maximum-security prisons found that 43 percent committed animal cruelty. Another study found animal cruelty to be especially prevalent among the most violent criminals. The investigators of this study divided 117 inmates into violent and nonviolent offenders. The violent offenders engaged in animal abuse significantly more often than the non-violent offenders (63 percent versus 11 percent).

The Massachusetts Society for the Prevention of Cruelty to Animals (MSPCA) and psychologists from Northeastern University jointly published one of the most notable studies depicting the connection between animal cruelty and other crimes. The researchers identified 153 convicted animal abusers prosecuted by the MSPCA between 1975 and 1986 and examined whether they had histories of other criminal behavior. They found that in comparison with a control group, 70 percent of animal abusers had also committed other crimes within the prior ten years, including interpersonal violence, property damage, and drug offenses. The study authors concluded that animal abusers are three times more likely to commit drunken or disorderly offenses; four times more likely to commit property crimes; and five times more likely to inflict violence on people.

The Chicago Police Department found similar results in a more recent study. Of 332 animal cruelty arrests, 86 percent of suspects had histories of multiple arrests. Seventy percent had prior felony charges; 68 percent had prior drug or trafficking arrests; 65 percent had been charged with battery against another person; 59 percent were suspected gang members; 27 percent had firearm charges; and 13 percent had arrests for sex crimes. The study, the investigators stated, "revealed a startling propensity for offenders charged with crimes against animals to commit other violent offenses toward human victims."

The connection between violence against animals and other crimes is so firmly established that the FBI recently made major changes to how it tracks animal abuse. Previously, when local police throughout the United States reported cases of animal cruelty to the FBI's National Incident-Based Reporting System, these crimes were lumped into the "other" category. As a result, minimal data were collected on animal abuse, if at all. With its recent changes, the FBI now collects data on animal cruelty like it does on murder and rape. Animal cruelty is categorized as a Group A offense and includes four subcategories: simple/gross neglect, intentional abuse and torture, organized abuse such as dogfighting, and animal sexual abuse. With these new categories, the FBI can get richer, granular data on the circumstances of the abuse.

Perhaps what is most heartening for me to hear from the ASPCA's Howard Lawrence is not just that law enforcement is increasingly aware of the strong connection between crimes against animals and humans but that cops are concerned for animals for *their sake* too. More than ever before, police officers are bringing animals of all kinds to the ASPCA for help. Dogs, cats, chickens, guinea pigs, hamsters, birds, you name it. And often, the cops end up taking many of the animals home as new members of their families.

But I learn that some changes within the police force are still slow to come. When Lisa Bergen presents later in the afternoon, she shows a series of photos, each titled "Animal Abusers." Many of the photos are of the same serial killers that Mike Murphy showed in the morning. Dahmer, Bundy. But then Bergen shows a photo of former Atlanta Falcons quarterback Michael Vick and the audience breaks out laughing. I look around, bewildered, not understanding why there's laughter this time. In 2007, Vick was convicted of the brutal treatment and killing of dogs whom he "trained" for his animal fighting ring. Vick starved dogs to make them more aggressive and dogfights ended when a dog gave up or died. Vick executed dogs who underperformed by hanging, drowning, strangulation, electrocution, shooting, or slamming them on the ground. A search of Vick's property uncovered the remains of seven of the dogs killed. After pleading guilty, Vick spent less than two years in a federal prison before rejoining the National Football League (NFL) with the Philadelphia Eagles. Vick went on to play for several other teams before leaving the NFL in 2016.

On the stage, Bergen points out that there's a new era in animal fighting. It's not just a few individuals holding a fight in their back-yards. As Vick illustrates, she says, wealthy individuals from the sports and entertainment worlds are jumping in.

After several more talks, the ending of the training is announced, which brings on applause, cheers, and whistles from the crowd. As everyone gets up to leave, I linger. There's something I have to find out. Why did everyone laugh at the photo of Michael Vick?

⁂

At five A.M., four months after the NYPD training session, Nick hands me a bulletproof vest and tells me we are heading out to make arrests. This is the first of my four days riding along with the NYPD's Animal Cruelty Investigation Squad. I put on the vest. It's about four sizes too large. Apologizing, Nick says, "It's all we have with us." I'm dubious, but as long as it doesn't slip down my waist, I guess I'm okay.

I slide into the backseat of an unmarked black Ford Explorer. Nick drives while Mike, a cadet, helps him navigate the congested streets. For such an early, dark hour, the traffic is heavy. We cross the Whitestone Bridge connecting Queens to the Bronx, past the New York Botanical gardens, and stop at a public housing development in the 40th Precinct in the South Bronx. Another black SUV carrying detectives Charlie, Tara, and Ron join us.

Nick, Mike, and I step out of our car and join the other detectives. Everyone is on alert and guarded. I watch the detectives secure their bulletproof vests and place their hands on the semiautomatics hol-stered to their hips. "Yesterday," one of the detectives tells me, "we dropped everything in the middle of the day to investigate a pos-sible dogfighting ring. Found cocaine, guns. It was a place like this."

The other three detectives enter the building while Nick, Mike, and I stand outside. I notice them closely watching the fourth-floor windows from the street. I turn to Nick and ask him why they are staring at the windows. Without taking his eyes off his target, he says, "In case, someone up there starts making trouble. Wants to start shooting."

I take a step back and look up at the windows. They're dark and still.

"Sometimes when they see us coming, they throw out their guns, crack, coke . . . out the window," Nick adds.

Is this a dogfighting gang we're about to bust? "Who are you arresting?" I ask, puffing myself up in anticipation.

"Elderly woman. Sixty-eight years old."

⬦

Who hurts animals?

The elderly woman, I learn, committed a misdemeanor for neglecting two water turtles. She turned them over to animal control because she no longer wanted them, unaware that she had committed a crime. Animal control called the police.

"One turtle lost a leg," Nick tells me. "The other's shell flattened out." The water turtles were so sick, animal control euthanized them. One turtle's limb turned black and fell off, a common scenario when people buy aquatic turtles from pet stores without knowing how to care for them. Forced to live twenty-four hours a day in filthy water without a place to dry off their limbs, turtles frequently contract infections. The second turtle whose shell flattened out probably suffered from softshell syndrome. A metabolic bone disease due to a lack of calcium in the diet from severe malnutrition or from insufficient sunlight exposure, softshell syndrome causes shell deformities. The turtle grows, but the shell does not. Over time, the turtle becomes weak and has trouble walking due to the softened bones, which easily fracture. Both diseases, especially the deformed shell, take days, months, even years to develop. And both cause tremendous pain. The woman could not have failed to notice that the animals were severely sick. She would have walked by the two small turtles languishing in their dirty aquarium day after day, saw them literally rotting away before her eyes and done nothing.

The woman likely didn't hurt the turtles out of malicious intent. But did the suffering she caused these animals who were completely dependent on her care constitute abuse? To this woman and to many others, probably not.

It's easy to think of the serial killers, the severely mentally disturbed, the outliers, as perpetrators of violence. There is a twisted comfort in believing that monsters crouching in the shadowy underpasses of society are the problem; these are people who are clearly abnormal. But if "normal" people abuse animals, then what does that say about humanity?

At the end of the NYPD training session, as everyone was departing, I turned to several older cops and asked them why the audience laughed at Michael Vick's photo. They replied, "Here you have a photo of a professional football player up on the same slide with serial killers. You don't expect someone like him to abuse animals. They still don't believe it." Lisa Bergen echoed the two officers' response. "When I first started giving this lecture," she told me, "I was surprised that most people reacted the same way every time I put up Vick's picture. They see him as one of the guys. 'Yeah,' they would tell me, 'but he's such a good football player.'"

Cruelty is in the eyes of the beholder. Throughout the ages, cultures have shaped the definition of violence like bread dough. It's been pinched, stretched, punched, expanded. This has been especially true for definitions of domestic violence and abuse of children. How we define abuse is influenced by our beliefs, cultural mores, and, perhaps most importantly, the biases of those in power. For these reasons, domestic violence has been downplayed and only recognized as a legitimate concern, even by law enforcement, in recent decades. Men have historically determined what constitutes violence toward women. Adults decided what child abuse is. Worst of all, victims often believed these definitions.

For too long, people have buried any suggestion of sexual abuse of children, especially by family members (or in my case, by a close family friend). It was taboo. It was shushed. It was ignored. If you think getting recognition of familial child sexual abuse was bad in the Western world, imagine what it was like in a Pakistani family. My parents' radars were fixed on strangers, not on friends and family. My father continuously admonished me as a child every time I tried to sneak out the door wearing short sleeves and shorts. He genuinely believed that by telling me to cover up, he was protecting me from strange men's roving eyes. The irony was not lost on me, even as a child.

Though there is still a ways to go, much has been improved in how we look upon violence toward the less powerful. Women, people of color, gays, and sometimes children, are rightly calling violence as it is. But what about animal abuse? Humans define it. We decide whether an animal has been abused or not. As to determining who hurts an animal, we hold the paintbrushes. To many of the NYPD officers, a successful football player doesn't fit their portraits. To probably most of us, little old ladies who bake cookies don't fit our portraits. But give the paintbrushes to the dogs and turtles who suffered at their hands, and I think we would get a painting to rival that of Henry Fuseli's *The Nightmare*.

After ten minutes inside the public housing building in search of the elderly woman, Tara and the other detectives walk out, empty-handed. "The woman's not home," she explains to the rest of us waiting outside. "Already at work."

We get in our cars and drive half an hour through congestion to make the next arrest on the list. The woman is not there. We then drive another forty-five minutes to make a different arrest and . . . the person isn't home. He'd already left for work. In the movies, when they show detectives, chests swelling, kicking open the front door of a residence or warehouse to bust the bad guys, they never show the more mundane prior attempts the cops probably made.

We pile back into the cars. This time, I ride along with Tara. "Are we going to drive to their workplaces?" I ask about the offenders we didn't find at home.

"I don't have their addresses with me. We'll have to come out another day."

I mull this over as we drive through bumper-to-bumper traffic back to the satellite office in Queens. We drove all this way for nothing. Why don't the police keep the offenders' work addresses as well as their home addresses with them? I would think that would be an obvious thing to do. I keep my thoughts to myself.

In the afternoon, I accompany Sergeant Murphy, Mike the cadet, and Nick to the Queens District Attorney's Office in Kew Gardens to meet Nicoletta Caferri. An assistant district attorney (ADA) for twenty-seven years, Caferri is New York's first ADA working full-time on animal cruelty cases.

"I went last night to a screening of *Unlocking the Cage*," she tells me, after Murphy introduces us. "Do you know of it?" I do. The documentary follows animal rights attorney Steven Wise as he challenges the court system to recognize legal personhood status for chimpanzees. Personhood would allow lawyers and advocates to defend abused and confined chimpanzees through legal devices. Habeas corpus, for example, is a legal procedure through which a person can report unlawful detention or imprisonment and request that a prisoner be brought to court to determine whether the detention is lawful. This is a right that only humans currently hold. "There was a Q and A afterwards with Steven Wise," Caferri tells me. "The whole thing was fascinating."

Prior to 2015, Caferri would never have considered issues like animal personhood status, but that changed after she prosecuted her first animal cruelty case. Caferri tells me, "I was working on a case that went to the Court of Appeals, New York's highest court. It was a simple neglect case and, at first, everyone was asking me, 'Why are you taking this little misdemeanor case?'"

The 2015 appeals case concerned defendant Curtis Basile and a dog under his care. Acting on an anonymous tip, an agent for the

ASPCA discovered a long-haired, mixed-breed German shepherd confined to a garbage-strewn backyard by a four-foot leash tied to a fence. The agent found no food, water, or shelter nearby. The dog was so emaciated that the veterinarian who later examined him said he was "one step away from death." Basile was found guilty of a misdemeanor and was sentenced to three years of probation and forty-five days of community service. He appealed the conviction, arguing that the prosecution did not prove that he "knowingly deprived the dog of or neglected or refused to furnish the basic necessities required to maintain the animal's health." It's the "I didn't know I was doing anything wrong" argument.

Perhaps because of the ludicrousness of the defense, this case garnered a lot of public attention. "It was the first time the Appeals Court heard an animal cruelty case," Caferri says. "Lawyers don't normally help each other on cases, and, all of a sudden, everyone was helping out with the case. Lawyers, animal protection folks, cops."

Basile's defense did not work. He lost the appeal. Afterward, Caferri went to the DA and said they should do this full-time. The DA agreed and created an Animal Cruelty Prosecutions Unit in the Investigations Division of the Queens County District Attorney's Office. It's the first of its kind in New York. Caferri now serves as the Inaugural Chief and her enthusiasm fills the room. "I never saw myself doing this. I was going to retire. But now I'm really excited to be doing something that's so new and innovative. It's like a second career."

Nick nods his head. "I think we all feel that way."

Murphy adds, "It's like a breath of fresh air. Everyone cares. Everyone bands together to help."

"Now people are recognizing that this is necessary," Caferri says.

Caferri is aware of the studies connecting violence toward animals and humans. In addition to other crimes, animal cruelty is associated with antisocial behaviors and personality traits, and noncriminal but destructive behaviors, such as substance abuse. Using the results from the National Epidemiological Survey on

Alcohol and Related Conditions (NESARC), investigators examined the sociodemographic, psychiatric, and behavioral correlates of cruelty to animals. NESARC is a nationally representative sample of more than forty-three thousand adults who were interviewed face-to-face. One of the questions asked was: "In your entire life, did you ever hurt or be cruel to an animal or pet on purpose?" The investigators found that cruelty to animals was significantly associated with all assessed antisocial behaviors, particularly robbery, harassment, and threat of violence. In addition, pathological gambling, history of conduct disorder in childhood, obsessive-compulsive and histrionic personality disorders, and lifetime alcohol abuse were strongly associated with a history of animal cruelty.

Another study looked at age of onset of substance abuse and its association with animal cruelty. The researchers interviewed 193 adolescents entering outpatient substance abuse treatment centers. Their study found a significant association between early onset of substance abuse or criminal involvement and cruelty toward both animals and humans.

Perhaps the strongest association between violence against animals and against humans is in domestic violence and in child abuse. Animal cruelty, particularly abuse of companion animals, occurs disproportionately in households with interhuman violence. In one study, 60 percent of those who either witnessed or committed violence against animals as children reported histories of child maltreatment or domestic violence. This includes child physical and sexual abuse, intersibling abuse, and partner abuse (same sex or heterosexual). In a study in North Carolina, investigators compared police reports for disturbances and domestic violence and assault, with animal cruelty reports. They found that almost all of the animal cruelty reports came from the same residences as the police reports.

"People don't feel safe in their communities if an animal crime is happening," Caferri says, "and if you build it, they will use it. We didn't have a lot of cases when we first started, but now we do. People are reporting. They know that we will look into it."

Murphy nods. "Since we took over, it's like a 500 percent increase in arrests."

Caferri says, "A lot of people just love animals. We have so much support now. From the public. From cops. I think it's because of the vulnerability of animals. They're so completely innocent."

Caferri tells me about other DAs working full-time on animal cruelty. There's one in Oregon and one in Texas. "But they don't have a special squad of detectives to work with and don't have the phenomenal ASPCA and their forensic work," she says. "New York is the biggest jurisdiction that's set up a model. And we've devoted a lot of resources to this. Many years ago, people didn't get arrested for DV [domestic violence] cases. Now we have a whole bureau. I think it's going to be similar with animal crimes. All eyes are on this model."

⌒∽⌒

As we drive out to Brooklyn to investigate a complaint, Murphy tells me a little more about his squad. "Right now, we have eight detectives, one supervisor—me—and one civilian," he says. He nods to Mike the cadet sitting beside me. "I get calls all the time from cops who want to join us because they're animal lovers. But they have to be trained investigators. I only recruit experienced detectives." When a 911 call about animal cruelty comes in, local street cops will go out first to inspect the case. If the case looks to be complex and more involved, it will be turned over to Murphy's squad. His cadre of detectives covers all of New York.

When we arrive at our destination, Murphy tells me that this next case concerns a raccoon. "So, Doc, about this case we're seeing. Someone had called 911 for a different animal-related case. An anonymous call came in saying the superintendent was burning rats. When the cops got there, they found a raccoon's body in a trap, bloody with what looked like some kind of liquid over him."

"What happened to the raccoon?" I ask.

"It's been sent to the vet. We're waiting for the pathology report to see if he was burned with acid."

Oh no, that poor, poor animal.

Nick parks the SUV in front of an apartment building on a busy street. A locked, grilled screen door blocks our entry into the brownstone. Murphy tries several methods to open the door but to no avail. A driver sitting in a Chinese food delivery truck parked on the curb watches us with interest before he points us toward an alley on the building's left side. The four of us follow the narrow alley, climb over a tall pile of flattened boxes and a large dumpster, and make our way around to the back.

A small yard of sorts frames the back of the building, though it looks more like a junkyard. Given how busy the front street was, it's amazingly quiet back here. We walk around to the other side of the building and see a small door, opened onto a short staircase into a curving hallway. To Mike and me, Murphy commands, "Stay back."

With his hand on the black Glock on his hip, Murphy enters the basement, followed by Nick. Mike and I watch them round the bend, then disappear. Several minutes go by. We look at each other then back toward the hallway, trying to see what's going on. Suddenly, we hear raised voices coming from inside. Someone is yelling. I can't make out most of his words, but his profanities are clear. "Fuck! . . . Fucking . . . you fuck! . . ." I hear Murphy's voice roar something back. Several more minutes go by and then Murphy, Nick, and a tall, skinny man emerge. He's dressed in baggy slacks, a dirty T-shirt, and a baseball cap. The Super.

The Super paces about the small yard. His body is never still. Neither is his voice. He doesn't talk. He rants. His frenetic pacing sharply contrasts with Murphy's calmness. I really like Murphy. He has an easy, modest nature. But his gentle voice can quickly turn and command authority. Murphy calms the Super down and asks him about the raccoon.

"Yeah, man," the Super says, "I trap coons. Possums. Gotta keep the building clean, know what I mean? Had one tenant, a woman, she says a raccoon climbed to her third-floor window and attacked her. Can't let that happen, you understand? Coons got rabies. Been working here steady now."

"There's been no rabies here for a long time," Murphy tells him, but the Super still jabbers.

"I gotta job here. Gottta keep the place clean, you know what I mean? Got rabies, you hear me? Can't have that."

"Look at me," Murphy says. "There have been no reports of rabies here. *No rabies*."

"Yeah, well, if you say so, but I got to do my job. Yeah, I trap coons. Burn 'em. Stab 'em. But kept that last one there." He points to a small metal trap lying on its side in the corner of the yard.

"You kept him in the trap?" Murphy asks him.

"Yeah, yeah, done nothing . . . he died in the trap. Done nothing to him."

"How long was he alive in the trap?"

"Don't know how long he was alive, you know? I trapped him Saturday. When I come back to look yesterday, he was dead." Three days.

Nick proceeds to get the Super's contact information as Murphy and I inspect the trap. "It's actually sad, Doc," Murphy tells me. "An animal trapped in there, dying, going crazy. Maybe I'm becoming a liberal. I don't know." He looks at me and gives a half-hearted laugh. "It is really sad, though."

Murphy can arrest the Super today if he wants to. Keeping an animal unattended in a trap for more than twenty-four hours is a crime in New York. But Murphy wants to wait for the pathology results to learn how the raccoon died. Even if the report shows that the raccoon was burned alive with acid or by another means, it won't change what crime Murphy can charge the Super with. The reason why is not because of how the raccoon was killed, but because of something far more fickle.

❧

Who is an animal?

Humans are, of course. Though we do our best to deny this. Putting that aside, who an animal is depends in part on what state he or she happens to live in.

155

Oregon says an animal is "any nonhuman mammal, bird, reptile, amphibian or fish." Missouri defines them as "every living vertebrate except a human being." That leaves out crabs, octopi, and lobsters, who are animals the last time I checked my biology books. I can't figure out the rationale behind Texas's definition: "a domesticated living creature, including any stray or feral cat or dog, and a wild living creature previously captured." Not included are never-captured wild living animals (basically all wildlife) or cows, goats, pigs, and chickens, who are defined not as animals but as "livestock animals."

We can't really blame the states for being so confused in determining just who is an animal. The writers of the Animal Welfare Act (AWA) can't figure this out either. The AWA is the "only Federal law in the United States that regulates the treatment of animals in research, exhibition, transport, and by dealers." The AWA defines an animal as "any live or dead dog, cat, monkey (nonhuman primate mammal), guinea pig, hamster, rabbit, or such other warm-blooded animal, as the Secretary may determine is being used, or is intended for use, for research, testing, experimentation, or exhibition purposes, or as a pet; but such term excludes (1) birds, rats of the genus Rattus, and mice of the genus Mus, bred for use in research, (2) horses not used for research purposes, and (3) other farm animals such as, but not limited to, livestock or poultry, used or intended for use as food or fiber, or livestock or poultry, used or intended for use for improving animal nutrition, breeding, management, or production efficiency, or for improving the quality of food or fiber." That's a brainteaser.

Fortunately, states may define animals more broadly than the authors of the AWA. New York defines animals as "every living creature except a human being." In New York, then, the raccoon that the Super allegedly killed is indeed an animal. That means the Super can be found to have broken the law.

The next question that follows is what kind of law did the Super break? According to New York State law, anyone who "tortures or cruelly beats or unjustifiably injures, maims, mutilates or kills

any animal, whether wild or tame . . ." is guilty of a class A misdemeanor. The penalty for a misdemeanor is up to one year in jail
and/or a fine not to exceed $1,000. Regardless of how the Super
may have hurt and killed the raccoon, the maximum offense he
could face is a misdemeanor.

Let's say the raccoon wasn't a raccoon, but a dog instead. In this
case, the Super could be charged with aggravated cruelty, which
occurs when a person "with no justifiable purpose . . . intentionally
kills or intentionally causes serious physical injury" to an animal.
Aggravated cruelty to animals is a felony with a maximum imprisonment of two years. The jail sentence is not much greater than that
of a misdemeanor, but with a felony charge, the court can choose
to impose a five year period of probation. This probation would
prohibit the Super from owning, living with, or having contact with
companion animals during that period.

Why is it that the Super could face a felony charge if he poured
acid over a dog but not a raccoon? It comes down to how we
define our relationships with animals. In New York, a raccoon is
just a raccoon, but a dog is placed into a special category. A dog
is automatically considered a companion animal. So is a cat. So is
potentially any "domesticated animal normally maintained in
or near the household of the owner or person who cares for such
other domesticated animal." Only harm to companion animals
can meet the criteria for aggravated cruelty to animals. Granted,
the definition of a companion animal can be expansive. Rabbits,
mice, gerbils, birds, or even raccoons could be included in this
definition if a human declares them to be companions.

It's possible that if someone housed and cared for this raccoon,
he could legally be considered a companion and his suffering
could lead to a felony charge. But since the raccoon was making
his way about this world on his own, retribution for his death
will not be as severe.

Similarly, if a woman intentionally poisons her friend's cat
because her friend angered her, she could find herself behind bars
for two years. If, though, she poisons a cat in the name of research

in a laboratory, she's protected. In New York and in every other state, no animal in experimental laboratories, including dogs and cats, is legally considered a companion animal.

Why should the laws protecting animals be based on whether or not a human deems them to be companions? Sure, the people who loved these animals are also harmed by their suffering. But is that a sufficient, logical reason for the discrepancy in laws protecting companion animals versus other animals? If an orphaned child is killed, the criminal penalty for his murder wouldn't lessen because he had no family. The harm done to the child is what matters, not his relationship to others.

Why not simply base animal protection laws on the type of harm done to the animal? Regulations concerning animals are schizophrenic because, ultimately, all animals are considered legal property. Despite the progress made in recognizing crimes against animals, even today an animal is still just an animal. Whether or not he is afforded any legal protection and what form that protection takes depends on how we choose to use him. Is he a companion? An experimental tool? An afternoon snack?

I don't think a cat would care one whit whether a woman is poisoning him in the name of science or because he's a companion to the woman's friend who angered her. The effect on him is the same.

Let's tease apart the laws some more. Beyond New York, as we saw, many states omit altogether certain animals from inclusion in their animal protection laws. And the AWA excludes birds, rats, mice, all cold-blooded animals, and farm animals. This begs the question: When is an animal not an animal?

The answer is both simple and complex. The easy answer is an animal is not an animal if the people writing the laws decide an animal is not an animal. The thorny answer is an animal is not an animal if it's convenient to define an animal as not an animal.

By denying an animal even that most basic identity, we drop that animal into a hazy, vague void where the animal is not quite a thing, but also not quite *not* a thing. By placing animals into this other category, we can ensure that the activities we want to continue, no matter how much harm they cause those animals, continue. Things or almost-things don't need to eat, don't need to have room to move, don't feel pleasure in the sun's warmth, don't feel pain when injured, don't feel anxiety, sadness, love. Or, we might confess to one another, these almost-things do have the above needs and the ability to feel pleasure and pain, but not *that* much.

It's a handy "alternative fact" we tell our children and ourselves.

By the third of my four days riding with Murphy's squad, I have an easy relationship with the detectives, as though we've known each other for a lot longer. There's friendly banter. Today, I'm in a Dodge SUV driving with Charlie and Chris. As we drive, we talk about recent movies we've seen and books we enjoy. Since I can talk about food all day, our discussion inevitably turns to that topic. I mention some of the great restaurants in Manhattan that I have been meaning to visit. "Now that you've been in New York for a few days," Charlie asks me, "what restaurants have you been to?"

I laugh. I'm so tired at the end of the day that I look for what's quick and nearby. "Taco Bell!" I reply.

I ask Chris how he became involved with this squad. "I'm an animal lover," he says immediately. "My boy cat and I bonded." The detectives in the squad all have their own story of animals they have loved.

The case we are working this morning is on the other side of town. Charlie tells me, "The complaint comes from a woman. Says one of her neighbors got into an argument with her and snatched her dog from her and threw it on the ground."

When we park in front of an apartment complex in the Bronx, a woman sticks her face against a barred first-floor window. She then opens the door and introduces herself as Aida. Dressed in slippers and a robe, she welcomes us into her apartment where we find a small, timid Chihuahua scrambling under her feet. Another little floppy-eared dog sits on the couch, watching us and yapping away. We can hear birds chirping in the back room. "I have little parakeets," Aida tells us. "I have five. But I used to have seven. They like to get out of their cage."

"So do I," Charlie mutters.

This woman is the image of the crazy cat lady, except with birds and dogs. Boxes and knickknacks cram her apartment. Despite the disorganization, though, she's prepared. "I have the paperwork from the vet of his injuries," she tells us, as she takes out a folder from a kitchen drawer and hands it to Charlie.

As I stand outside the tiny kitchen watching, the Chihuahua walks up to me with a limp and sniffs my leg. "Hi little guy!" I say and then turn my attention to Charlie and Aida. I catch snippets of their conversation as she shows Charlie the veterinarian's report: "SPCA wants X-rays . . . anesthesia . . . might not wake up . . ." Through this conversation, my mind registers that Chris is trying to get my attention. "Uh, I think . . ." I hear him say, but I'm too focused on the woman to hear the rest of what Chris is telling me.

Aida takes us to a little park across the road. "I was sitting over here with my dog," she says, pointing to a park bench. "She comes across here. She says, 'If your dog bites me, I'm going to bite you.' Why would she say that? My dog wasn't even near her. She kept coming towards me. I kept walking backwards with my dog. She comes, grabbed my dog's leash, swings it like this (she motions with her arms), and throws the dog over here." That would explain why the Chihuahua is limping.

"The woman's boyfriend," Aida says. "He's been causing me trouble. Why? I got a lot on my plate!"

"How do you know them?" Chris asks her.

"I don't. They're just here. You keep a watch on people around here. I put a flag on my door the other day and then it was gone. You have to keep watch here in this place."

"This is a drug area," Charlie says to Chris.

Charlie looks about and notices two security cameras at each end of the apartment building. "Let's see if the cameras caught the incident."

As Charlie wanders off, Chris walks over to me and says, "I think the dog peed on you." I look down my left leg. Damn.

After getting all the needed information from Aida, we head back to the 105th Precinct. As soon as we walk into the satellite office, Murphy leaves his desk and walks up to me. "Doc, I hear you got peed on."

"What?" I respond. "We just got here! And I never heard the others with me tell you over the phone. How did you find out so fast?" But he just chuckles and walks back into his office. Within an hour, all of the detectives have heard that "a dog peed on the doctor."

⬥

Since there are no other complaints to investigate this afternoon, I have some free time. I call Dr. Robert Reisman, whom I first met at the NYPD training session months earlier. A veterinarian, Reisman is the ASPCA's forensic science supervisor. I ask if he has any interesting cases today.

"We are going to do a necropsy that might interest you. It's of a dog that was handed over by its owner. But it's suspicious. We are starting just after lunch. One-ish."

It's now twelve thirty. There is no way I can make it from Queens to downtown Manhattan in half an hour. But I jump into my car and drive as fast as I legally can.

By the time I arrive in the necropsy room in the basement of the ASPCA's clinical center, Reisman has just begun. Dressed in surgical scrubs, he's looking over the body of a small Chihuahua that was laid out on a gray rubber mat on top of a steel table. "Come in, come in," he says when I enter the room. "You're lucky. We got started a little late."

He introduces me to two veterinary students interning with him from Ohio State University. An ASPCA employee, Javier, enters data into the desktop computer and takes photos. "Roxanne" by The Police plays in the background.

The body on the table is tiny. Emaciated. Patches of raw skin on the neck and matted fur on the flank look like they must have been painful. The dog's prominent ribs glare back at us, challenging us to expose a story of abuse. "The dog was brought into the city shelter as an abandoned stray," Reisman informs me. "They euthanized it. The more they talked with the woman who brought the dog in, the more the story changed. She first said she found the dog near her home. Later, she admitted she and her husband had the dog for two to four years. She guessed the dog was ten years old. If I had a dog for two to four years, I would know if it was two or four years. They probably had the dog all ten years."

Reisman is one of a handful of veterinarians who conducts formalized forensic investigations on animals. A graduate from Cornell University College of Veterinary Medicine, Reisman practiced as a general veterinarian for many years before joining the ASPCA in the 1990s. At the ASPCA's Manhattan hospital, Reisman took care of numerous animals who were brought in by the NYPD or ASPCA investigators after suspicion of abuses. But Reisman quickly realized that he and the other veterinarians could be doing much more to support the cruelty investigations.

"So law enforcement would bring animals and we would provide them care," Riesman tells me, "but there wasn't any sense that we had any responsibility to participate in the process of an actual criminal case. So there was, like, one handwritten sheet that would basically say the animal's underweight, it needs to be fed. That was it. There was nothing else."

Although many veterinarians have been practicing forensic work of sorts for decades, there is no formalized training and no distinct field. Reisman taught himself by studying texts on human forensics, looking to child abuse cases for parallels. Like animals, children are often unable to voice their stories. Using guidance manuals explaining how to investigate child abuse cases, Reisman created a similar process for animal cruelty examinations. Among other things, Reisman and his team now document the animal's general body condition, matting of hair, weight, physical injuries, and signs of dehydration and starvation. Their job is to find any and every clue that the body reveals that can help them determine if an animal was abused and, if so, how and for how long.

Reisman places the dog's body on a scale: 1.2 kilograms (2.6 pounds). The average weight of an adult Chihuahua is five to six pounds. This dog weighed at best about half his normal weight. Reisman opens the jaw. "All of his teeth are gone. Part of his lower jaw . . . rostral aspect of mandible is missing." He picks up a small instrument and punches out a piece of skin. As he collects skin specimens from different parts of the body, he drops them into sterile jars of formaldehyde. He calls aloud to Javier the labels to be written on each jar. "Right lateral thorax." *Plop* goes one piece of tissue into a jar. "Dorsal lumbar." *Plop.* "Right inguinal." *Plop.*

Reisman then takes a scalpel and slices a long slit up the length of the body. He wipes away the fluids and blood oozing out with a piece of gauze. "One of the differences between a forensic necropsy and a regular necropsy is we do a lot of photography," he tells the students. "So we clean up the blood as we go so that we can take clear photos." The dog's body is so tiny, I don't smell anything emanating from its exposed cavity. By this point, whenever I've participated in human autopsies, I would have to hold my breath for long stretches of time.

As Reisman plunges his gloved hands through the long incision and wriggles out part of a back leg, he says, "Significant loss of muscle mass for me to expose the head of the femur like that." He shakes his head. "He has no subcutaneous fat."

He looks up at the students. "This is my own playlist," he says referring to the unfamiliar music playing in the background. "Do you know whose music this is?" Both students look perplexed. "You don't? They're from Ohio." He turns and looks at me.

"I have no idea who they are," I tell him.

"They're the Black Keys." Reisman's deep voice is disapproving as he turns back to the tiny body.

Reisman pulls open the dog's mandible and cuts it free. "Look at this," he says. "The jaw is not even connected. There's only soft tissue here." He shows me the jaw—it's practically nonexistent. "Probably osteomyelitis from severe neglect," he says. "You know how much it hurts to have a toothache? Can you imagine going through this? I'm going to submit this for histopathology. They won't like it."

"Who won't like it?" I ask

"Cornell. I send all the tissues there. They don't it like when we send big chunks of tissue. Here, let's take another photo." Reisman lays the mandible down on the mat alongside a small ruler to document its size. As Javier photographs the mandible, Reisman says, "Sometimes we see evidence in bones. There was a dogfighting case where there were punctures in a dog's skull."

Reisman holds the entire mandible as Javier now videotapes. "This is what the dog lived with," he says as he moves the jawbone back and forth. "Nothing is attached. It's more like cartilage. There's no strength. No substance. A lot of disease in this jaw. I don't think this dog could eat well. If this case goes to trial, can you imagine how powerful this video will be?"

Reisman and other ASPCA veterinarians routinely testify on animal cruelty cases, providing a strong medical arm that was previously missing. Now with the partnership between the ASPCA's forensic team, the Animal Cruelty Investigation Squad, and the district attorneys, the triad of medical, enforcement, and prosecution form a powerful team that exists nowhere else in the country.

Veterinary forensics continues to evolve. Reisman often partners with human forensic scientists on more complicated cases. "There was a case of a deceased dog. She had been starved to death," Reisman tells me, "but that's difficult to prove in some cases. She was severely decomposed to the point where she was mummified. Depending on the environmental condition where an animal dies, their body will decompose in different ways. Mummification happens in very dry areas. The skin becomes taut and everything dries out like a mummy. You could see it was a dog, but all that was left was skin and bones. So we reached out to a forensic anthropologist for help." Reisman contacted Amanda Fitch, both a crime scene analyst with years of experience investigating human crimes and a forensic anthropologist. They radiographed the body. "What we found was the dog was eating broken glass. They'll eat anything to stay alive and the stomach was literally full of broken glass."

When examining animal remains, sometimes Reisman calls on Dr. Jason Byrd, a forensic entomologist at the University of Florida in Gainesville. Byrd studies insect patterns on human remains to help decipher the location of death (different insect patterns will appear in different climate regions), the time of death, and sometimes, the underlying cause. Lately, Byrd has been using his knowledge to help with animal cases. In 2008, in partnership with Byrd and other forensic scientists at the University of Florida, the ASPCA held the nation's first veterinary forensics conference. Reisman tells me that they were expecting about forty attendees. They got almost two hundred. "There was so much more interest than we could have imagined. And it's just growing." The conference led to the formation of the International Veterinary Forensic Sciences Association, which now holds annual events.

Javier finishes videotaping the mandible, and Reisman drops it into a clean specimen jar. "Cornell vet school is looking into having a one-year vet fellowship in forensics," he tells me. "It's not available anywhere so far."

Reisman next picks up a Stryker saw (named after the surgeon who invented it), which has a motor that oscillates at high speed. "So the next thing I do is cut through the femur for Cornell to do a bone marrow to show there's no fat. The bone marrow is the last place for fat to disappear. I assume when they look, they'll find most of the fat gone. So it's a way to say that this was a chronic process if even the bone marrow fat content was affected."

With the Stryker saw, Reisman cuts through the right femur. Now comes the smell. Patrick has an oscillating saw, which he uses for woodworking. But where Patrick's saw produces the clean smell of oak, cedar, and pine, this saw releases a stench that's similar to burnt hair.

Reisman then uses a pair of scissors to fully separate the femur from the surrounding tissues.

"Can I see that?" the female student asks.

"What?" Reisman answers.

"Bone marrow. Some people eat that, don't they?"

Ignoring her question, Reisman next cuts through the ribs and pulls apart the underlying omentum, a fold of tissue covering the abdominal organs. He peers at the intestines. "Looks normal." He grabs several teal-colored plastic cutting boards from a nearby shelf and places them onto the table in front of him. "I get these from IKEA's kitchen department," he says when he sees the question on my face.

He pulls out the internal organs one by one and displays them on the cutting boards. Kidneys, lungs, heart, intestines, liver, spleen, stomach, gallbladder. I can't get over how small they are. They look like toy organs from the board game *Operation*.

A song by k.d. lang comes on. "Do you know who sings this song?" Reisman asks his students. When they say nothing, he adds, "You guys aren't doing that well. It's going to affect your grade." Even though he's joking, his voice never changes to reflect this. He dissects each organ on the cutting boards. As he does so, he continually wipes clean the blood that seeps out. He says aloud to anyone in the room. "Do you cook?"

"Sometimes," one of the students replies.

"Do you clean up as you go along? Or do you let it all pile up? I can't stand piling up the mess. I have to clean up along the way." *So do I*, I think to myself. But I—and I'm certain the students watching—don't have much of an appetite at present.

Reisman discards the esophagus into a jar. When he slices open the stomach and intestines, he says, "There's nothing in there. No food. That's not normal. I think this guy was so compromised. He couldn't eat right, not with that jaw. The owners would have known. They should have brought him in for care." *Plop* goes a slice of intestine into a jar. "Hunger pain is real. Based on the research. This animal has always been in pain."

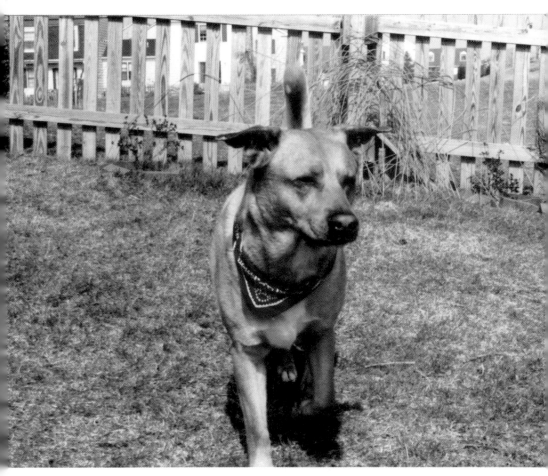

Sylvester at four years old after he and I spent the afternoon romping through the woods. *Photograph from the author's collection.*

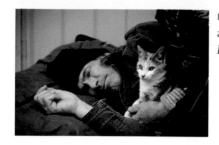

LEFT: One of the many homeless with their animal families. *Photograph courtesy of Feeding Pets of the Homeless.*

RIGHT: This man brings his dog every year to a free veterinary clinic sponsored by Feeding Pets of the Homeless. The dog will growl at anyone who comes too close to his beloved human companion. *Photograph courtesy of Feeding Pets of the Homeless.*

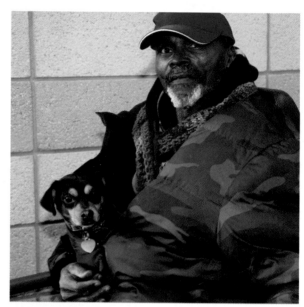

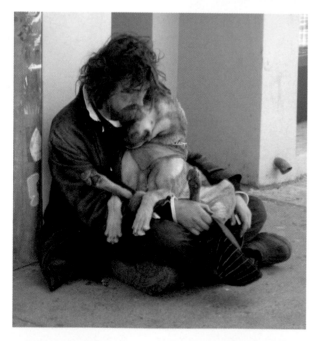

LEFT: This photo brought a lot of public attention to the plight of the homeless and their animal companions. *Photograph courtesy of Feeding Pets of the Homeless.*

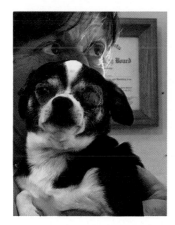

LEFT: A man who has been homeless for twenty-three years lives with Matty in a tent in Santa Rosa, California. The man called Feeding Pets of the Homeless for help after Matty badly injured her eye. *Photograph courtesy of Feeding Pets of the Homeless.* BELOW: James Guiliani at Brooklyn's The Diamond Collar boutique holding Boots, a rescued cat. *Photograph from the author's collection.*

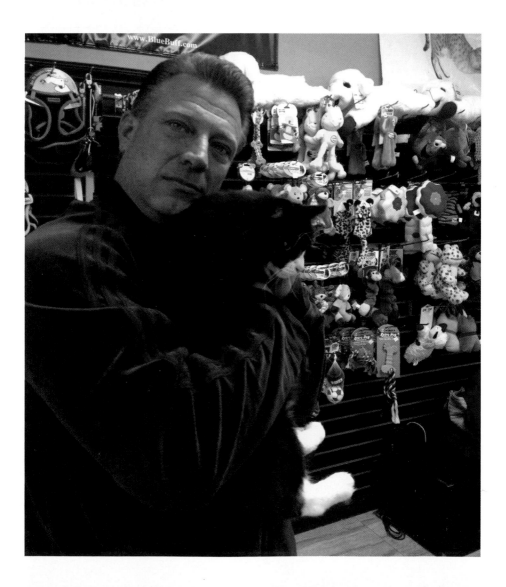

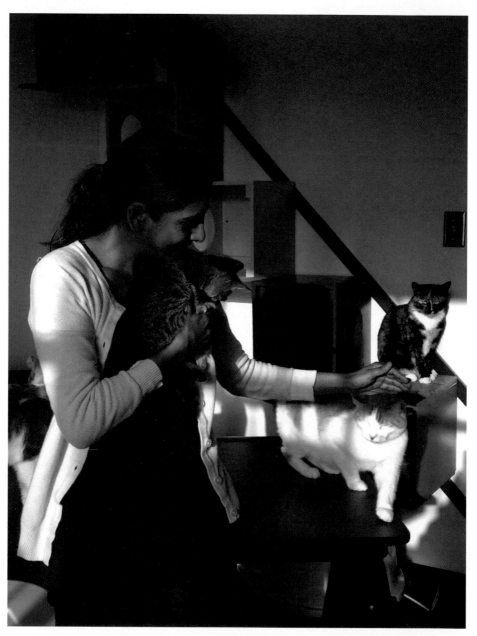

I'm happily ensconced in cats at the Pendleton Correctional Facility's cat sanctuary in Indiana. *Photograph from the author's collection.*

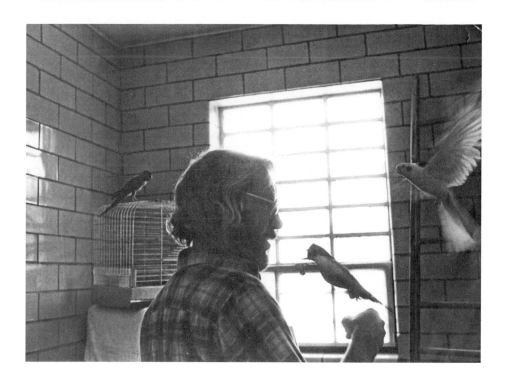

ABOVE: Social worker David Lee at the Lima State Hospital in Ohio in 1979. *Photograph courtesy of David Lee.* BELOW LEFT AND RIGHT: A few of the many critters cheering up the lives of patients at the Lima State Hospital. *Photographs courtesy of David Lee.*

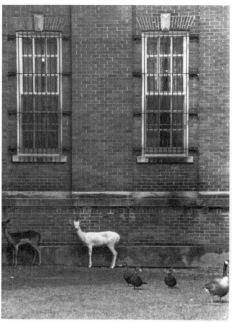

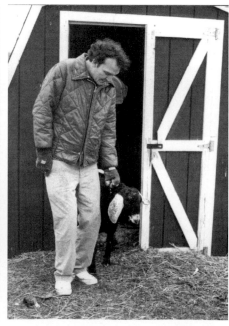

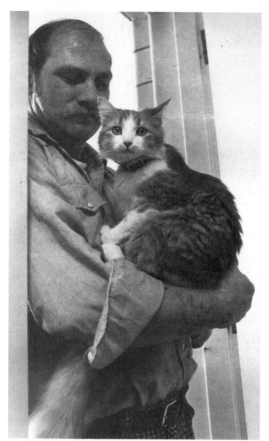

LEFT: This patient at Lima State Hospital refused to leave without his beloved cat companion. *Photograph courtesy of David Lee.* BELOW: One of the "FBI" men at Lima State Hospital with his cherished feline friend. *Photograph courtesy of David Lee.*

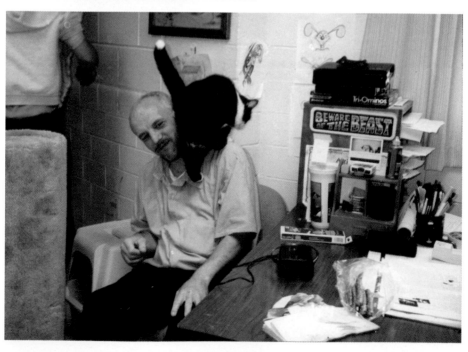

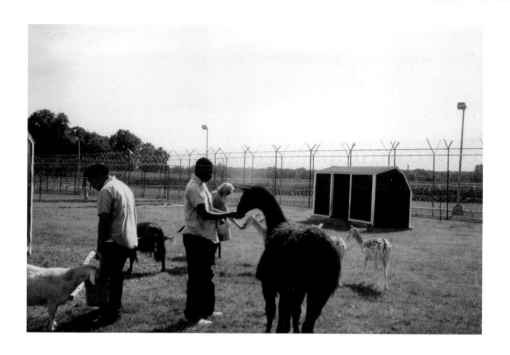

ABOVE: The animals were some of the best "therapists" for the patients at Lima State Hospital. *Photograph courtesy of David Lee.* BELOW: Grave of unclaimed patient at Lima State Hospital's cemetery. *Photograph from the author's collection.*

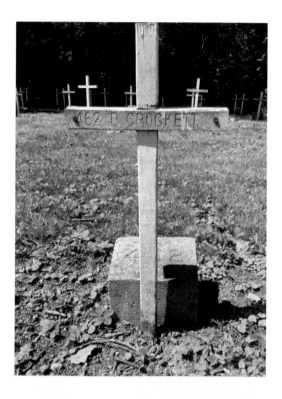

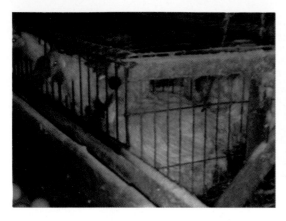
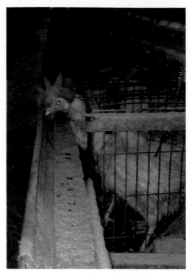

ABOVE LEFT AND RIGHT: Chickens at the Wendell egg farm. These hens live their entire lives in the space of a sheet of paper. I named the hen on the right Clover Meadow. *Photographs from the author's collection.* BELOW: Hens at the Wendell farm. This is what passes as "free range." *Photograph from the author's collection.*

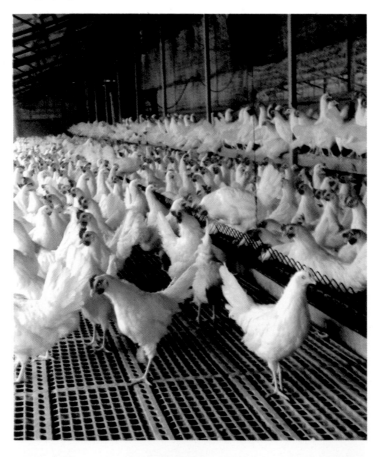

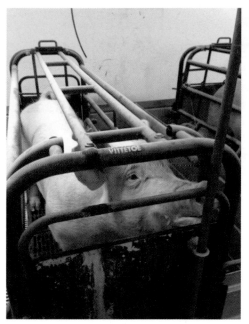

LEFT: I named this girl Petunia. Her daughters will be brought to this room at Oklahoma State University to live in separate gestation crates. Her sons will be turned into bacon and sausage. *Photograph from the author's collection.* BELOW: Like me, Gizmo takes food seriously. Unlike me (well sort of) he will knock you down to be the first in line at feeding time. *Photograph courtesy of the Rowdy Girl Sanctuary.*

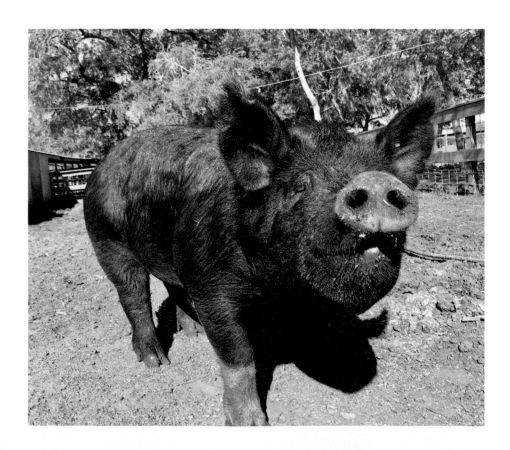

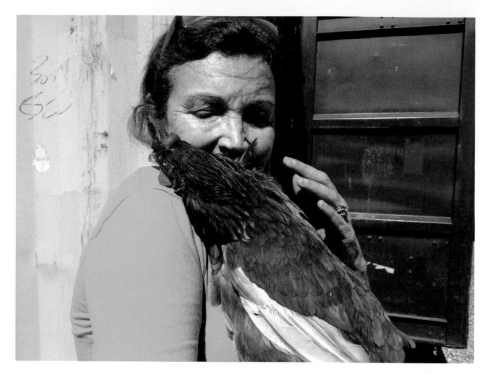

ABOVE: Renee King-Sonnen with Lulu at the Rowdy Girl Sanctuary before Lulu passed away. Lulu loved to be held and would nestle her head into your shoulder. *Photograph from the author's collection.* BELOW: Tommy trying to calm Muley, who's foot was stuck deep in the water. Muley, at 21 years old, is the sanctuary's oldest cow and the mother of three. *Photograph courtesy of the Rowdy Girl Sanctuary.*

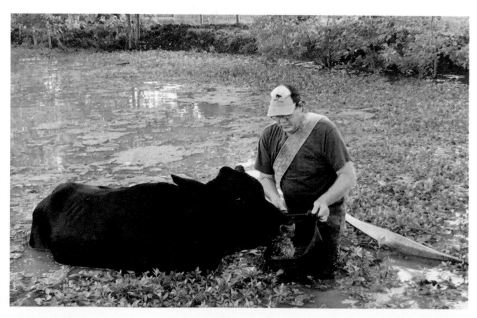

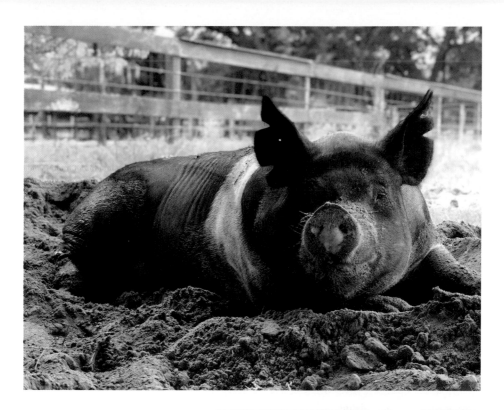

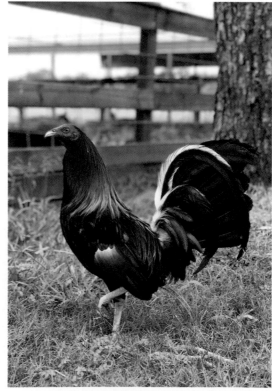

ABOVE: Roux is best friends with Gizmo and Penny. She loves playing chase with visitors. *Photograph courtesy of the Rowdy Girl Sanctuary.* RIGHT: Sunrise was rescued from a cockfighting ring. He is very popular amongst and protective of his lady friends (eleven hens!). *Photograph courtesy of the Rowdy Girl Sanctuary.*

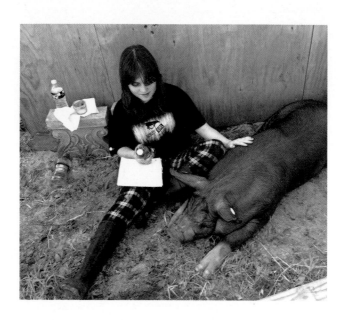

ABOVE: Alena Hidalgo with Gizmo. Alena holds annual birthday parties for Gizmo and dresses him up in party hats. Gizmo loves his birthday cakes! *Photograph courtesy of the Rowdy Girl Sanctuary.* BELOW: You give Ivy some treats and you have a friend for life. *Photograph courtesy of the Rowdy Girl Sanctuary.*

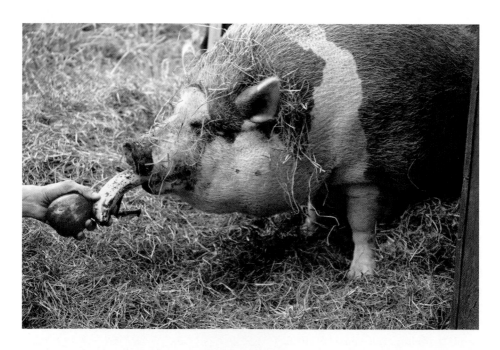

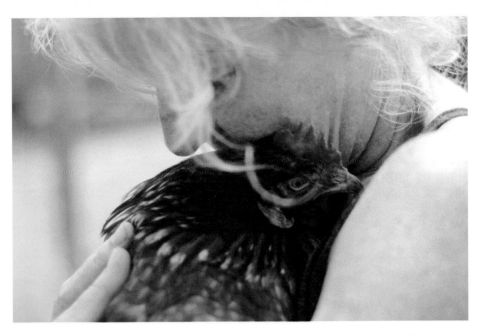

ABOVE: Sanctuary volunteer with Lulu, who would run up to greet all visitors. *Photograph courtesy of Molly Colvin.* BELOW: Pepper, on top of his soapbox, loves to watch everyone else at the sanctuary. *Photograph courtesy of the Rowdy Girl Sanctuary.*

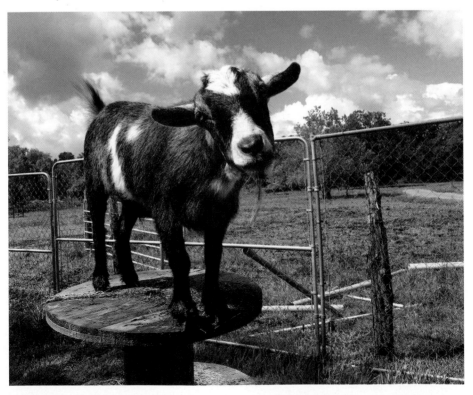

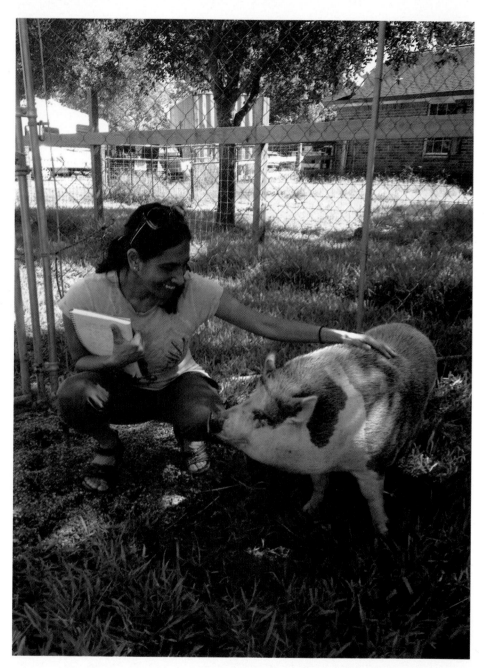

The first time I met Ivy. *Photograph from the author's collection.*

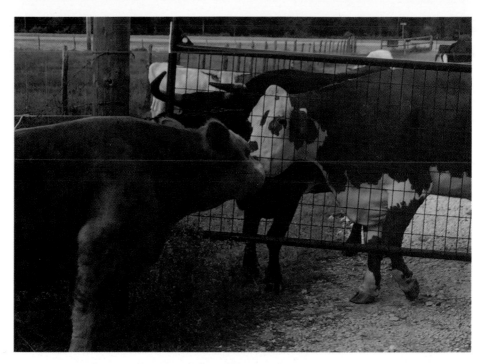

ABOVE: Charger (on left) being greeted by other sanctuary cows. *Photograph from the author's collection.* BELOW: The sanctuary cows lined up along the fence to touch noses with the newly arrived Charger (on left) and to welcome him. *Photograph from the author's collection.*

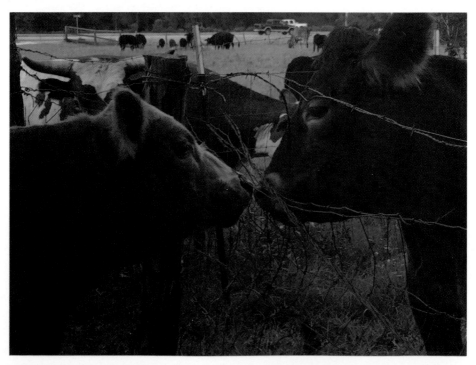

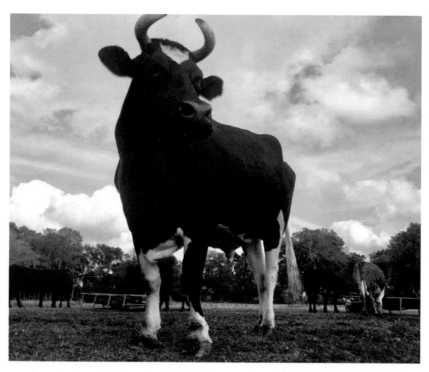

Murray, who was rescued from a cruelty case in Florida, adores bananas.
Photograph courtesy of the Rowdy Girl Sanctuary.

For the first time since he started the necropsy, Reisman stops and stands still. He looks down at the small body on the table. The dispassionate, clinical demeanor he held throughout the procedure is suddenly replaced by unguarded emotion.

But just as quickly that hint of sorrow dissolves and he's back to business. After he removes the internal abdominal organs and slices and dices them for analysis, he cuts through the skull using the Stryker saw and a chisel. Strong burnt-hair smell now. He lifts open the top of the skull. Immediately, I see problems. The brain's right hemisphere is shrunken with significantly fewer overlying blood vessels compared with the left hemisphere.

"Can I take a look at the brain?" I ask as Reisman removes it. He nods. I pull on a pair of gloves and take the brain into my hands. The left hemisphere is softer and somewhat gelatinous. The right is hard. The atrophied right hemisphere could be due to underlying natural diseases, but it could also be due to an old traumatic brain injury. What happened to this dog?

⚬

At night, back at the hotel, I can't sleep. I lie on the sheets awake, my mind racing, thinking about the dog Reisman autopsied and the other animals in the cases I've witnessed. What suffering did they endure?

Until a decade or so ago, these animals would have been overlooked. They would have fallen through the cracks with barely a whimper. I think about how grateful I am to have met Murphy's team, Reisman, and the other wonderful people making sure that no harm to an animal is too small to notice. Even two little turtles who lived sad, short lives capture their attention.

Our legal system no doubt needs improvement in recognizing crimes against animals. Even though laws exist to protect many animals from at least some forms of mistreatment, they nevertheless treat different animals differently. We elevate animals we define as companions and lessen those we do not. Companions or not, however, animals are legally considered things, possessions not unlike cars, watches, and chairs. Animals have fewer protections in the United States than even corporations, to which the US Supreme Court affirmed "corporate personhood" status in 2010. Corporations have a legal identity separate from their shareholders. In general, animal protection laws have not considered animals independent from their human relationships. They have yet to grant animals their own individuality. Until we universally acknowledge animals as the living beings they are, the laws will remain confused.

There are inklings of change. Throughout the country, the animals' interests are being increasingly considered. Thanks to a million-dollar donation from Bob Barker from *The Price Is Right* TV show, the University of Virginia law school opened its first program in 2009 to exclusively cover animal law. More law schools now teach animal law.

In some cases, the courts are slowly viewing animals not as property, but as something akin to persons. Since 2000, some states have begun allowing people to leave estates or trusts to care for their beloved companions. In custody battles over animals, courts have traditionally treated companion animals as possessions, but this is changing. Courts have awarded shared custody, visitation, and alimony payments to animal guardians. In a 2013 divorce proceeding in New York, a divorced couple fought a custody battle over a dachshund named Joey. The plaintiff argued that Joey was her property because she bought him with her own funds prior to the marriage. The judge ruling on this dispute, Mathew F. Cooper, rejected applying a property analysis to the dog, as virtually every court had done before. Instead, Cooper used a standard akin to the "best interests of the child" analysis that is used in child custody battles in granting a hearing on the case. Before the hearing date, however, the couple came to an agreement.

In January 2016, Alaska became the first state to enact "pet custody" legislation. This allows a court to consider the animal's well-being when deciding who, in divorce cases, should be allowed to care for the family dog, cat, African grey parrot, iguana, turtle, and even a python. Rhode Island is considering similar legislation.

Outside of the court, the recognition of animal individuality is occurring more rapidly. A few months ago, my stepbrother in Charlottesville, Virginia, was surprised when his television viewing was interrupted to announce an amber alert for a lost dog. And in 2017, police in Boston urged the public's help in locating a lost dog and, months later, a lost puppy, by placing pleas in the *Boston Globe.*

We are slowly acknowledging animals as their own, unique selves. We are starting to recognize animals not as what, but as who.

And it isn't just the companion animals who will one day be given back the selfhoods we took away from them. In 2013, attorney and president of the Nonhuman Rights Project, Steven Wise, began a series of lawsuits filed on behalf of four New York chimpanzees. Two of the chimpanzees, Tommy and Kiko, were privately owned. Tommy was first found living alone in a cage in a shed on a used-trailer lot. Kiko was being held in a cage in a cement storefront. The two other chimpanzees, Hercules and Leo, were formerly used in experiments and held by Stony Brook University. In an attempt to release the four chimpanzees to a sanctuary, Wise filed lawsuits to have them declared "legal persons." In a New York Supreme Court hearing in 2015 concerning the two chimpanzees used by Stony Brook, Justice Barbara Jaffe ruled against Wise and the chimpanzees. She felt bound by legal precedent from an earlier case involving the chimpanzee Tommy.

However, her ruling was not a complete blow. Indirectly, she left a challenge for future judges. Jaffe expressed sympathy for Wise's arguments. She wrote that in the eyes of the law, something does not have to be a human being to be treated like a person, noting the personhood status given to corporations. Jaffe also stated that the concept of legal personhood continues to evolve: "Not very long ago, only Caucasian male, property-owning citizens were entitled to the full panoply of legal rights under the United States Constitution."

Notably, in her conclusion, Jaffe wrote, "Courts, however, are slow to embrace change, and occasionally seem reluctant to engage in broader, more inclusive interpretations of the law. . . . As Justice Kennedy aptly observed in Lawrence v Texas [a 2003 gay rights case], "Times can blind us to certain truths and later generations can see that laws once thought necessary and proper in fact serve only to oppress."

⁂

On my last day with the NYPD, I head out to Manhattan with detectives John and Tara. We arrive at a modern, upscale high-rise apartment building called the Sky Towers. As we enter the lobby, I'm astounded. It looks more like a swanky hotel than an apartment building. The building houses indoor and outdoor pools, basketball court, daycare, physical therapy center, yoga room, billiards room, and pet spa. Gold and marble flank the foyer's gas fireplaces, sparkling chandeliers, and a large oblong-shaped concierge desk where staff greets us. After John explains the reason for our visit, a staff member calls up a security guard to take us to a small back room in the building's basement.

We came to watch a video that the security cameras captured a week ago behind the building. The security guard displays the video for us on a small TV. Tara, John, and I crowd around and watch the image of a garbage collector opening the lid of one of the dumpsters, then stumbling backward with shock on his face. He looks about, bewildered, and hurries out of view of the camera.

The security guard rewinds the tape for us and nods his head toward the image of the man in the video. "He called you guys, huh?"

"Yeah," John replies.

The building worker had called the police immediately. What he saw when he lifted the dumpster lid was a ripped, opened garbage bag with the bloodied head of a small dog sticking out. The police who first responded to the call tracked down the dog's "guardian," who freely admitted that he stabbed the dog in his chest with a knife, put the body in a garbage bag, then tossed it down the garbage chute.

The twenty-four-year-old research analyst claimed self-defense for killing the dog—a sixteen-pound terrier. The terrier, he said, was "acting irrational" and scratched his arms. Later, after a court hearing for charges of aggravated cruelty and torturing animals, the prosecutor would deem the defendant's scratches to be "very small and minor." Forensics would reveal that along with stab wounds, the dog suffered from "bruising, hip dislocation, and a broken pelvis due to blunt force trauma." But the defendant apparently did not believe there was a thing wrong with his treatment of the dog. Fortunately, many others do.

After showing us the video again, the security guard says, "I've been at this job for fifteen years. You find a lot of crazy things, but never anything this bad." He leans back in his chair and adds, "You guys arrest the guy?"

"Yes," John answers.

"Yeah? Good."

SIX

Do We Hurt with Animals?

I tried to reconcile my inaction with what Dave was doing to Sylvester. I convinced myself that Sylvester's body didn't feel a lot of pain when it hit the walls. That I mistook my misery for his. Maybe, I thought, he just doesn't suffer that much. Maybe animals are different from humans in that way.

It was a reassuring tale I spun for months. Until one day, something happened that loosened the thread.

After a week of torrential storms, the sky sparkled as if scoured clean. I begged Aunt Fiza to take Sylvester and me down to the creek a few miles away from our apartments. The stream was more like a small river. It was so wide and deep, the water came up to my chin in places. Sylvester and I frequently swam there. On this glorious day, the three of us walked down the hill, across the busy avenues, and into the green oasis that sat in the middle of the trash-strewn streets. Sylvester, not on a leash as usual, bound ahead of us and then looped back, ran ahead and looped back. I think he and I must have had the same silly grins on our faces, in anticipation. I looked forward to the creek's cool current slipping over me like my mom's chiffon scarves.

However, when we arrived, the stream was swollen and turbulent. So we walked along the water instead. Sylvester wasn't satisfied with walking. He kept trying to dodge into the water, and Aunt Fiza and I kept holding him back as best as we could. After about a half hour, we saw a man up the embankment walking a leashed dog. To our horror, Sylvester chased after the dog. But he didn't stop there. Perhaps frustrated from not being allowed in the creek, he kept running. In less than a minute, he disappeared into the thick woods.

Fiza and I wandered about the creek, calling Sylvester. We walked from business to business, house to house, asking if anyone had seen a brown puppy. We searched all afternoon. Sylvester was lost.

We returned home, depressed. I curled up on my bed crying my heart out. My baby was gone. And it was my fault. My greatest fear was that Sylvester tried to swim in the creek and drowned. Grief distorted my perception. To my nine-year-old mind, the stream was akin to a rapid river. I envisioned Sylvester tumbling and rolling in the rough water, his little body hitting against the rocks while he struggled to stay afloat. As I imagined Sylvester's pain and panic, my stomach felt as though a giant hand had pinched it in two. I couldn't get out of bed for the pain. I lie there clutching my belly and I realized that I had deceived myself. Over the months as Dave hit Sylvester, I wasn't merely suffering *for* Sylvester, I was suffering *with* him.

❧

About a decade ago I was listening to a talk on spinal cord injury at a neuroscience conference. There were about three hundred neuroscientists and neurologists like myself sitting in the audience. When one of the panelists stood up to give his talk, he showed a brief video clip that haunts me still.

The researcher presented a video of his experiment in which he had crushed a cat's spinal cord and was recording her movements on a small treadmill. In the clip, I saw the orange tabby cat, with electrodes implanted in her brain, struggling to keep upright. She was dragging her paralyzed back legs on the moving treadmill. She kept falling off and the researcher kept putting her back on.

At one point, the experimenter lifted the cat up to reposition her on the treadmill and she did something that was utterly unexpected. She rubbed her head against his hand.

I sat up straight in my seat. I looked to the presenter to see if he would acknowledge in any way what had happened in the video. But he kept on, steady in his talk, seemingly failing to notice any ethical question or implication that might arise from what was depicted in the video. I then looked about the room to see if anyone else in the audience noticed what I did. Even at the peak of her suffering, the cat was seeking comfort from the very hand that caused it.

Since that day I often wondered: Did the experimenter, in his quietest, most private moments, ever ache from the pain he caused that cat?

When visiting my parents, I drive an hour over winding rivers, through forested hills, and by historic villages. As I near my parents' home, there is a large lot with four long buildings set back from the road. The gray, rectangular buildings show no trimming, no windows. No architectural features to draw a person's eyes. That's on purpose. Over the many years of driving that country route, I never once gave a thought about what's inside those unmarked sheds. Until one day I wished I could forget.

I was giving a talk at a conference in Oklahoma about the public health dangers of industrial animal farming, or "factory farming" as it is commonly called. Each year, more than 64 billion animals are raised and killed for food globally. In the United States alone, 1 million animals are slaughtered every hour. Largely because of increased demand for cheap animal products, intensive animal operations have replaced most traditional farming practices worldwide. The transformation of animal agriculture is so dramatic that it has been dubbed the "livestock revolution." This unprecedented change in the human relationship with animals has led to not only more animal suffering than ever before in human history but also to devastating harms to human health.

At the conference, I presented data showing how animal agriculture (and the resultant high consumption of animal products) causes more greenhouse gas emissions than the entire transportation sector. It also pollutes our land and water and increases our risks of cancers, obesity, strokes, and infectious diseases like salmonella, E. coli, and bird flus. Throughout my presentation, a solemn-looking woman with short, auburn hair and glasses kept shaking her head in disagreement. When I ended my talk and opened the floor for questions, the woman went on the attack. She disputed everything I said. There are no environmental hazards, no infectious disease risks, no animal welfare problems.

"Have you ever visited one of these farms?" she demanded, with evident anger.

I told her I had not because these places are not open for the public's viewing. But my data came from reputable studies published by institutions like the Johns Hopkins Bloomberg School of Public Health and the Food and Agriculture Organization of the United Nations. The evidence is so strong, the American Public Health Association called for a moratorium on factory farms.

The woman, Jean Sander, was dean of the Oklahoma State University's Center for Veterinary Health Sciences. "You need to visit our farms," she replied. "They are nothing like what you say."

Three months later, I take Jean up on her offer. The farms are worse than anything I've read.

On a dismal morning in late November, I meet Dr. Sander at the parking lot of a Sonic fast food restaurant in Bristow, Oklahoma. After we greet each other and complain about the weather, I get into her car. We head out to visit an egg-laying farm about a half hour away. This farm is not the place Jean initially set up for my visit. She was originally going to take me to see a "broiler" farm, where chickens are produced for meat, which is contracted by Tyson Foods. The Tyson chicken facility is one of Oklahoma's largest.

But a few days before my flight to Tulsa, the Tyson facility manager backed out. He informed Jean that an undercover investigation at a chicken facility in Tennessee recently caught the attention of news reporters. As a result, he was not letting any outsiders in his buildings. The undercover investigators videotaped farm employees beating sick chickens with spiked clubs. Like the Oklahoma facility, the one in Tennessee was also contracted by and supplied chickens to Tyson Foods.

It's a wonder that the Tyson manager was initially willing to let me in at all. When I told Jean during my earlier presentation that factory farms don't allow visitors from the public, I wasn't exaggerating. Over the past decade, states have enacted laws to protect animal agricultural farms from outside attention. "Ag-gag" laws, in particular, criminalize journalists and animal protection groups, and they prevent just about anyone from taking undercover videos documenting what occurs within. These investigations have revealed not only rampant animal cruelty but also violations that have led to some of the largest meat recalls in the United States. As an editorial in *The Atlantic* stated, Ag-gag "illustrates just how desperate these industries are to keep this information from getting out."

The only reason I am being allowed in is because of Jean. Her affiliation with Oklahoma State University, one of the largest agricultural schools in the country, has placed Jean in a position to know many of the animal farm managers in Oklahoma. They view her as an ally. And thanks to my connection with Jean, they must have seen me as nonthreatening. Even so, it took months for Jean to find facilities that would open their doors to us.

As she drives, Jean describes this first facility that we are visiting as a smaller, family-run farm. She has never met this farmer before or visited his farm. But this independent farmer is very willing to let us visit. Jean and I chat about our families, our careers. She's friendly and warm. Still, I brace myself for the visit. I've seen photos and videos of what these places are like and I have no desire to see them up close. But Jean had a point. If I am permitted to personally see what factory farms are like, I should.

We follow the driving instructions Mr. Wendell provided. After miscalculating our turn several times, we find the "large boulder on the right corner" where we turn left and drive down a hill. We can see the long sheds up ahead alongside a white, two-story clapboard house. As we pull into the driveway, we see a slightly stooped, gray-haired man carefully making his way toward us, as though his knees bother him. When we step out of Jean's car, the first thing I notice is the calling of a mob of chickens from inside the shed in front of us. Next, I'm confronted by a familiar smell. Have I been transported back in time to the apartment buildings in Arlington? The odor of sweat, onions, and backed-up toilets shrouds the air.

Herbert Wendell walks up to us and shakes our hands with fervor. With his ruddy cheeks and cheerful welcome, he immediately reminds me of my father-in-law. He introduces Jean and me to some of his family members. Unlike his two shy sons, his granddaughter is talkative. She recently graduated from veterinary school and came to the farm today to help Herbert show us around. Herbert comes from a family of crop farmers and was the first to move into animal agriculture. In 1957, he bought one chicken that started his egg-laying business. Since then, the number of chickens has grown to about thirty thousand.

After a few minutes of greeting, Jean hands me a disposable coverall, pair of booties, and gloves. They are meant to keep us from inadvertently introducing infectious agents into the facility as part of a biocontainment plan—methods that clearly don't work, given how often bird and swine flu epidemics sweep across industrial farms in the United States. Jean and I cover ourselves. We then follow Herbert and his granddaughter inside the nearest of the two animal sheds and . . . oh my god!

The smell that hovered outside drops hard and tries to smother me. I immediately turn away from the others, hold onto my knees, and gag. My head heaves. I'm so nauseated I think I'm going to throw up. As a doctor, I've been around plenty of bad smells. Nothing comes close to this. The best way I can describe the smell is this: Don't clean a cat's litter box for a month. Then add to it the litter from ten other cats, whose litter you also had not changed in a month. Then add a rotting egg. Then a decomposing body. And, just for good measure, add a healthy dose of sulfur. Now stick your head inside this giant litter box, and that will give you an inkling of the smell inside this facility. Just an inkling.

I hide my face so the others don't see me gag. I'm worried I'll offend Herbert if I vomit. I'm amazed that no one else is bothered by the smell. The stink of ammonia and feces fill my mouth like a balloon. It rises into my nose, oozes down my throat, bloats up my lungs. I can't taste anything but that smell. I don't know anything but that smell.

With great effort, I swallow the bile pooling at the back of my throat and straighten up. Slowly, my other senses kick in. Touch first. Flies land on my face. I swat ineffectually at my forehead, nose, ears. Next comes sound. Not the individual noises of calls, clucks, and squawks. But a roar. A singular shout.

Then sight. Through the dim lighting, I see rows and rows of wire cages stacked two stories high. Each holding five hens. Twenty-five thousand birds kept in this building alone. The hens are so jam-packed that their heads stick out above, along the sides, even below the cages. Their feet stand on wire grids. They have nowhere to go. They can't even stretch their wings.

Jean tells me that the standard of practice used to be to allow 54 square inches per bird in a cage. Now they're moving to 60 to 65 square inches per bird as an animal welfare gesture. Sixty-five square inches is about two-thirds the dimension of a single sheet of letter-sized paper. A hen is forced to live her entire life in the space of my laptop screen, but this is considered, by the agricultural industry, as progress.

Plastic sheeting comprises the walls of the building, providing barely any insulation from the cold outside. Despite the chill, the air inside is moist. As we walk down the rows, I breathe through my mouth to somewhat ease the stench. The birds scurry and climb on top of one another to hide near the back of the cages. They're terrified of us. I'm scared too. Scared that they will crush one another, which Herbert tells me, has happened. Up closer, I see raw, red exposed areas on most of the birds, where their feathers rubbed off against the wires entrapping them. I can't imagine how painful that must be.

"I'm sorry," I whisper to them. "I'm so sorry."

Since birds crowded like this commonly go mad and peck one another to death, these birds were debeaked, a practice whereby workers grab baby chicks in one hand and thrust their beaks between hot, steaming blades. Workers cut off anywhere from one-third to two-thirds of chicks' beaks while they're fully conscious. The industry calls this "trimming their beaks." But slicing chickens' beaks off with a heated blade or a scissor device, as is frequently done, is not like trimming your nails. Birds' beaks are sensitive, highly innervated and able to feel pain and other sensations. It would be like having your toes cut off without anesthesia. Not only do chickens rely on their beaks for many functions, having their beaks severed causes them immense, acute, and, often, lifelong pain.

As we walk about, Herbert describes how the facility functions. Conveyer belts run along the span of the building, automatically collecting the eggs that fall under the chickens. Trenches alongside the cages hold feed pellets. It's all mechanized. No human hand need ever touch a bird until the time of her death. This, then, is a chicken's life. To huddle in a cage cowering on top of another for one and a half years until someone kills you.

Jean reminds me this is a small facility. Average-size farms house 100,000 birds. The largest may contain 200,000. I am so over-whelmed by the smell of filth and fear, I can't fathom what those larger factories must be like.

"We keep the top and bottom rows of cages stacked," Herbert says, breaking into my thoughts, "so that all of their droppings fall through the cages onto the floor below." For the first time, I peer below the cages at the floor. It's alive.

Maggots. Hundreds, thousands of maggots squirming about the ground. I jump and lift my legs. Squashed maggots are stuck on the bottom of my bootie-covered sneakers. As I hop on each leg to inspect my feet, I slip.

And down I go.

When I look back at this moment, the image that comes to mind is a scene in the movie *Poltergeist* (the original, of course), when the earth beneath the haunted family's house erupts and releases the screaming skeletons and gaping skulls buried beneath. In the downpour of a raging storm, the mother desperately tries to rescue her children trapped inside the house. As she runs into their backyard screaming for help, her foot slips along the edge of a large, muddy pit. She slides into a pool of death.

My fall isn't as dramatic, but if this place isn't haunted by anguished souls, what is?

⬥

I have a neighbor who calls himself a documentary filmmaker. When I asked him about the films he makes, he told me that he creates video advertisements for biological supply companies that sell animals to laboratories. Not just animals, though. Their catalogs also offer stereotaxic instruments, decapicones, irradiation chambers, fear-conditioning packages, and shock chambers. Farm supply catalogs sell shackles, gestation stalls, electric prods, poultry scalding machines, bloodletting tables, and skinning conveyers. I have often wondered, when someone sits down and orders from a catalog a bloodletting table, is this not premeditated violence?

The most common relationship humans have with animals is that we eat them. This is followed by wearing animals, experimenting on them, and trading them for profit. Most animal abuse occurs not by rogue killers, violent spouses, or drug gangs, but by industry and government. Research labs, fur farms, hunting ranches, animal trades, puppy mills, factory farms. These institutionalized forms of violence are more treacherous than any other kind because they have become normalized. By eating animals, experimenting on them, and wearing them, we have embedded the practice of violence into our everyday routines. With our tax dollars, our purchases, and our appetites, we have told our governments and businesses to go ahead and hurt animals. We'll just look the other way.

We have to look the other way, otherwise our natural empathy for animals will be confronted. These institutionalized practices are hidden from our view precisely because the suffering they cause distresses us. We tuck these forms of animal cruelty away from our day-to-day reality in order to feel comfortable. But we don't stop there. We have to think the other way too. Words matter. They not only reflect how we think, they influence it. We use language to develop mental models that become the lens through which we perceive, interpret, and respond to the world. To sever our inherent emotional bond with animals, we practice a form of linguistic deception.

Through words, we classify animals into fabricated categories. The tendency to classify concepts, objects, and living beings is ingrained in human nature. It's how we make sense of the world. The danger of our schemas though is that they don't just organize information; they filter it. When we think about an object or a being through the lens of categories, we latch onto a few preconceived pieces of information that dictate how we should feel about it or her. Every word is a schema unto itself. If I say I saw a squirrel, what immediate thoughts and feelings come to your mind? What pops up when you see the words Arab? Australian? Vegan? Woman? Rat? Dog? Republican? Atheist?

Categorization boxes in our thinking. It can lead to stereotyping and prejudice. Studies reveal that with categorization, we stereotype subconsciously and immediately. Consider skin color, one of our most troublesome categories. Why not instead group people by the lengths of their lashes or shapes of their ears? They're just as arbitrary. Psychologist Joshua Correll studied how skin color affects real-life decisions. In his study, participants played a video game in which they encountered armed and unarmed targets, who were either black or white, and had to quickly decide whether or not to shoot the target. The participants, all non-black, shot more quickly if the armed targets were black and took a little bit longer to shoot if the targets were white.

Black. White. Our simplest classification systems are binary ones that create stark divisions. Good, evil. Smart, dumb. Male, female. Me, you. Human, animal. Us, them. Simple divisions between groups affect our empathy in ways we are just beginning to understand. There is mounting evidence that empathy can be modulated by our categorization of another. Imaging studies show that the executive functions of the brain (i.e., our "thinking part") can dampen our empathetic responses depending on our inherent attitudes toward other groups. A study published in 2011, for example, showed that how we identify social groups—as either us or them—directly activates the parts of our brains that influence our empathy for another. Studying "avid fans" of the Red Sox and Yankee baseball teams, the investigators found that the fans experienced pleasure in response to their rival team's misfortunes (and pain in response to their successes). When perpetuating the "us versus them" mentality, our minds generate an empathy gap.

When we categorize, we polarize. How many times have we followed the "us versus them" mentality to justify violence against another? At its most extreme, bias for the "us" group leads to dehumanization of other people. Dehumanization has produced some of the darkest chapters in human history. In almost all cases, people have been devalued by being compared with animals. Portraying the "out group" as animal-like and less capable of emotions and thought render them less deserving of compassion.

Dehumanization only works, though, when we deanimalize animals. When we strip animals of their being-ness, we turn them into objects, into brutes acting merely on instinct, incapable of experiencing pain or pleasure, incapable of thinking. In this way, antipathy and empathy alike for other humans and animals share a strong commonality. The more "other" we perceive another, the more comfortable we are to disregard their suffering. Our categorizations of living beings, be they human or nonhuman, prevent us from seeing the interconnectedness of our lives.

A study conducted at Brock University examined how beliefs about nonhuman animals affected people's tendencies to dehumanize and reject immigrants. The investigators found that the participants who viewed humans and animals as being more dissimilar had more negative attitudes toward immigrants. However, when participants read stories that emphasized similarities between humans and animals, they developed greater empathy toward immigrants. The findings suggest that not only do our mental categorizations of animals influence how we perceive other humans, but also that our categorizations can dissolve. That's the good news.

The bad news is that, without effort to alter them, our schemas are self-sustaining and so are our beliefs that stem from them. In his book *On Being Certain*, neurologist Robert Burton provides a compelling case that most of what we think we know is not based on conscious rational thought, but on involuntary, subconscious impulses. In the face of disconfirming evidence, we instinctually grasp on to our schemas and beliefs even harder. If something does not match our preconception, such as evidence against it, that information is suppressed, ignored, discounted, or revised. Burton cites, for example, an observation made by social psychology professor Leon Festinger, who described a cult that believed that a flood was going to destroy earth. When the flood didn't happen, the more invested cult members who had given up their jobs and homes reinterpreted the evidence to show that they were right all along, but that earth wasn't destroyed because of their faithfulness. As Burton writes:

> The more committed we are to a belief, the harder it is to relinquish, even in the face of overwhelming contradictory evidence. Instead of acknowledging an error in judgment

and abandoning the opinion, we tend to develop a new attitude or belief that will justify retaining it.

When it comes to our beliefs about animals, we are Olympic gymnasts. The mental acrobatics we perform to convince ourselves that monkeys in labs don't suffer, that cows in California are happy, and that fox trim is not real fur, is nothing short of remarkable. And when old stunts no longer impress, we come up with new ones.

Historically, sharply dividing humans and animals might have been sufficient to dull our empathy toward animals. This might have been helpful to our survival—hunters needed to put aside their empathy to feed their families. Today, though, we don't need to hurt animals. We have options. And as most people now have companion animals, it is more difficult to lull ourselves with the simple binary belief model. From firsthand experience and the growing evidence from animal behavioral studies, we know that animals aren't as distinct from humans as we once believed. How, then, do we reconcile cherishing some animals and hurting others?

We divide animals into groups. When I was in high school, I worked weekends at an emergency veterinary hospital. On one slow afternoon, I was chatting with a technician when I learned that on Mondays through Fridays, she experimented on dogs and cats in a research lab. I was, frankly, shocked. I asked her how she was able to work at the hospital on weekends easing the pain suffered by dogs and cats and on weekdays causing it. She looked at me as though the answer was obvious. "Those animals are bred for research."

Today, we categorize animals as lab animals, food animals, fur animals, game animals, wild animals, labor animals, and companion animals. The labels dictate the narratives we assign them. A lab cat? Well, he was born to have electrodes implanted in his brain. A food lamb? To be carved at our Easter dinner tables. A fur mink? To have her skin peeled away to decorate our coats. You get the idea. There's no need to question. The labels tell us all we need to know, think, and feel about those animals.

In a 2011 study, a group of psychologists found that the simple identification of animals as "food" has a significant effect on how we think of those animals. The psychologists asked participants to read about animals being harmed in different scenarios. Labeling animals as food substantially reduced their perceived capacity to suffer and diminished the reader's moral concern about those animals.

But our labels are artificial—schemas based on our current knowledge of the world, on our biases, and on whim. Increasingly, even those labels we attach to different groups of animals aren't enough to numb our empathy. People have started to learn that pigs can be pessimistic or optimistic, cows show excitement when they learn something new, chickens share and tell one another when there is food, monkeys help one another give birth, and rats enjoy being tickled. Confronted with this knowledge, we are forced to devise ever more tortuous mental contortions.

A seminal study looked at how different ways of presenting information influence altruism. The researchers examined how people donate money to a hunger-relief charity through three different appeals. The first appeal was a story of a starving girl, Rokia. The second appeal presented facts and statistics of the millions of starving children. The third appeal mixed stories with statistics. Which appeal do you think resulted in more charitable donations? It was the first. People donated twice as much after reading Rokia's story than after reading the second appeal, which presented only facts. Even the third appeal did not fare much better. The findings suggest that abstractions like statistics decrease our empathy. Stories, on the other hand, make the abstract concrete. They turn a number into a relatable individual.

A study looking at people's willingness to eat meat found that the less we are reminded of the individuality of animals, the lesser our empathy and greater our willingness to eat them. So, to further remove who animals are, we slice and dice them into pieces. Cows, hens, turkeys, and pigs become steaks, veal, beef, filets, ribs, nuggets, wings, thighs, breasts, bacon, ham, sausage, joints, loins. Or we rename animals altogether. Experimenters refer to animals in laboratories as models, tools, systems, and preparations.

Our truths about animals are a creation of language. We have divided animals into separate categories, broken them down into parts, and reduced them into abstractions. All so that we can ease our conscience. Does it really work?

⁂

Down on the ground in the chicken shed, I get a much better view of what else is here. In the seconds before I manage to steady myself, I glimpse feces, feathers, grubs, other bugs, and suspicious-looking pools of liquid. I jump up as fast as I can, shudder, and tear off my coverall. I look around, embarrassed, expecting the others to laugh at my folly. They have already moved on, though. Over the birds' clamor, I hear Herbert chatting to Jean down another row. He has to yell to be heard. I look around for a place to put my coverall. Seeing no trash can, I ball it up in a corner on the ground, along with my gloves. The disposable clothing had a purpose after all. To protect me. A little. My jeans are gooey. And I don't want to know what's wetting my backside.

I hurry over to join the others and ask about the largest larvae I saw crawling on the floor. The granddaughter explains that they are wasp larvae. They buy the wasps to eat the flies in the building. It's not working. The air is so humid with ammonia and filth; flies must love it here. By this time, I feel a headache coming on and my throat and eyes burn. I want so desperately to rub my eyes, but I don't know what I touched in here. I'm not letting my hands anywhere near my face.

Herbert says something to me that I can't hear.

"I'm sorry?" I reply.

"*I said, You ever hear about* The China Study?"

"Sure." *The China Study* is a book written by T. Colin Campbell, professor emeritus of Nutritional Biochemistry at Cornell

University. It was based on his twenty-year study that evaluated death rates from cancer and other chronic diseases in China.

"How much do you know about it?" Herbert asks.

"Uh . . . it's been a while since I've read it." I'm too embarrassed to admit I don't recall the details.

"They looked at different groups and what they ate. Do you know which group lived the longest?"

"Um . . ." I don't know what Herbert's point is. Why is he talking about *The China Study*, of all things? My head is pounding now. "I don't. . . ."

"The peasants!" he yells triumphantly. "And you know why?" This time he doesn't wait for an answer. "Because they hardly ate any animal products. We're here dying from strokes, cancers, heart attacks—because of eating too much meat!" He scratches his chin. "I'm vegetarian. Well," he pauses, "I'm more vegan now. I used to drink milk three times a day. But cut that out. Because of joint problems. You know that milk and animal products increase the inflammation in your body? Had to cut down on eggs too. I love eggs, but now I'm seeing how it's affecting me."

"How is it affecting you?" I ask. This is one of the strangest conversations I have ever had. Never would I have predicted that an egg producer would be describing to me the ills of eggs.

"My cholesterol was high until I went vegan, and my cholesterol now is about 140. I love eggs, but as long as my cholesterol stays down to 140, well . . . I may slip a few eggs here and there . . . but nobody thinks about that anymore. They just eat the way they please and go to the doctor and get a pill that cures whatever ails them. I have several friends I went to college with that became doctors and specialized in open-heart surgery. Do you know what they do in open-heart surgery?"

"Yes, I do."

"They just cut right down the middle of your breast bone and pry your ribs open and get right down to your heart. I can hardly bear to think about that, and that's one of the bigger reasons I decided to be vegan. I don't want to endure open-heart surgery."

I gape at Herbert, looking like an idiot.

Herbert leads us into the next building, which houses five thousand of what he calls his "free-range, organic hens." Because the public has become increasingly uneasy at the images of chickens and turkeys crowded into factory cages, free-range has become a hot selling point for marketers. But what does free-range mean? If you ask most people, they would probably paint a bucolic scene of chickens roaming about green, sunny pastures living lives according to strict governmental standards and free from pain and suffering (that is until they are hoisted up by their feet and have their throats sliced at slaughter time).

The reality is often far different. According to the US Department of Agriculture, free-range simply means "producers must demonstrate to the Agency that the poultry has been allowed access to the outside." The definition of *outside* is shaky and up to interpretation by the producers. Outside could be rolling grassland or a slab of concrete. Access is also loosely defined. It might mean a window chickens could theoretically squeeze through, or a small opening to a fenced-in section of open concrete that only a few birds can enter at one time. The organic label is even more vague.

For Herbert, *free-range* means living in a shed that is split into two. Half of the chickens live in the right side, and half in the left side of the building. For each group, there is a wooden beam that runs down the middle. Some of the birds are perched on the beams, but they can't all fit. Most of them stand on the same metal wiring that encloses the birds in the other building. They don't even have that minimal criterion of "access to the outside." Their urine and feces drop into the dark nether regions below. Even though there are far fewer chickens in this building, the stench is almost as strong as in the first and maggots squirm below us. In the very back of each "room," there is a long row of nesting boxes where some of the birds can go inside.

"When they're ready to lay their eggs, they like to nest in the boxes where it's darker," Herbert says.

There's nothing else for the birds. Nothing else to enrich their lives. These chickens aren't just denied a life free from daily pain, but also any joy. I once argued with my high school biology teacher that keeping frogs in tiny glass jars, about the size of twelve-ounce cups, was harmful to them. He countered that the frogs were fed, protected from the cold, and safe from predators (other than humans). They preferred the glass jars, he said. I suggested we lift up the jars and see what the frogs decide. The teacher wasn't keen on trying that experiment.

It's taken a long time for biologists and animal behaviorists to admit that animals actually like to have things to do. Being protected from the elements isn't enough. As biologist Jonathan Balcombe wrote, "Just thirty years ago it was scientific heresy to ascribe such emotions as delight, boredom, or joy to a non-human. . . . Researchers around the world have found that there is more thought and feeling in animals than humans have ever imagined." Nature is thrifty. She doesn't like to throw out things that work like the basic neurologic wiring that causes pain, grief, anxiety, joy, loneliness, boredom, and delight. To repurpose a phrase from Carl Sagan, we are made from the same stuff. With animals, we share far more than we don't share.

These "free range, organic" hens don't have the chance to show what they share with us. Their enclosures are a step up of sorts from those in the first building, but essentially these birds just live in larger cages.

I've seen enough. We have been here only a half hour, but I feel as though the maggots have crawled up my legs, bored their way through my skull, and wiggled inside the folds of my brain. I want to drive back to my hotel room, take a shower and an aspirin, and curl up in the dark. But Herbert wants to show us something about the fan systems in the first building, so we slog back through the muck into the larger shed. Here I notice something that I didn't before. When I ask Herbert about it, his response and the conversation that follows shocks me more than anything he's said so far.

In a corner of the larger shed, a makeshift chicken-wire fence encloses about fifteen square feet of ground and five hens. The hens walk not on wire mesh, but on real, dirt ground. They nest in fresh hay and eat from a bowl of hand-delivered food.

"What are the chickens in here for?" I ask Herbert.

"See that hen over there?" he points to the hen holding one foot up. "Got something wrong with her feet. All of them do. I don't have the heart to put them in a cage."

"Why not?" I ask watching a second hen snuggle into the hay.

"If anything happens to a chicken, she's not able to defend herself against the others in the cage."

Herbert calls this pen his medical unit, where he sequesters sick birds and cares for them personally. This confuses me. It's nice of Herbert to take these injured birds aside and give them special treatment, but what about the rest? Although they may not be noticeably limping, how can you tell they are not maimed when they are jammed into cages where they can barely move? Herbert's sentiment to help these few hens ignores the larger issue of how he's treating all the birds. I ask him further about his sick unit.

"Anyone that can't stand up in the cage we put in here. Twenty-five percent of them are weak, probably."

"But you don't see anything wrong with keeping the rest of the chickens in those cages?"

Herbert's defenses suddenly rise. "This gets into all kinds of hysteria. That's baseless. The most efficient way to raise chickens is in a cage. We had no problem with that forty years ago. Everybody in America had roosts in the country. And they knew about chickens out in the farm, chickens out in the barnyard. They'd run around and eat manure and they wanted caged eggs because the chickens were sanitary. Caged eggs were premium. But now animal rights people come along and convince people that this is inhumane to chickens to put them in a cage; it's inhumane to chickens to lock them up in a house. Now we're cruel because we don't let them run free out on the range. As soon as you let them run free on the range you have to start worrying about worms, you have to start worrying about them getting mites and all these other kinds of problems. And they're not very comfortable when it gets cold outside." His words remind me of those of my biology teacher.

"Well, Herbert, I noticed that the hens' feet are all resting on wire. You don't—"

Herbert anticipates what I'm about to say. "That's hard on their feet all right, but it doesn't really deform their feet that much."

"You don't think it does? You don't think standing on a wire for months would be painful?"

"It's not as comfortable as being on the ground, but as soon as you take them out of there you've got to worm them for intestinal parasites."

"You don't have to worm them in cages?"

"In cages you don't ever have to worm them."

I'm not ready to let this go. I recall the dogs and cats I saw running around his front yard and ask him about them. "Let me ask you a question. You have dogs and you have cats—"

"I love cats and dogs."

"Would you ever put them in cages like you do your chickens?"

"No."

"Why not?"

"Let me ask *you* a question," Herbert replies. "How do we decide which creatures to eat and which creatures to pet?"

"I don't know."

"Well, there you go."

He leaves it at that as though my three-worded answer explains it all. Maybe in a sense it does. Do any of us know?

Our conversation takes an even more interesting turn when Herbert's granddaughter, who had left, rejoins us. Herbert buys his birds from a breeder when they are eighteen weeks old. At about eighteen months, the hens' usefulness is spent. They don't produce enough eggs to justify the expense of keeping them alive.

"We used to sell the hens to a rendering plant and get a nickel a pound," Herbert says. "They would be rendered down to bonemeal and things like that. I think they were being fed to other chickens. But now if you take them to the rendering plant, they charge you."

"So what do you do with the chickens now?" I ask.

"So we had to start killing them ourselves and we got permission to bury the birds on our property. We would take the birds in large groups and put them into a dump truck where we gas them with CO2. But they get so terrified when we put them in the dump truck. So terrified that they climb on top of each other. They just start panicking and climbing on top of each other. Ninety percent of them die from smothering themselves before the CO2 is even turned on."

This scene Herbert describes horrifies me. I am surprised, though, how much it horrifies Herbert and his family.

"We can't bear to kill them," he says. "My sons, my granddaughter, we just can't bear it. My sons absolutely refuse to kill them."

"If it bothers you so much, how are you able to kill them?"

"We just shut our eyes and we just don't think. We can't bear to think."

The granddaughter nods her head in agreement. "The last time, we were lucky. Another farmer bought two thousand birds in one go. We didn't have to kill them. We were so happy that we all celebrated that night by going out to dinner."

⁂

In her book *Perpetration-Induced Traumatic Stress*, psychologist Rachel MacNair first proposed that the act of inflicting trauma on another causes in the perpetrator a constellation of symptoms that overlap with PTSD. Symptoms include drug and alcohol abuse, paranoia, anxiety, panic, depression, and disassociation. MacNair defined *perpetration-induced traumatic stress* or PITS as a form of PTSD that arises when people are required to perform actions, including socially sanctioned actions, that go against their natural inclination to not harm or kill another. Many soldiers, she found, report deep discomfort with killing and only do so under pressure.

Analysis of WWII soldiers found that most soldiers did not fire their weapons because of an innate resistance to killing. What's more, many studies suggest that soldiers in combat who have killed, like Capt. Jason Haag, who I met earlier, suffer more severe PTSD than those who have not killed. MacNair's theory proved so compelling that psychiatrists added to the DSM-5 that active participation in harming another is a cause of PTSD.

Although MacNair focused on combat veterans, Nazis, policemen, executioners, and torturers, she wondered, do people who harm animals in culturally accepted ways experience PITS?

At first glance, MacNair's question might seem odd. After all, humans have been killing animals for food, labor, and for their skins for centuries. Killing animals is nothing new. So why should humans feel trauma when doing so?

In 1972, the television drama *The Waltons* illustrated the conflict many families have faced concerning the animals under their care. In the episode "The Calf," after the family cow gives birth, the children become attached to the newborn calf. They are devastated when, to raise much-needed funds, their father sells the calf to a neighbor farmer, who intends to slaughter the calf. Eventually, the father recognizes the children's loss and that of the mother cow, Chance, who moans for days lamenting her baby. At the end of the show, the father approaches the other farmer and pleads, "You see, to you this calf is just meat on the table, but to my children, he's become a playmate and part of the family." The father negotiates a deal with the farmer and buys back the calf, ending the show on a happy note.

For the Walton family and the two cows, empathy wins. Most of the time, though, humans have stamped down their empathy as a way to resolve any conflict about harming animals. We convince ourselves that empathy is a weakness and we harden our hearts. The problem with trying to suppress a natural response is that it doesn't really go away. Like a weed we may think we killed, empathy sprouts roots that dive deep underground, waiting for the right time and place to resurface. The more we try to poison that weed, the more likely it will return in an unruly form.

It's well known that slaughterhouses have high employee turn-over rates, as high as 200 percent in the first year of operation. While most sociologists point to the dangerous nature of the work, the high risk of injuries, the low wages, and the terrible treatment of employees, several investigators asked whether the psychological impact of killing animals could also contribute to high turnover.

In one study, investigators asked slaughterhouse workers which was the worst section to work in. The choices were the receiving room (where workers first receive the birds), the cutting room (where workers kill the chickens), evisceration (where workers remove the chickens' entrails), the bleeding sectors (where workers drain the birds' blood), plucking (where workers remove the chickens' feathers), packaging (where workers package the chickens for consumers), and freezing (where workers cool the birds' bodies). First place was given to the room where workers kill chickens. "Aha!" you might say. The kill room was chosen because it was the most dangerous. Maybe. There could be another explanation, though.

Two psychologists who conducted in-depth interviews with slaughterhouse employees noted that "Slaughter employees inevi-tably remember their first encounter with the slaughterfloor and having to slaughter. They recall vivid images of blood and describe the experience as traumatic. . . ." Employees reported feeling pained, saddened, and ashamed. Many experienced recurring nightmares filled with fear and anxiety. They reported dreams of fleeing from vengeful cows, being confronted by slaughtered cows who failed to die, seeing animals in pain, and fighting with and being watched by animals.

In his blog, the late Virgil Butler, a Tyson slaughterhouse worker for nine years, describes the mental trauma he experienced long after leaving the job. In one confession, he describes a night on the kill floor:

> The chickens are panicking. Many of them are squawking loudly, some are just sitting there trembling. Sometimes you catch one looking up at you, eye to eye, and you

know it's terrified. . . . No one can convince me that that
chicken did not know what was about to happen.

How do slaughterhouse workers cope with this anguish? Many
quit. But some can't afford to. As one psychologist put it, "The
industry has become quite adept at recruiting the most marginalized populations that are quite vulnerable." Slaughterhouses tend to
employ migrant workers, many here illegally, and others desperate
for work. To stay employed, their survival depends on detachment
from the reality of the situation. Temple Grandin found that the
most common psychological approach workers use is what she calls
the "mechanical approach," during which "the person doing the
killing approaches his job as if he were stapling boxes moving along
a conveyer belt. He has no emotions about his act." She found that
the second most common approach is sadistic: the worker enjoys
killing and causing more suffering. "By devaluing the animal," she
wrote, "the person justifies in his mind the cruel things he does to it."

In her 1997 book *Slaughterhouse*, Gail Eisnitz interviewed dozens
of slaughterhouse workers in the United States about their experiences. Among the workers, she encountered numerous instances of
both detachment and sadism. One worker described:

The worst thing, worse than the physical danger, is the
emotional toll. If you work in that stick pit [where the
pigs are killed] for any period of time, you develop an
attitude that lets you kill things but doesn't let you care.
You may look a hog in the eye that's walking around
down in the blood pit with you and think, God, that
really isn't a bad-looking animal. You may want to pet it.
Pigs down on the kill floor have come up and nuzzled me
like a puppy. Two minutes later I had to kill them—beat
them to death with a pipe. I can't care.

Nothing takes more energy than that which we suppress. As with
soldiers who have killed, there is compelling evidence to suggest

that slaughterhouse workers suffer from harming animals. Signs of PITS, like substance abuse, occur frequently in slaughterhouse workers. There have been several cases of workers taken to the mental hospital for treatment of recurring dreams of violence. A large study of almost one thousand employees in Brazil found higher rates of anxiety, depression, and other mood problems among slaughterhouse workers compared with employees who worked in other types of stressful situations. Mental disturbances were highest among the slaughterhouse employees who worked on the kill floor. Many employees had mutilated themselves in fits of rage and were suicidal.

There aren't enough studies to conclusively state that slaughterhouse workers commonly suffer from PITS, but examination of other types of workers add support to the idea. Among employees who routinely kill animals in shelters and laboratories, 39 percent have mild symptoms suggestive of PITS and 11 percent have moderate symptoms. Although it's been a hush topic for decades, evidence is emerging that many laboratory workers who directly handle and experiment on animals suffer deep emotional trauma. They report experiencing guilt, grief, sadness, anger, anxiety, headaches, sleeplessness, despair, overeating, and rage. Scarred by the suffering they caused animals, a team of former laboratory workers created a support group for researchers traumatized by their work.

A growing unease is developing. Hurting animals in ways that may have been tolerated in the past are slowly becoming harder to endure. Could our empathy for animals be getting stronger?

⁂

Before heading off, Jean and I wash our hands with soap. I scrub my face too, hoping to leave the stench behind me. We thank Herbert and his family for the tour of their facility, then hop into Jean's car to drive to our next destination. To my dismay, the smell follows me. It won't let me go. My jeans, my sweater, my hair, my skin. Everything reeks.

I ask Jean if the smell bothered her. It didn't. Not one bit. I then ask her how Herbert's facility compares to the more modern facilities she has seen. She says the newer facilities are a bit cleaner, but admits that the conditions of the birds themselves are similar. Debeaked birds with raw, exposed skin and swollen legs. In other words, the same miserable animals, only in much greater numbers.

Jean hopes that our next stop will show me what state-of-the-art facilities are like. We drive to Oklahoma State University's Department of Animal & Food Sciences in the town of Stillwater. Jean tells me that these are research and teaching facilities. They are very small-scale versions of what I could expect to see at commercial establishments.

The manager of the swine facility—a tall, large man—is not happy about our being here. With his legs set in a wide stance and his fists at his side, he looks me over, in particular, with great suspicion. I fight my frown and smile up at him. He heaves a great sigh to let us know how much we are putting him out. "Okay. Justin here will show you," he points to the college student in the room. "But don't touch anything." He points at me. "You hear?"

"Of course," I say. When we enter the first room housing pigs, I immediately start snapping photos.

The noise in this room rattles me. It's as though a group of fifty cultists are beating drums and shrieking around a fire. About twenty pigs stand upright in crates, facing the center aisle. Their bodies fill up these gestation crates from side to side, front to back. All they can do is stand. They can't turn around. Not even to scratch an itch. Each pig is barking and beating her head and snout against the cage, up and down, up and down. That's about the only movement they can make.

The pigs stand on slatted metal flooring, so that their wastes drop beneath. Even with only twenty or so pigs, the stench is strong. Jean tells me that what I smell here is hydrogen sulfide, as opposed to ammonia back in the chicken sheds. My untrained nose can't discern the difference between this stink and the other stink.

This room looks like a modern facility. Sterile, lifeless. Like a laboratory. There's nothing in the room except the pigs. But it's just a taste of what the average-size facility is like, where thousands may be confined to a single shed. Ninety-seven percent of pigs are imprisoned in factory farms.

I remove my right glove, crouch down in front of the pig nearest me, gaze into her eyes, caress her snout, and say, "You poor baby. What a sweet little girl." But human comfort is not something she recognizes. Her eyes look to someplace beyond me. She jams her head against the bars, up and down, foam frothing around her mouth, like the other pigs. In concert, they produce an almost deafening thumping that ping-pongs off the barren walls. No one in her right mind could look at these pigs and not immediately see that they had gone mad.

Justin informs us that Tyson Foods funds the school's program in researching infection control measures and breeding fatter pigs. Before workers kill them, the pigs stand in gestation crates for a total of three to four years. In this first room, workers inseminate the female pigs with pig semen about twice a year. Justin leads us into the next room where the mothers give birth. Farm workers allow the moms to stay here for two weeks to nurse their young. In this room, the crates that imprison the pigs are called a different name. These farrowing cages are a little larger than gestation crates, but not by much. They have small side aisles to accommodate the litter of six to nine piglets per mother pig. Justin tells me that the side aisles prevent the mothers from crushing their babies. Something, he says, that inevitably occurs otherwise.

Even if that is occasionally the case, Justin's argument is misleading. These pigs are primarily kept in crates to save money. I push Justin further.

"Do you think these crates are cruel?"

"You know there's animal rights and welfare groups who get all upset about gestation crates. But it's actually much more humane to keep these animals in these crates. This way, we can see each one and watch for diseases." Like keeping frogs in jars.

The third room is the nursing facility. Ten to fifteen pigs live in a cage, without their mothers. The moms were put back in the gestation room, where they will be inseminated and recycled again through the rooms. When I kneel down, these piglets rush to my hand, allowing me to rub their noses and stroke their silky ears through the cage bars. These boys and girls are still young. Insanity hasn't set in, yet.

From here, the pigs move from room to room down along the assembly line into increasingly smaller groups per cage. When they are about 280 pounds, the pigs are selected for either further breeding or to be killed.

"The ones that get sold for slaughter end up going into things like sausage, bacon, and other processed pork products," Justin says. They send the breeding pigs to the gestation crates in the first room, to live side by side, but in separate cages, with their mothers. There they remain until it's time to move to the farrowing room to give birth.

I ask Justin, "How do you get the pigs from the gestation room to the farrowing room? Wouldn't it be hard for them—who haven't exercised their legs in months—to move into the next room?"

He chuckles and says one of the saddest things I've ever heard. "Well it's actually quite easy. You'd be surprised how much they like to walk."

⌘

Biologist and author Rachel Carson once said, "Until we have the courage to recognize cruelty for what it is—whether its victim is human or animal—we cannot expect things to be much better in this world."

Ignoring our treatment of animals has far-reaching implications. In the 1980s, a team of sociologists examined whether socially sanctioned violence can "spill over" into other spheres of life. The team's theory was based on previous studies showing that cultural support for killing during wartime coincides with higher murder and child abuse rates. To test their theory, the sociologists measured sanctioned violence in all fifty US states and in Washington, DC. They looked at factors like public approval for the death penalty, the number of hunting licenses, the popularity of violent media, and approval of police violence. The results were troubling. In the states where there was great support for legal forms of violence, incidence of rape was especially high. The study did not asses causality, therefore it could not prove that the higher rates of rape were specifically due to acceptance of other forms of violence. It did, however, add weight to the theory of cultural spillover: the more a society legitimates the use of violence to attain ends for which there is widespread social approval, the greater the likelihood of illegitimate violence.

Does spillover violence occur with cruelty to animals? For decades, sociologists have noted that when slaughterhouses move into town, rates of violent crimes—including property damage, drug-related crimes, spousal and child abuse—go up. Finney County, Kansas, for example, experienced a 130 percent increase in violent crimes within five years after two slaughterhouses opened, which could only be partly accounted for by the 33 percent increase in population. Several reasons have been offered as the cause for the increased crime rates, which include the demographic characteristics of workers (often used to justify racism against immigrants), social disorganization resulting from the sudden population boom, unemployment rates secondary to high turnover, and physically stressful and demanding jobs.

Psychologist Amy Fitzgerald had a different idea. Many interviews with slaughterhouse workers suggest that the violence they inflict on animals seeps into other parts of their lives. From one worker, who described his thoughts of killing his wife:

> I've got the short temper. When I'm alone sitting, thinking . . . I'm killing thousands of cattle; hey I kill 800 or 900 cattle, it's nothing that's gonna stop me to shoot only one person.

From another worker, who identifies himself as a hog sticker, one who stabs and bleeds pigs to death:

> Every sticker I know carries a gun, and every one of them would shoot you. Most stickers I know have been arrested for assault. A lot of them have problems with alcohol. They *have to* drink, they have no other way of dealing with killing live, kicking animals all day long. If you stop and think about it, you're killing several thousand beings a day.

Based on anecdotes like these, Fitzgerald wondered if the increase in crime associated with slaughterhouses has to do with the theory she calls the Sinclair Effect. In his groundbreaking book *The Jungle*, Upton Sinclair observed a connection between the routine slaughter of animals and other forms of violence. To test the Sinclair Effect, Fitzgerald compiled information from the FBI's Uniform Crime Report database, census data, and police records from 581 US counties from 1994 to 2002. She looked at the crime rates in counties with slaughterhouses and compared them to rates in counties with comparable populations employed in factory-like operations, such as motor vehicle manufacturing and the steel industry. These counties had similar labor force composition and injury and illness rates. But the industries in these comparable counties had one key difference: they didn't involve the killing of living beings.

After crunching the numbers, Fitzgerald found that a slaughterhouse employing 175 people would be expected to increase the number of arrests by 2.24 and the number of police reports by 4.69. In counties with 7,500 slaughterhouse employees, the arrests and report rates of crimes like property damage, child abuse, and sex offences were more than double the values where there were no slaughterhouse workers. Fitzgerald's study strongly indicates that it is not repetitive and dangerous work that causes increased crimes, but the killing of animals.

Particularly telling were the high rates of child abuse and rape in counties with slaughterhouses. Iron and steel forging also had a significant effect on arrests for rape, but a negative one. Employment in these industries was associated with a *decrease* in arrests for rape. Fitzgerald surmised that the high rates of violence against children and women might come down to how slaughterhouse workers come to perceive the less powerful, including animals.

A more recent study in Australia tested levels of aggression in slaughterhouse workers. The investigators found that aggression levels in slaughterhouse workers were "so high they're similar to the scores . . . for incarcerated populations." Interestingly, aggression was highest among women workers.

The obvious question that follows this and Fitzgerald's study is, Do slaughterhouses desensitize people, or do they attract less empathetic people in the first place? Fitzgerald doesn't believe it's the latter. "The one thing slaughterhouse workers have in common is a kind of desperation for work," she tells me. The studies mentioned earlier by Temple Grandin and others certainly suggest that for many workers, their empathy is squeezed out of them by the business.

Most scholars have overlooked the potential spillover of sanctioned violence against animals into other forms of violence, perhaps because they are afraid of the conclusions that that might follow this line of study. To date, Fitzgerald's study is the only one to systematically do so. But given that individual cruelty to animals strongly links with other forms of violence, is it so far-fetched to think this could be the case with systemic abuse of animals as well?

⁂

By the end of the day, I feel hollowed out and exhausted. On our ride back to the Sonic parking lot, Jean is just as energetic as she was this morning. With obvious pride, she tells me how the university facilities are doing cutting-edge research into increasing the efficiency of meat and milk production and are models of animal welfare. I don't understand her. I can only imagine the mental contortions Jean is making. She thought she was driving me around today to dispel the "myths" I read. Instead, I am more convinced than ever that these facilities are cruel to animals and threaten human health. The fumes alone from the animal buildings still dance like evil sprites in my head.

The moment I step into my hotel room, the cage I held around my emotions shatters. I tear off my clothes, grab a plastic trash bag lining one of the bins, and tie the bag around my clothes, as though I can package away the day's stink and misery. In the scalding shower, I wash my hair three times and scrub my skin raw. With a spare, unused toothbrush, I scour under my nails. Get off! Get off! I yell at the smell, which I swear taunts me still.

Afterward, dressed in clean clothes, I text Patrick, who has been waiting all day to hear how things went. I let him know I'm done and will talk when I get home tomorrow. As I sit at the foot of the bed, staring at the blank TV in front of me, my stomach churns. I'm hungry. Not just hungry. Ravenous. I'm not surprised. When I am upset, I eat. When Patrick lost his job, I ate. When my dad got pancreatic cancer, I ate. When my grandmother died, I ate. I want to eat.

I get into my car and drive toward a Taco Bell near the hotel. No, I want a drink, too. I see a chain restaurant and swing into the parking lot. When I walk into the restaurant, no person stands at the front desk to greet me. I look about the room. A bartender is busy preparing a drink, and I don't see any other staff. I seat myself at a booth and wait. Only a few people are dining on this Monday night. Three men sit in the booth behind me, talking in hushed tones. One of them turns to me, gives a nod, and says, "Hi."

"Hi," I say and turn my head facing forward. That's the extent of the conversation I want to have. I sit and look ahead until a waiter notices me. "Gosh, you're so quiet back here," he says, "I didn't see you!"

When my meal arrives—a veggie burger, a glass of red house wine, and two sides of fries—I consume it within ten minutes. I hail the waiter again and ask for my check.

"You must be in a hurry to get out of here!" he laughs. When he returns with my check, I look over the price, and then look up at him with a question on my face.

"Yeah," he says, "that guy sitting behind you paid for your wine. He didn't want me to tell you until after he left, but I thought you would want to know."

I turn to the man behind me to thank him as he's getting up to leave with his friends. I get a better look at him this time. Dark eyes, long, straight raven hair lands on his shoulders.

I begin, "Mr. ummmm—"

"Tom Perry," he says.

"Thank you very much for the wine. That was really nice of you."

He nods. "You just looked so sad." With that, he walks out the door with his friends.

I take the earliest flight out the next morning. With only six other people on the plane, I have the row to myself. As I sit there, in the dark predawn, I try to make sense of yesterday. I recall one of the last things Herbert had said to me when I asked him if he could start over and do things differently, would he?

"I probably would have loved to farm big," he replied. "A few thousand acres of crops and not have to worry about . . . this . . . killing chickens."

I think about Tom Perry's words. How did he know? I *am* sad. I'm sad for the animals whose lives will never be their own. I'm sad for Herbert who feels trapped in a grim business. I'm sad for Jean who believes in this twisted relationship with animals. I'm sad for me to have witnessed such cruelty. I'm sad for the whole damned world.

In the warm, dark, thrumming of the plane, I quietly cry.

When I get home, I cry. And I cry. For two weeks, three, four. I plummet into this depression. As with every depressive episode before, I keep it from others, from friends, from co-workers. I fight to keep my knees, shoulders, spine erect—to not allow my body to crumple into itself. Especially this time. How many would empathize with my despair over the lowliest of creatures? I weep when alone. In the shower. In the car. In the closet. But I don't fool Patrick. One day, he finds me huddled on the bathroom floor, sobbing. He looks at me with pain in his eyes. Without a word, he scoops me up in his arms, carries me to the bed, and holds me as my tears fall free.

⤬

Grief, despair, and trauma are contagious. In 1981, a psychologist published a review of the emotional reactions of therapists who worked with Holocaust survivors. The therapists, she wrote, often "found themselves sharing the nightmares of the survivors they were treating." Vicarious trauma was a new idea at the time, but there have since been many indications that people suffer by hearing about, witnessing, and even reading about the violence inflicted on others.

Aid workers commonly suffer emotional health problems. A survey by *The Guardian* revealed that almost 80 percent of humanitarian workers experience mental health problems, with almost half having been diagnosed with depression. Some of the symptoms the aid workers experience may be due to threats to their own personal security and to working in dangerous, under-resourced areas. But the respondents frequently cited witnessing human tragedy as a cause of their own suffering.

Vicarious traumatization causes high risk of burnout.

Journalists comprise another group that experiences vicarious trauma. The more time journalists spend combing through violent images and videos—such as those showing the aftermath of earthquakes, car bombs, and mass rape—the greater their likelihood of having symptoms of PTSD. It's now coming to light that military drone pilots experience vicarious trauma. These are the pilots who "fly missions" over different parts of the world, collecting photos and video feeds, flying bombs, conducting deadly strikes in warfare, and carrying out CIA assassination missions. They do these tasks from the comfort of their desks and are far removed from any danger. It came, then, as a real surprise when some investigators learned that drone pilots suffer from anxiety, depression, substance abuse, and thoughts of suicide as much as combat pilots do.

Why would drone pilots suffer trauma? There are two lines of thought. The first is that long hours and frequent shift changes cause burnout. The second is that that, unlike combat pilots who fly into an area, drop a bomb, then fly out as quickly as possible, drone pilots witness the resulting carnage. They spend hours each day in front of video screens. They get up close and personal in a way that combat pilots do not. The violence drone pilots witness is, ironically, more real to them.

Drone pilots may suffer from "moral injury," which overlaps with perpetration-induced traumatic stress. Defined as "perpetrating, failing to prevent, bearing witness to, or learning about acts that transgress deeply held moral beliefs and expectations," moral injury may cause long-term suffering, "emotionally, psychologically, behaviorally, spiritually, and socially." Drone pilots watching the aftermath of men, women, and children impacted by their actions may experience psychological damage because their acts violated their conception of right and wrong. As one drone pilot put it, "A predator [drone] pilot has been watching his target[s], knows them intimately, knows where they are, and knows what's around them." Knowing their targets—seeing them as individuals and not merely as the collective category of "them"—may cause in drone pilots a moral trauma that confronts their innate empathy.

Trauma is not just a private problem. It's the consequence of civilization gone wrong and arises from the collective cruelties of humanity. Studies on media exposure to tragedies like the Boston Marathon bombings and 9/11 show that we are emotionally affected by the suffering of others. Repeated media exposure significantly increases the risk of suffering from collective trauma, which occurs to a group of individuals or an entire society. Trauma is global. Cruelties against others root themselves into our own consciousness. Even the cruelties inflicted on animals.

We are naturally inclined to connect with animals and yet we continually act against this inclination. When we go against our natural empathy for animals and inflict violence on them, either individually or systemically, we open ourselves to all forms of violence. And as our understanding of who animals are continues to evolve, so too does our empathy. We suffer when animals suffer.

One day I was talking with Dr. John Gluck, psychologist and professor emeritus at the University of New Mexico, about his past experiments on monkeys with Harry Harlow. Although Gluck grew up loving animals, he had systematically desensitized himself in order to experiment on them. While working with Harlow as a PhD student, Gluck assisted with behavioral experiments in which they put baby monkeys into isolation chambers for up to two years to study the effects of social deprivation (no surprise, the monkeys became deeply disturbed). Although considered a respected authority figure among his colleagues, Harlow's cruel experiments drew the ire of the public. In the 1970s, people started sending Gluck letters protesting the experiments. Most of the letters didn't sway Gluck. But there were some that shocked his sensibilities and started him on a journey into animal advocacy. "People wrote to me saying, 'Knowing you're there doing what you do . . . it has harmed me,'" Gluck tells me. "I got into this work to alleviate harm, not create it."

⁂

In high school, my brother introduced me to Mozart. I fell deeply, passionately in love with Mozart. I mentioned long ago that most of my depressions feed off of news of human brutality and injustice. During countless depressive episodes, Mozart would come to my rescue. Don't despair, his music would sing to me. Don't lose hope! And he would convince me. Humanity can't be so bad if it can create music of such magnificence that it can tug from me tears not of sadness but of utter bliss.

It's not just Mozart. It's my husband, who would wrap me in his arms forever if they could shield me from grief. It's the Tom Perrys who would buy a stranger a glass of wine because she looks sad. It's the humanitarians who would risk their lives to heal refugees. It's the boys who would stop traffic to rescue a turtle. It's the makers of *Seinfeld*.

It's those who give to the world beauty, kindness, and laughs who save me. Ultimately, they save us all.

Every time I've come out of a depressive episode, I felt as though I crawled through a gauntlet. Worries, fears, sorrows, and doubts throw their best at me. But I scrabble to the other side, bruised yet feeling a little stronger, a little more powerful. I survived.

I emerge from this depression with a weapon of my own—a new understanding. The mental convolutions we go through to anesthetize our empathy for animals isn't a reason for dismay. It's a reason for hope. Our compassion is so strong that we have to go to great lengths to override it. These convolutions want to right themselves. To make us ask if there is another way. And as I came to know about my and Sylvester's abuse, someday we will also come to know as a society that there is indeed another way. If we are brave enough to look for it.

Until then, I can't give the animals I met in Oklahoma a better life. But I can give them something else. I can give each of them a name. And with a name, I give back life stories that we stole from them. I take out the pictures I took from the facilities. In this photo before me from Herbert's farm, I name the first five hens Henrietta, Geraldine, Hilda, Ethel, and Isabella. In the stories of my imagination, these animals never knew lives in a cage. They grew up together in a sanctuary, rarely leaving each other's sides. Henrietta wakes up first from their nest of soft hay, steps out into the sunshine, and stretches her wings. Geraldine and Isabella soon emerge, call to her, and join her in exploring the fields.

With a name pronounced, a light in a dark corner of the world sings. There's Trixie, Kamala, Sir Foggington-Smythe, Gertrude, Ramsey, Cedric, Yoshi, Angelica, Oscar, Bacchus, Ms. Mabel, Asami, Felix, Snowy, Licorice, Mr. Wellington, Raj, Edwina, Winston, Buttercup, Willow Tree, Earl Grey, Sparkles, Miss Matilda, Esther, Peanuts, Olaf, Bongo, Eduardo, Loki, Wally, Beatrice, Suki, Yvonne, Sir McCutcheon, Fenton, Big Blanche, Magnolia, Keiko, Blackbeard, Napoleon, Juan, Arya, Gandhi, Veronica, Petunia, Nicholas, Milton, Mortimer, Clover Meadow, Romeo, Dr. Zhivago, Wenona, Princess Kwame, Chamomile, Sage, Bruno the Magnificent . . . .

PART THREE

Joining with Animals

SEVEN

Standing with Animals

S ylvester.

He was missing. I couldn't sleep. I didn't want to go to school. I wanted to spend every possible hour searching for him. Was he still alive? Was he hungry? Was he scared? After school, I went around with my aunt, my brother, or with Dave knocking door-to-door asking if anyone saw a little dog who loved to give you his paw if you asked for it.

At night, my greatest fear churned in my head. Did Sylvester run away because Dave was hurting him? As this question taunted me, the worse thought was not about what Dave did to Sylvester, but what I *did not do* for him. When Sylvester needed me most, I failed to stand with him.

In August 2004, six cows escaped from the Nebraska Beef, Ltd. slaughterhouse in Omaha and made a dash for freedom. Omaha police and slaughterhouse workers quickly caught four of them, but two cows proved more elusive. The fifth animal galloped down the main boulevard to the railroad yards, and a cream-colored cow charged down Thirty-first Street, causing pedestrians in his path to scatter. Traffic slowed and crowds gathered to watch the spectacle as police and plant workers matched wills against the two cows who would not easily be corralled onto the trailer that would return them to the slaughterhouse. Meanwhile, as one reporter put it, nearby cows mooed loudly in the background as though to cheer on the escapees.

"It's an ornery one," said Police Sgt. Deb Campbell of one of the escaped cows. "It has a mind of its own."

After almost an hour, police cornered the fifth cow against a chain-link fence. Three officers with shotguns fired six shots. The cow ran a little more, then collapsed and died. The crowd groaned. Soon after, the police shot and killed the remaining cow. The shooting took place during a ten-minute afternoon break, when slaughterhouse workers stepped outside for fresh air and a cigarette. Many of the workers watched as the cops killed the cows.

This story in itself isn't remarkable. News sites frequently report of pigs, cows, and other animals making desperate dashes to escape their fates. What is curious, though, is that the day after the police shot the cows, news spread rapidly among the slaughterhouse employees, fueled by the graphic retelling of one worker who witnessed the events. "They shot it, like, ten times," she said. She was angry and so were many of the other employees. She compared the shooting of the cow to the recent shooting of an unarmed man from Mexico by the Omaha police. Many of the slaughterhouse workers were immigrants and worried about prejudice and threats from the police. To the workers, the police killing of a defenseless cow was unjust—even though the cow was escaping from a place that was going to do just that.

Oftentimes, the ground that buries our deep-rooted empathy cracks open just enough to let a tendril or two escape. For the slaughterhouse workers, whose collective empathy was numbed by the routine, normalcy of killing, it took taking a few cows out of their usual context to break ground. Seeing and hearing about cows not carved up on the killing floor, but instead shot in the city streets by police, jolted the workers into a new narrative, however briefly, about the cows and themselves. That day, as angry stories passed from one worker's ear to another, they felt solidarity with the cows.

∽

Nothing beckons fellowship with another as much as a shared fight for survival. For Steven Peterson, it happened as he crawled across a river of ice that threatened to split at any moment.

In Steven's family, hunting is a tradition. Hunting deer since childhood, Steven never paused to reconsider his activity. Until one winter afternoon when he risked his life to save a deer.

When Steven's car crossed over the Kettle River south of Duluth, Minnesota, he noticed something strange. On that frigid December day, fifty-year-old Steven was returning to his home in Duluth after spending the Christmas holidays with his family in Missouri. Steven had been recently laid off as a woodworking instructor at the Michigan School for the Deaf and had moved to Minnesota to start a new life. On his drive home, with no job to rush to, he leisurely scanned the snowy panorama. As he passed over the Kettle River Bridge on Interstate 35, he spotted movement in the river far below and saw what looked like a rock bobbing up and down in the water. Not sure what he was seeing, he continued to drive on.

"I tried to forget what I saw," Steven tells me, "but as I continued to drive, all I kept thinking was that something wasn't right." No longer able to ignore the growing doubt, Steven pressed on his gas pedal and turned around at the next exit. When he returned to the bridge and got out of his car, he clearly saw the top half of a fawn. "Its back legs and most of its body was invisible beneath the river's surface. It was trapped in an ice hole in the river and was struggling again and again with its front hooves to pull itself out. But it wasn't able to get traction."

Steven's immediate reaction was to call 911, but being deaf, he believed the effort to communicate with the operator would take too long. The temperature that day was just above the teens and the deer looked as though she was ready to collapse from exhaustion and drown at any moment. "Time was of the essence," he says to me. "So I thought, Forget 911. I knew it's going to be on me."

He reached for a trailer strap inside the truck, left the bridge, and scuttled about a quarter of a mile down the steep bank, slipping and sliding through the tangled bushes. When he got to the quiet, still river, he hesitated by what he saw. The river was about as wide as a football field and was covered with a thin layer of ice. In the river's center, water that the deer had splashed from her struggles was chilled into small mountains on top of the ice sheet. The icicles hanging from the fawn's eyelashes, cheeks, and chin had etched her face into a frozen landscape.

"The deer was so exhausted," Steven says. "It had probably been struggling in the river since the early-morning hours. It was afternoon now and the water was getting colder and the hole was shrinking. The deer was going to go under at any moment. And I thought, If I step on the wrong place, I could be in the water, too."

But then the deer turned her head and looked him in the eyes. And that's when Steven turned on the video feature on his phone and in sign language left a message to his family and friends telling them that he was going to risk his life to try to rescue the deer. He put his phone away and grabbed the strap and a large log. Using his body as a vertical line, Steven made a T with the log to help with balance, and shimmied inch by inch across the ice. As he crawled closer to the center of the river, he saw water moving beneath him. The ice was getting thinner.

The further he crawled toward the center, the more translucent the ice became. When he neared the deer, she ceased struggling and gazed at Steven. "It wanted to escape," he tells me, "but there was nowhere for it to go. The ice formed a perfect circle around it. The deer was just looking at me in the eyes and trembling. I almost felt like it was asking for help." As Steven mentally repeated to the deer that he was here to help, he threw the strap he was carrying around the deer's head, careful not to let it loop around her neck for fear it would choke her. After several attempts, he caught the rope around the deer's back and right shoulder. As soon as he saw her chest rise as she heaved a deep breath, he pulled. Hard. And he pulled the fawn right out of the hole.

She was out, but she wasn't safe from drowning until she was off the ice. Neither was Steven. Except for her trembling, the deer did not move. Steven tried to push her along the ice. But that wasn't getting them very far. It was like pushing a forty-pound sandbag across a dirt road. He then sat on the ice and again waited for the deer to take a deep breath. Using his legs to propel him backward, he pulled at the strap. That seemed to work. So he kept at it, syncing his movements with her breathing. Chests heaved, legs pushed, arms pulled. It was as if they labored in unison. The only sounds heard deep in the valley were theirs. "Each time I grunted and pulled," Steven says, "she bellowed."

Bit by bit, Steven got the deer up to the bank. He was thrilled. Then he glanced up and his heart fell. The bank on this side of the river climbed almost twenty-five feet to the top. It was steep—dangerously so. The deer, who was showing more life by now, crawled up the bank, only to immediately tumble back down onto the ice. "She got up onto land again and fell right back down," Steven says. "Again and again, she climbed up the hill only to slip back down. I thought, Any moment now, she will end up breaking the ice and plunging into another hole." Steven was worn out. His hands quivered from the cold. There was no strength left in them. How was he going to get her off the ice? After all his effort, was he going to watch her die?

No, he told himself. That's not going to happen. Gripping the loose end of the strap, he crawled up to near the top of the hill. When he looked down, he felt despair descend again. It was so far down to the river! With his waning strength, he tried one last effort. Taking off his wet gloves, which were by now adding to his misery, he pulled the strap with everything he had. And he pulled and pulled until the deer, lying on her side and giving no resistance, was yanked onto dry land and to safety.

After describing this scene to me, Steven takes a long pause as if to brace himself for a memory that remains especially poignant for him. When he resumes, he says, "I stumbled to the deer and collapsed beside her. We were both cold, exhausted, soaking wet, breathing heavily. She kept looking at me and I kept looking at her. We just lay there with each other."

Time stilled. And in that hush, fawn and man were the same.

❧

There is a memorable episode of *Star Trek: The Next Generation* called "The Measure of a Man," a play on the title of Stephen Jay Gould's *The Mismeasure of Man*, which critiques the use of biological heredity to support racism, sexism, and class boundaries. In the *Star Trek* episode, a scientist wants to dismantle the android Data to learn what makes him tick, in a procedure that may cost Data's life. Data has no desire to be taken apart and killed, but the scientist argues that Data is merely a machine and has no rights in the matter. Throughout the episode, in accordance with his view that Data is insentient, the scientist refers to Data as "it."

Data's fate is decided during a climactic trial before a judge. Defending Data, Captain Picard builds a case around Data's personal possessions and his sentimental attachment to them: his Starfleet medals, a book that Picard gave him, a hologram of a shipmate and his former lover. (Data also cared for a cat he named Spot—another sign of his humanity.) These displays of Data's personality surprise not only the judge but also the scientist. Picard then challenges the scientist to prove that the captain is sentient while Data is not, which the scientist is unable to do.

The judge rules in Data's favor. When she walks up to the disappointed scientist, he states of Data, "He's remarkable."

The astute judge looks at him and says, "You didn't call him 'it.'"

This was a pivotal moment, not only for Data, but also the scientist. Little did he know that from the moment he met Data, somewhere deep down within, he was gently erasing the sharp line that divided them. With each revelation of Data's sentience, the scientist's opinion of Data changed. By the trial's culmination, Data ceased being an inanimate object. He was a person.

Sometimes the ability to see another not as an abstract, but as an individual not so different from ourselves requires a lifetime of lessons. Sometimes, it just needs an afternoon.

I notice that as Steven tells me his story, at some point he ceased referring to the deer as "it" and instead as "she." I don't think he recognized his change in language. It wasn't a conscious decision on his part; it just developed naturally. As if reliving the rescue transformed his perception of the deer.

We empathize with others' struggles for life. When I ask Steven why, given that he often killed deer, he went to such great lengths to stop and save this one, he simply replied, "She was fighting for her life." The ability to recognize oneself in the other and vice versa is deeply democratizing. It cuts through social barriers, wealth, education, gender, professional status, and even species. With a healthy use of empathy, the barriers between "you" and "I" melt away. Not so much that you or I get lost in the process (that would be unhealthy), but enough so that we become more than just ourselves. We become, quite literally, "we." Empathy harmonizes our separate rhythms.

As Steven lay beside the deer, he touched her face. He brushed snow off her face and body and, one by one, lifted her legs and shoulders to inspect for injury. He found several bleeding cuts, but none looked deep. Finding no serious injury, Steven lightly lifted the deer onto her legs. She wobbled like a newborn calf, took a few unsteady steps, circled back, and crouched onto the ground on her elbows. For almost an hour, Steven stayed by her side, gently stroking her as she recovered her energy. Finally, when her legs found their footing, he caressed her one last time and said, "Farewell."

Steven named the deer Miss Ice River, and his rescue may have sparked a radical change. When I ask him about his hunting, he tells me, "I think I will take my gun to a blacksmith, forge its barrel closed into a knot and put it up on my wall as my last trophy."

⚬

Will Steven stick to his self-pledge not to hunt anymore? I don't know if his single encounter with the fawn will be enough to alter a lifelong habit. But tales abound in which seemingly tiny, trifling moments in time ripple into something momentous. As it did with James Guiliani.

I first meet James Guiliani at his pet store, the Diamond Collar in Brooklyn, New York. The shop consists of two short aisles, with merchandise packed from floor to ceiling. Pet food, collars, litter boxes, beds, clothes, bows—but no animals, or at least no animals in cages. James and his co-owner and love of his life, Lena Perrelli, will never sell animals. The critters roaming about the shop are rescues for adoption. Three cats—Boots, Oreo, Lexi—are sleeping in various places among the shelves and bedding materials. Three dogs of different shapes and sizes stand behind a doggie fence at the sales counter.

The doorbell rings every few minutes as customers walk in, most of them towing dogs with them. Bouffant-haired, little old ladies in pumps; tattooed-covered, dentured men; yoga-suited women; diva men carrying pocket-size diva dogs. James greets them all like he knows them. He calls everyone baby, sweetie, and mamma—no matter if they're young or old, female or male. Washstands, clippers, brushes, shampoos, blow dryers, and towels wait in the back of the room, ready for use. On this crisp, Saturday morning, within an hour's time, more than twenty-five people bring their dogs in for a wash and a haircut. This might be the busiest salon in all of New York.

If you are ever lucky enough to meet James, chances are you will have the same initial impression I did. He swaggers and boasts and yet inside that puffed-up exterior lies a hard-as-rock gentleness.

James stands behind the cashier counter. He's six feet, two inches tall and weighs about 250 pounds. Dressed in a blue velvet jumpsuit and a white tank top, he has slicked brown hair, a cleft square chin, a chain-link tattoo around his neck, and a lighted Marlboro silver in his right hand. Just what I pictured a former mobster to look like.

James is blowing his nose and apologizing to me. "I feel miserable and I can't afford to get sick, mamma," he says. "I'm going on day three hundred in a row. Not even a day off for Christmas. No. I'm sorry, I did have one day. There's no one else who's gonna do this, mamma." The "this" isn't the Diamond Collar. The income the store brings in supports James's real passion: his animal shelter. Today he gushes over his "babies." In the past, though, he would have told you that he did not like animals. Saw no reason for them. Dirty, smelly nuisances they are. Yet it was one of these nuisances who taught him a lesson that changed his life.

James didn't grow up with animals. Born in 1967 to a mother of German descent and a father of Italian descent, he was the fourth of five boys and an older sister. They lived in Richmond Hills, commonly known as Jamaica, in the borough of Queens, New York. They were a close-knit, blue-collar Catholic family. Finances were always a struggle. Their father was frequently laid off in the 1980s because there was little work for union carpenters then. Without much in the way of games and TV, the five brothers looked for entertainment elsewhere.

Guiliani and his brothers joined the 112 Nutso Park street gang, whose overarching purpose seems to have been to spray graffiti as extensively as possible to mark their territory, and to defend their turf, mostly by fistfighting, from other street gangs. Occasional black eyes, stitches, and arrests for disorderly conduct and petty burglary were small prices to pay for a life of drinking, smoking, and respect from other kids. In less than a year, however, James's street gang life was cut short when a man named "Fat George" DiBello introduced him to the son of John Gotti Sr., one of America's most powerful and dangerous crime bosses.

At seventeen, James joined John Gotti Jr.'s crew as an enforcer, "making threats and breaking legs." "I had to go out with someone to collect, bust up a slow pay or someone who disrespected somebody connected," James says. Much of the time James served as a gofer, running errands for senior members; dealing illegal cigarettes, steroids, and narcotics; and robbing houses, especially those of single women. "It wasn't hard for me to meet (women)," he tells me. "I would coax them into taking me back to their houses with them; and then when they were sleeping, I'd rob their house." The mafia took a ten percent cut of everything James "earned." In return, it made an oath to back James up if he ever got into trouble. As James took to the mafia, his brothers left their lives of small crimes to pursue respectable careers. James became a social outcast among his siblings. He turned to the Gotti crew as his new family.

In December 1985, John Gotti Sr. organized the murder of Paul Castellano, then head of the Gambino family (named after former boss Carlo Gambino). John Sr.'s subsequent reign over the Gambino family—the best known of the "Five Families" that dominated organized crime in New York throughout most of the 20th century—made way for the cream years for the Gotti crew. Money rolled in and so did the good times. When James wasn't on a job, he hung out with other Gotti members at the Our Friends Social Club, where mobsters regularly conducted business. The club had a list of rules to follow. First, no mustaches. "Rats and cops have mustaches," John Jr. told James when he saw his mustache and ordered it shaved. Also, no earrings. Never discuss anything that goes on inside the club outside the club. And never mention the word *drug*.

John Jr. had zero tolerance for drug use. This proved to be the most challenging rule for James to follow. He had turned into a full-blown cocaine addict and alcoholic. He would sneak into John Jr.'s bathroom to snort cocaine. "If he had ever caught me," James says, "he would have killed me on the spot." If other crew members noticed James's addictions, they looked the other way. It was a forgiving time.

The Gotti party ended when John Sr. was arrested in December 1990. It would take two more years before he would be convicted of five murders, extortion, racketeering, and other crimes. But with the loss of the powerful Gambino boss, the high times were over, in more ways than one. In 1993, James got sloppy. "I was coked up for a hijacking on the far end of Long Island," he recalls. Two other members were with him. They were each carrying a loaded gun, "which made absolutely no fucking sense because the hijacking was supposed to be an inside job. We would be moving a truck-load of very popular Game Boys, a huge score if everything went as planned." When, at midnight, they arrived at the loading dock where they expected the truck, Suffolk County policemen surrounded their car and pointed shotguns at their heads. Their inside guy for the hijacking had been caught a few weeks earlier in a drug bust and "had offered us up on a silver platter for his own deal."

It was a "kidnapping kit" that did James in—a bag with gloves, tape, ski masks, and handcuffs—along with burglary tools and the guns they were carrying. James was charged with conspiracy to commit burglary, kidnapping, and murder. He was convicted and sent to the Riverhead Correctional Facility. Two years later, when James walked out of the prison doors, Fat George was there to pick him up in "one of the biggest, longest stretch limousines I'd ever seen." Fat George handed James an eight ball of cocaine and a rolled-up wad of twenty-dollar bills. James was back in with the Gotti crew and into his old habits. He became an even bigger junkie, so much so that within a year, John Gotti Jr. got fed up with him and gave James the boot.

With nowhere to go, James returned to the streets where he continued to deal in crack cocaine, marijuana, and anabolic steroids to support his own addictions. He bummed from place to place. After the glamorous life of a mobster, his new life was downright depressing. He would look at the men and women in their sixties and seventies who lived from drink to drink and wondered if that was his future. For the first time, James took a hard look at his life. At thirty-five, he recalls, "I had nothing to show for my time on this planet except heartache for those who loved me, prison tattoos, and a conviction record." So on a hot August evening in 2002, he drove to Rockaway Beach in Queens with a "cheap .25 Raven" he kept under his bed. Far enough away from the lingering beachgoers, he walked up to the sea, closed his eyes, and said some prayers to pay penance for the last crime he intended to commit: "my own murder."

Two things would turn his life around: the love of a good woman and a little dog.

⁂

At the beach, as James whispered his prayers, he heard giggling behind him. A group of young women invited him to join them and, being that they were pretty, he felt he couldn't turn them down. As he partied with them that night, one pulled him aside and told him that she noticed his gun. She had a hunch about what he was going to do when they met and she begged him to make one promise to her before they parted. "I want you to talk to a friend of mine." When this friend, Lena Perelli, called James on his cell phone several hours later, they hit it off. For the first time, James opened up about his life to another person. They began dating and a week later, he moved from the streets of Queens into Brooklyn—and into a house of five dogs and about a dozen cats.

Lena Perrelli was known as the Crazy Cat Lady of Brooklyn. Lena loved animals and could not turn her back on any animal in need. When she first bought her house in Brooklyn, she noticed a litter of kittens in her backyard. After she started feeding them, more hungry cats and dogs found their way to her garden and often into her home and onto her couches, chairs, and beds.

Lena took in James like she did other strays, but James didn't give up his street life. He continued to drink and dope and hustle drugs. For the next two years, he would binge and disappear for a few days at a time, only to return, find his belongings on the front yard, and beg forgiveness from Lena. They also fought about the animals.

"I wasn't having it," James says. "I chased all the animals out of the bedroom. I didn't want them where I was sleeping. I didn't want them were I was eating. I just didn't like them. They were dirty. Lena kept pushing me to love them, and I was like screw that." When Lena teased that he would one day fall in love with a dog, James mockingly paraphrased a line out of a Bugs Bunny cartoon: "Oh what a cute little doggie. Just what I always wanted. My own little doggie. I will name him Bruno and I will hug him and pet him and squeeze him." Little did James know how foretelling his words were.

In 2006, Lena left her job to open a pet boutique. She offered James a partnership in the business. "A pet boutique?" he asked her. "What the fuck is that?" The Diamond Collar was to be a place that sold "high-quality products. From leashes to foods to outfits to beddings." Knowing that Lena was getting fed up with him, James reluctantly agreed to the partnership.

On a fine spring day, James and Lena were sipping coffee at an outdoor café, blocks from their newly built pet shop, when Lena noticed something odd outside of the veterinary hospital across the street. "She sees something," James tells me, "and she says, 'Oh my god! What is that?' I say, 'It's a rug,' because it looked like a rug. She goes, 'That ain't a rug! That ain't a rug! Go look and see what it is.' So I walk across the street and see that it's a dog. A fucked-up dog."

The dog was a small, emaciated shih tzu. His fur was so matted into knots that James winced thinking how painful it must be. The dog's jaw was crooked and his fur was a putrid color from diarrhea and vomit. "The dog was green and yellow," James tells me, "I swear to God." Maggots writhed over open sores and a thick rope was wrapped around the dog's neck. The other end was tied to a parking meter. The dog was barely moving.

James figured someone dumped the dog in front of the hospital to be euthanized, but the staff in the veterinary office had so far either not seen the dog or was ignoring him. James picked up the inert dog. He felt his skin moving from the maggots. When he carried the dog into the hospital, the veterinarian walked up to him and asked, "Is he your dog?" When James said no, the vet replied, "Then get it out unless you're going to pay for it."

As James cursed the vet, Lena begged him to cover the charges. James reluctantly handed the dog over to the vet. They would return after the vet's examination. Back at home, James fumed, first at the vet and then at the person who left the dog behind. How could anybody leave him alone like that, he thought, as sick as he was?

Although James didn't realize this at the time, anger gave his stalled empathy its wheels. Empathy isn't limited to experiencing another's sadness and joy. It can be an emotional response to someone else's distress that results in anger rather than grief. Anger is a strong motivator. College students, for example, who feel more empathetic anger concerning various social issues are more likely to take action and advocate for change in unjust systems. Perhaps more than any other emotion, empathetic anger expresses fellowship with another. It says, "I stand with you."

All James's empathy needed now was a little shove. Several hours later, the news from the vet was, as expected, not good. After hospital workers shaved the dog's hair, they found him riddled with tumors. Someone had also broken the dog's jaw and left it to reset, unaligned. The dog would not live long. When James and Lena returned to pick up the seven-pound shih tzu, they found him cleaned, shaved, and with life in his eyes. A technician handed James the dog, and that's when the push happened.

The dog licked his face.

Without thinking, James kissed his head. The dog wagged his tail and kept licking his face. "You like me?" he asked the dog. In reply, the dog licked him on the mouth and James laughed. His own reaction confused him. "He's licking his ass," he tells me. "He's licking his balls, and I let him lick me in the face. I would never before have let an animal lick my face."

As Lena looked at James hugging the dog, she said, "I guess you know what we're naming him."

"You bet your ass you know. We're naming him Bruno."

❧

James's newfound empathy for Bruno sent him into an alternate existence, one bound not by self-absorption, but by kindness and a desire to do good. Does empathy have a downside, though? It's now well established that empathy shapes our morality as it relates to the desire to prevent suffering in others. It is what compels people to run into a burning building to save another. Seeing a terrified person trapped in a burning building arouses our emotions and empathetic concern. But empathy can be fickle. It can be easily swayed by trends and by the here-and-now. If an issue or a person in need is out of sight, then they are also, all too frequently, out of mind. That's why charities constantly flood airtime with images of children starving around the world, of cats huddling in the cold, and of families toiling in refugee camps. Charities need to continuously remind us and pull on our heartstrings.

Tug too hard on our heartstrings, though, and that can lead to ineffective altruism. As an example, when Hurricane Katrina hit, many people rushed to adopt abandoned animals whose sad faces were plastered all over the web. While a compassionate move, helicoptering these animals all over the country to their new homes may not have been the best use of those dollars. A more lasting, effective use of resources that would have helped far more animals would have been to use that money on spay-neuter campaigns and on educating animal guardians on how to care for animals during emergencies. Philosopher Peter Singer refers to this more impulsive act of charity as warm-glow altruism, which causes a temporary rush or buzz that makes people feel good about themselves. In contrast, effective altruism, Singer argues, relies more on reason rather than emotion to use resources to the best end possible. Because of the lack of immediacy of impact, it may not feel as personally rewarding to give to an educational campaign rather than open your home to a puppy. But that educational campaign can possibly save thousands of puppies.

Another limitation with empathy is that knee-jerk emotional reactions can cause in-group bias, as discussed previously, rather than fairness and justice. It's what leads many to wave national flags during wartime and overlook the suffering caused to "enemy" civilian populations. We've coined a term that helps us overcome this cognitive dissonance: collateral damage. In-group bias also explains why we can lavishly care for our companion animals while we munch down on a chicken's wing. Our partiality can blind us to the needs of others.

For these and other reasons, the use of empathy as a moral guide, particularly as it pertains to emotionality, is often criticized. However, without empathy, the concepts of morality, ethics, justice, fairness, and equity would not exist in the first place. As much as many of us may aspire to become more cerebral, we are emotional creatures. That's not always a bad thing. Think of how boring watching the Olympics would be without that emotional connection with the athletes. Without empathy, we would not share in a figure skater's joy when he lands a quadruple axel. Or his disappointment when he falls.

Additionally, recall that the most advanced forms of empathy require both an emotional and a cognitive component. Our use of reason, insight, and imagination allow us to understand another's experiences and needs, while the emotional component of empathy compels us into action. When used in combination with our rational faculties, our emotions can help us best take in the perspective of another and foster the most effective altruism possible.

The answer then to how to create an ethical world is not to uproot empathy, but to nourish its tender sprouts to become strong—unbending to the winds of fashion, impulsivity, and bias. Rather than faulting the emotional warm glow we feel when we help another, embrace it as the start of a larger journey. Those folks who adopted Katrina animals may very well have followed up by funding educational campaigns. Oftentimes, it takes an emotional connection with one individual to extend empathy to an entire group. As it did with James.

When James named the dog, he had with his heart and mind committed himself not only to Bruno but also to other animals in the same plight. *I see you*, James pledged, *not as a nuisance, nor a category, nor a number. I see you as you. And I am with you.*

James was with Bruno through health and through sickness. That first night, he took Bruno to the pet shop because Lena's pug, Brock, did not take kindly to the new canine addition. At the shop, James spoon-fed Bruno, gave him his medicines, made him a bed of towels, and left him a bowl of water. When it was time to leave, Bruno walked him to the door. When James stepped out and looked through the storefront window, Bruno was standing there still, wagging his tail.

They kept Bruno at the store the next night and James felt like he was abandoning Bruno all over again. But when he woke up early the third morning, his thoughts weren't on Bruno, but on drugs. Jittering like a junkie, he needed to get his hands on more steroids. First, though, he had to feed Bruno. When he went back to the store, he found Bruno waiting for him with his tail wagging, "Like I was the best thing he'd ever seen in his life." James forgot all about drugs and spent the rest of the day with Bruno. He never touched drugs or alcohol again.

"That's my baby," James interrupts his story and points to a photo on the wall behind him of a small grizzle-chinned dog, spotted with patches of clipped gray and tan fur. James then continues with his story. "So now I'm walking around with this little bruised, seven-pound shih tzu with a tit hanging off his chest, bleeding out of his ass, and a crooked face. And loving it. And this should not be happening, mamma, do you understand?"

When I ask him why not, he replies, "I'm supposed to be this tough guy, this gangster, this badass."

Bruno lived only two more months. "It was Memorial Day weekend when I walked into the store," James says. "He didn't come running to me and I knew something was wrong." He and Lena rushed Bruno to the emergency animal hospital. After examining Bruno, the vet told James that the dog would have to stay in the hospital for at least three days, which would cost $3,000 to $4,000. "I had a ton of steroid money on me," James says. "I go, 'Here.' I pull about $10,000 out of my pocket and put it on the counter. She looks at me like I'm nuts. I said, 'Keep it. Keep it all. When I come back in three days'"—James chokes up—"I said . . . I said, 'Bruno better come back to me 100 percent healthy.'"

Bruno could not be saved. Lymphoma took over his vital organs. After Bruno died, James washed his body and buried him in their backyard.

I ask James why, of all the dogs and cats he lived with, did Bruno move him so deeply?

"He was beaten down." James blows his nose. I'm not sure if his sniffles are from the cold or his emotions. "He was broken. He was abused. I walked into the vet, and they gave him to me and he licked my face. You would think he would bite me. A human did this to him. Yet he forgave me."

As I watch James continually blow his nose, greet his customers, and walk about with one cat or another in his arms, it dawns on me why Bruno impacted him like no other animal had. Like the slaughterhouse workers who saw something of themselves in the escaped cows, James identified with Bruno. They were both bruised. In different ways, of course, but like Bruno, James had been beaten down to a nearly lifeless mat. Except, in his case, James had stepped all over himself.

Social theorist Jeremy Rifkin wrote, "One can't truly empathize with the vulnerability and struggle of another unless he is able to acknowledge the same vulnerabilities and struggles in himself." To understand the feelings of another, we need to be able to do so for ourselves. Business leaders with good self-awareness, for example, have more committed employees and are more successful. Those leaders have a good understanding of their own needs and emotions and are better able to empathize with others.

When Bruno first licked his face, James experienced a profound insight, even if subconsciously. He had lived a life that caused him great shame. A junkie living day-to-day for the next fix, an ex-henchman, a failed mobster. When Bruno forgave James for the hurt caused by another, James learned to forgive himself.

With forgiveness, his empathy took off at full speed. James has been drug- and alcohol-free for more than ten years and has no intention of sliding back; animals are his new addiction. He now runs Keno's Animal Sanctuary, named after another abused dog he loved. People from all over Brooklyn and farther call him when there is an animal in need. He has rescued hundreds of neglected, hurt, and abused dogs, cats, pigeons, raccoons, rabbits, squirrels, lizards, opossums, and pigs. James is busy. Every morning he wakes to feed his new gang of critters meowing and barking for his attention. He then cleans the rooms, one floor devoted to cats, another to dogs. The animals run about the sanctuary, where the motto is "couches not cages." In the evenings, he's back at it all over again.

When not actively rescuing and caring for animals, James does TV and radio interviews and speaks at libraries and schools, teaching others compassion for animals. No longer passively drifting through what life had to offer him, he now dictates his own course.

"I banged more girls, sniffed more coke, drank more beer, enjoyed more life in thirty-nine years than anybody will ever do," James tells me. "I don't want it no more. You know what I want to do? I want to give back a little something because I took so much. You understand? It's crazy. I've been bitten, scratched, peed on, puked on. I don't mind it a bit. I like getting bit. I like getting scratched. It makes it real. I love interacting with the animals. I love cleaning up their shit, as crazy as it sounds. We need each other. Because let me tell you, honey, if I didn't have them, I wouldn't be here. I'd be in a mental institution or I'd be in jail. Or I'd end up like Charlie Sheen."

❧

He came back!

Three nights later, Dave found Sylvester, shivering and bedraggled behind a bush near the apartments. Knowing that I was sitting in my apartment with my face buried in a pillow, Dave immediately brought Sylvester to me. When they stepped through our front door, Sylvester wriggled out of Dave's arms and threw himself at me. We hugged as though pledging never to fail each other again. As I kissed his furry face and inspected each paw for cuts and bruises, a decision was made, if not in my mind, then in my heart.

On a Friday afternoon, I fritted and fretted in my apartment until Dave would return home from bagging groceries for customers. When I mustered enough courage to walk into my grandparents' apartment, I found Dave alone in his bedroom, twirling his nunchucks.

"Dave," I began, "Sylvester is almost my dog, too. He *is* my dog, too. You can't hurt him anymore. If you do, I will tell my mom. I will tell."

Dave never hit Sylvester again.

❧

It's quite amazing how the most defenseless of beings can possess the power to utterly transform us. One little dog propelled James Guiliani into a changed man, who now devotes his life to saving animals. Sylvester would change me from a passive girl into one who took charge. The union I felt with Sylvester, both of us struggling against our own evils, would commit me to a lifelong battle against cruelty in any form.

We need empathy. It gives us the courage to command our fates. In countries ravaged by the littered remains of destruction, empathy is a stance against the very nature of violence and suffering. Since the Syrian civil war broke out in 2011, an estimated 6.5 million people have been displaced, with the city of Aleppo suffering from some of the worst devastation. While most residents have deserted the area, some Syrians have braved bullets and bombs to care for those left behind, including the thousands of animals caught in the war's crossfire. Like the handful of volunteers for the Syrian Association for Rescuing Animals (SARA) who risk their lives every day "for the outcasts, for the needy, for the forgotten ones." And like the Cat Man of Aleppo, ambulance driver Mohammed Alaa al-Jaleel who stayed to feed and doctor hundreds of starving and injured animals. For these individuals, caring for animal victims of war is their personal protest against the cruelty that surrounds them.

It is that solidarity with animals that led Naoto Matsumura to willingly sentence himself to death. In 2011, an earthquake and subsequent tsunami caused a radioactive meltdown at Japan's Fukushima Daiichi Nuclear Power Plant. It was the worst nuclear disaster since Chernobyl in 1986. Nearly 57,000 people in the radiation zone fled and never came back. But Matsumura, a former rice farmer, returned and has not left since. Matsumura lives without electricity and gets water from a nearby well. He's been tested for radiation contamination and the results, he says, show that his body is "completely contaminated." Although the effects of radiation exposure aren't evident, changes are happening deep in his cells as they slowly divide into cancerous mutants that will one day hijack his body—that is, if he lives long enough.

Matsumura doesn't let the radiation bother him. He stays behind because he loves the animals. When he returned to the small town of Tomioka, just ten miles from the power plant, he didn't find a ghost town as expected. He found a bevy of cows, pigs, dogs, cats, horses, chickens, and even ostriches. When the villagers abandoned the town, they left behind thousands of animals. Matsumura found dead and dying animals trapped in their barns or chained without food and water. The worst scene he remembered was of a mother cow who was just skin and bones. Her calf, starving for milk, was crying. "The calf was sucking on straw, as if it were the mother's teat," Matsumura says. The next day, the mom and her baby were dead.

The scene of dying animals angered Matsumura. The Japanese government, he says, has abandoned them and left the village to rot. "We're the victims," he told reporters. Matsumura has joined the animals in an act of brotherhood. Years have passed since the disaster and he is doing his best to give the surviving animals a better life by feeding them and taking care of them, particularly the cows, whom the government wants killed. "I couldn't leave the animals behind," Matsumura told reporters. "To me, animals and people are equal."

If death is a great equalizer, so too is empathy.

Empathy is powerful. It punches holes through mental walls and unites the seemingly distinct. It shows us that our individual struggles are not so different from one another's, even from that of animals. We share the same fight.

⁂

Uncle Talup arrived last night. I was already asleep when he flew in from London. Yet I knew he slept in the bed next to mine, in the room I shared with my sister Sahar and my brother, Kamran. Before he arrived, Sahar and I played rock–paper–scissors to decide who would give up her bed for Talup and sleep, instead, with our parents. I lost. I got to keep my bed.

With the late-morning sun streaming through the blinds, I got out of bed and looked over at the empty one beside me. The bed that Talup slept in last night was neat and tidy, just like him. I changed out of my nightgown—yellow polyester with ruffles at the bottom—and tucked it under my pillow. I washed up in the bathroom and walked into the sitting room. The room was empty. Maybe everyone was with my grandparents next door. The smell of tea and toast with marmalade lingered in the air. I walked into the kitchen looking for food and stopped. Talup was there.

With his back to me, he fiddled with the teapot on the counter. He turned when he heard me. He was wearing Western clothes: dark gray slacks and a light blue, long-sleeved collared shirt. Oddly, in the midst of my growing panic, I thought that he looked handsome. Full, dark hair, clean-shaven, Jimmy Stewart face.

"Kanwal!" he said. He still called me by the name I was born with. Since the English had so much trouble pronouncing it, we changed my name to Aysha when we moved to America. A new name, my mother told me, and a new start.

"I was hoping you would be awake when I came last night," Talup said.

I stood there, chilled with dread.

"Aren't you happy to see me? Your brother and sisters are happy. Won't you come say hello?" He opened his arms.

I still didn't move. I kept hoping someone would burst through the front door. That someone would rescue me.

"Come now," he said. "I am hurt."

As though hypnotized, I walked into his arms. He smelled of his usual citrusy aftershave. He put his arms around me, pulled me close to him, and kissed me, deep and long. Two seconds, three . . . five. When he let me go, he said, "You will not go to sleep? You will wait for me tonight?"

I didn't answer. I looked down at my bare feet. Why didn't I put sneakers on?

His grip on my arm tightened.

"Yes," I mumbled, "I will wait for you."

He released my arm. I ran to the shoe closet. Hurry. Hurry. Before he comes out of the kitchen. Before he wants more.

I slipped my feet into my sneakers. No time for socks. No time to tie laces. I rushed out of the apartment, into the hallway, down the stairs, into the lobby, out of the building. With my arm, I viciously rubbed his slobber off my face. Almost safe. But I needed one thing more.

I stopped by my grandparents' apartment, said a quick hello, and left with my companion. We walked to my playhouse, hidden from adults at the edge of the twin-apartment complex, at the bottom of the hill, below the swing sets. Through an opening in the trees and bushes that framed it, we entered the largest room, the "living room." Our footsteps crunched and snapped the browned leaves, pebbles, and twigs that carpeted the floor. In the left corner of the living room was a small kitchen pantry where the thorny blackberry branches densely crisscrossed. Although the weather was warm for mid-October, the blackberries were long gone and my stomach growled.

I held back the branches, ignoring the pain as they tugged and scratched my arms. I knelt down in the center of the thicket and pushed a boulder back and forth, back and forth. Until it moved just enough to uncover the small hole that I had dug with a sharp rock in the spring. I pulled out a can of purple soda. I played frequently in this imaginary house with my sisters, but I never told them about my secret pantry. I rolled the boulder back over the hole and walked into my "bedroom." My bed was high up in the tallest oak tree. I monkeyed up to the branch that had the best seat in the house. I must have been thirty feet high. I popped open the soda can and took a greedy swallow. It was like having the air trapped inside a balloon flow back down my throat. Stale and hot. The fizz was gone, but that was okay. The sweet grape flavor calmed my stomach. I must remember to put another can under the rock for the next time.

Perched atop this tree limb, I watched the other kids at the playground, undisturbed. The only friend I needed patiently waited and guarded me by the thick tree roots until I was ready to come back down.

EIGHT

Friends

T he smells of smoked meats, funnel cake, grilled corn, sweaty humans, animal musk, and manure mingled at the annual Houston Livestock Show and Rodeo in Texas. During a span of three weeks in March, more than two million visitors descended upon the many stages and arenas to watch live music concerts, tractor shows, animal auctions, and rodeos. Children with sticky hands, men in tight jeans, and women in cowboy hats roamed the grounds in search of another snack or the next event. In the main arena, thousands of patrons sat in the bleachers cheering the men and women taking their turns on a bucking bull. Away from the main festivities, a fifteen-year-old girl sat in a shadowed stable holding a three-hundred-pound pig and cried.

❧

An only child, Alena Hidalgo grew up around animals in her hometown of Pearland, Texas, with dreams of becoming a veterinarian. When her high school offered her an opportunity to participate with Future Farmers of America (FFA) and learn about animals in agriculture, she jumped at the opportunity. The FFA is the largest technical and career student-education program in the United States, with almost eight thousand chapters in schools in all fifty states, Puerto Rico, and the US Virgin Islands. Many schools revolve around their FFA programs, as did Alena's. She thought the FFA would teach her how to care for animals.

On her first day with the FFA, an instructor took Alena and her classmates to a nearby barn where young goats greeted them. Rather than being taught how to interact with and care for the animals, the teacher instead told the students to evaluate and judge the goats as if they were carcasses hanging upside down in a butcher shop. "They didn't teach us much about animals," Alena tells me, "but if they did teach anything, it was about animals being dead."

Despite this first introduction into animal husbandry, Alena was still excited about the chance to raise an animal, which came later in the course. A few days before this next phase of the program started, she ran home after school to tell her mother that she would get to raise a pig. When her mother replied that the pig will eventually be killed, Alena thought, *Well, that is the way of the world.* She told herself at least she would treat the pig kindly. *Giving a pig a few months of a good life would be good enough*, she thought. Then she met Chubbles.

Alena fell head over heels in love with the overweight pig. Chubbles was so large for his age that Alena's teachers put him on diets, though to no avail. He was a big boy and he relished the food Alena gave him just as he seemed to relish every other part of his relationship with her. Every afternoon for months, Alena was in the school's agriculture barn with Chubbles. If she wasn't bathing him or cleaning his pen, she was snuggling with him. Chubbles would put his head on her lap, giving gentle snorts as she scratched his head and belly. Often, Alena would let him out of his pen so that he could run. They played chase where she would begin by running after him until Chubbles turned and chased her, making barking noises like a dog, she says. Like he was laughing.

Alena's teachers weren't happy about the time she spent playing with Chubbles. The other students were getting ready for the Houston Livestock Show and Rodeo in the spring. The livestock show was the culmination of the year's course. At the show, FFA students would present their pigs before a panel of judges, who would score the pigs on their posture, build, and gait. The scores would influence the price the students could sell the animals for at the auction that followed. The higher the score, the higher the price.

In the weeks before the show, the students spent most of their days training the pigs in preparation for their thirty-second walk before the judges. The best way to train animals, according to the FFA teachers, was by whipping them. But Alena refused to whip Chubbles.

A few days before the show, one of Alena's teachers noticed that Chubbles was not walking as a trained pig should. "Here, let me help you," he said to Alena. He grabbed her whip, which she only pretended to use, and repeatedly beat Chubbles with the metal end. "He's whacking my pig really hard and my pig starts crying," Alena tells me. "I started crying and everyone was looking at me like, What is this girl doing because all these kids are so used to this." Furious, Alena grabbed back the whip and told her teacher she was done.

Alena never returned for the training sessions. As other students spent their afternoons whipping their pigs into proper postures, Alena sat in her pen, playing with Chubbles, trying to comfort herself. She knew what was coming and she lived in a mental cloud, cushioned by a vague belief that, somehow, everything would be okay. Even so, a lump of unease had formed.

On the day of the livestock show, the lump solidified into full-fledged dread. Things happened so quickly that even today, Alena has trouble making sense of them. When her turn came at the show, Alena led Chubbles in front of the judges. Unlike the other students, she never used her whip. "Chubbles trusted me so much that he just wanted to walk by me," Alena says. Despite his lack of training, Chubbles placed high in his category. Before Alena knew what happened, someone quickly bought Chubbles, handed her a check for $2,000, and took a group photo with Alena and Chubbles. "I didn't know what was going on. They took a photo of me holding this award. I'm crying in this photo and it's not a few tears—I mean like I'm crying. My parents are standing beside me, silently. I'm holding my pig, who's starting to panic now, and the people kept telling me not to touch my pig. It's not professional. So in the picture—the pig's in front so you can't see—but I'm touching him and petting him." Alena didn't have much time to comfort Chubbles. Immediately after the photo, Chubbles was taken onto a truck and driven away. That was the last time Alena saw him.

As Alena stood by her parents watching after the truck, another FFA student came up to her. "You got all this money and your pig was well placed," he said. "Why are you crying?" Alena could not understand how he needed to ask such a question. Through her tears, she replied, "I just lost my friend."

⌘

The FFA's mission is to make "a positive difference in the lives of students by developing their potential for premier leadership, personal growth, and career success through agricultural education." Alena's FFA experience transformed her into a leader, but not in the way her teachers anticipated.

After losing Chubbles, Alena didn't think she could continue with FFA. Her friend, however, convinced her that she would be giving an animal a better life than another student would. When the next school year started, Alena signed up with another piglet, whom she named Gizmo. Within the first week, Alena saw that there was something wrong with Gizmo. His bulging, red eyes oozed pus. She texted one of her teachers, pleading with him to take a look at Gizmo. The teacher didn't come and, instead, texted back that Gizmo probably had wood shavings in his eyes. He instructed Alena to wash Gizmo's eyes with water, which she did. The next day, there was no change in Gizmo's eyes. Alena texted her teacher again who gave the same instructions. For more than a week, Alena washed Gizmo's eyes repeatedly, yet the pus continued to flow. "I kept telling my teachers that they, you know, needed to come by and check on Gizmo," she says, "and they said just keep washing. But I kept insisting something was wrong." After a week, the teachers stopped answering Alena's texts altogether. Finally, one of the teachers decided to walk by and take a look at Gizmo's eyes. Alarm crossed the teacher's face. "We need to get your pig to the vet," she told Alena. "Immediately."

By the time they took Gizmo to the animal hospital, it was too late. The veterinarian diagnosed Gizmo with a severe allergic reaction to the wood shavings in his pen. The inflammation scarred his eyes. Gizmo was blind.

Although Alena was outraged at her teachers for ignoring her pleas, there was nothing she could do now. While Gizmo recovered at the hospital, she turned her attention to another pig who needed her help. Alena befriended the pig who lived in the pen next to Gizmo's and named her Kurtis. The student in charge of the pig's care was rarely seen. As the days passed, Alena noticed that Kurtis was sleeping in her own urine and feces. In the evenings, Alena could hear Kurtis cry from hunger.

Alena told the FFA teachers about the pig's neglect. They shrugged it off. One day, Alena found Kurtis lying in her pen, foaming at the mouth and panting heavily. She was overheating in the hot Texas sun. Fed up, Alena walked into the school building and confronted a teacher. "Mr. Ron, come look at this pig right now," she said. When they walked into the barn, Mr. Ron looked at Kurtis and said, "Yeah, it's overheating."

"I'm like, 'Yeah, I know,'" Alena tells me as her voice rises in remembered anger. "We need to do something. He says, 'Well are *you* going to do something about it?' And then he leaves. So I took this other pig out and I started giving her a bath and hosing her down. She was just the sweetest thing ever. I've never met a pig with that much personality. Her eyes were just so expressive." Alena took matters into her own hands from then on. Every day, she fed and bathed Kurtis and cleaned her pen. All the while, she mentally prepared for Gizmo's return from the animal hospital.

"Gizmo is usually so energetic," Alena says, "but that day when he came back, he just plopped down in his pen. He looked so tired. It was a hard moment for me too, because my pig is blind." Alena didn't know what to do for Gizmo, but it seemed that Kurtis did. "Kurtis must have sensed something. She walked into Gizmo's pen and started poking his belly with her snout. She lay beside him. It was obvious Gizmo was upset, and Kurtis just stayed with him the whole time."

After that day, Gizmo and Kurtis became fast friends. Whether taking naps or playing chase, they were together as often as Alena could allow. "There were times when one of them would lie down and the other would just lie right down, too. It was just like if you have a friend, and there's times when you could just chill out with them and you don't have to do anything. It wasn't easy for me to see because you're raised to believe these animals are food and stuff, but they really were snuggling together, taking naps. They were happy just being together."

As auction time neared, however, Alena panicked. Her loss of Chubbles still grieved her. She knew she would not sell Gizmo, but what about Kurtis? Kurtis was not her pig. She could not bear the idea of losing Kurtis or of separating her from Gizmo. Alena had approached the girl in charge of Kurtis and asked her not to sell the pig, but the girl refused. What was Alena to do?

Alena and her friend Kayree, who had also grown fond of Kurtis, made a decision. They were going to buy Kurtis. A few days before the livestock show, they started a crowdfunding page to raise money. The girls wrote on their page a heartfelt plea, asking for help to save their pig. In forty-eight hours, they raised $2,000. Just in time for the auction. Or so they thought.

At the show, rumors quickly spread about a girl who was trying to save a pig. Some people suspected the girl was Alena and did double takes when they saw her, whispering behind her back. Alena felt shunned, but her greater concern was for Kurtis. "I was sitting on the bleachers watching her turn in front of the judges," Alena says. "Her keeper starts walking her, but Kurtis doesn't know this girl. She never spent time with her pig. Since she was never trained, Kurtis isn't walking in proper form. The girl gets angry and starts whipping Kurtis. And you could see it on Kurtis's face. She was like, 'What are you doing?' The girl keeps hitting her so hard, and Kurtis is screaming." Alena's heart broke watching Kurtis cry. Immediately after the show, she ran up to the girl and implored her to let her buy Kurtis with the $2,000. It wasn't enough. The girl sold Kurtis to a breeder for a higher price.

Since Kurtis was alive as a breeding pig somewhere out there, Alena didn't give up. She still had the money. She and Kayree started a campaign to get Kurtis back. They emailed the FFA teachers, hoping to negotiate a way to buy Kurtis from the breeder. Their entreaties were ignored. Two weeks in, over the loudspeaker, the school principal called Alena into her office. "They never do that for any student over the whole intercom," Alena tells me. "When I get to the principal, the counselor was there too. The principal told me—and I'm not exaggerating, this is word for word—she told me all animals want to die."

Since that day, Alena felt the counselor's eyes were always on her. She tells me, "The counselor started calling me into her office for doodling on my papers. I doodle on my papers, but I've never been called to the office before. I drew this little alien thing, and she says this thing looks like it's going to touch itself inappropriately, and I just started laughing. I was like, 'What are you talking about?' They kept calling me down for stupid things after that. They kept a file on me."

The counselor and teachers bullied Alena. So did her classmates. They would snicker behind her back or outright call her names. But one classmate surprised her. "One of the kids came up to me, and he said, 'Did you hear about that girl in FFA who's trying to save a pig?' He did not know it was me. I was like, 'Oh yeah, what an idiot.' He was making fun of it, and I let him have his fun. Then I said that kid was me. He looks at me, like, 'Oh.' Then he started telling me that he understood and he kind of tears up about his pigs. All of his friends are in FFA, and he told me that he couldn't quit because he would lose his friends. It almost sounded like this kid was obligated to kill things to keep his way of life." Since that conversation, Alena often wondered, how many other kids wanted to save their animals but were afraid to say so?

Alena couldn't save Kurtis. However, she still had Gizmo to worry about. The school principal was not going to let her keep Gizmo at the barn much longer. Alena had to find Gizmo a permanent home. She and her friend Kayree contacted animal sanctuaries across the country to ask if any could take Gizmo. The sanctuaries were full. A month passed with no success. Alena was getting desperate.

One day, a church friend of Alena's mother told her about a newly formed sanctuary only forty-five minutes away. Accompanied by her parents who fully supported her, Alena visited the Rowdy Girl Sanctuary in Angleton, Texas, ready to beg, if needed. They were given a tour of the grounds and met the founder, Renee King-Sonnen. After hearing Alena's plea, Renee looked steadily at her and said, "We're going to take your pig. And we're going to love him."

❧

Dr. Anderson looks into a horse's mouth. "Limo looks okay," the veterinarian says aloud.

To me, Limo looks as nervous as a cat. The vet squeezes a dab of ivermectin dewormer paste into Limo's mouth, who spits his tongue back and forth like a child given a nasty-tasting medicine. In the adjoining stall, two steers warily watch. Next, with remarkable speed, Dr. Anderson injects a series of vaccines for tetanus, West Nile virus, and rabies into the side of Limo's neck. Limo buckles and neighs loudly. "For an alpha male, you're a big baby," Dr. Anderson says to him.

The first day of my weeklong stay at Rowdy Girl Sanctuary is a busy one. The veterinarian is making her quarterly visit to inspect, vaccinate, and treat the hodgepodge of animals who call these ninety-six acres home: one rooster, one goat, three ducks, four cats, four horses, nine dogs, twenty-four hens, forty-eight cows, and four pigs (including Gizmo). Add Renee King-Sonnen and her husband, Tommy, and you have one hundred domestic residents plus countless wild ones.

This morning, Kate, a sanctuary employee, Tommy, dogs Waylon and Sadie, and I are following the veterinarian as she examines each animal. After she's done with Limo, Tommy releases him. Limo bolts to the other corner of the stall, neighing the injustices of his ordeal to anyone who will listen. The next horse is calmer about her medical visit. Dr. Anderson rubs her hand over the horse's flank and abdomen. "She has a bit of a distended abdomen," she says, "A body wall hernia on her side, probably from a kick. It will heal itself."

After Dr. Anderson vaccinates the four horses, she turns her attention to the cows. As we enter the stall housing the two steers, Limo, who is still voicing his woes, quiets and turns back to watch us. It's as if he knows he's in the clear and can now watch the cows get tormented. The steers, one all black and the other with white legs, are big, weighing upward of 1,700 pounds each. I don't know cows. I know cats, I know dogs, I know squirrels. Not cows, especially not mammoth male cows. With their sharp horns, the steers kind of scare me. Murray was severely malnourished when he was first rescued. He's an old man of a steer now: ornery, distrustful. Still, Tommy smoothly encourages him into a corner of his stall. As Dr. Anderson injects Murray with several vaccines, Murray remains calm. His best friend, Big Bird, is another matter.

Somehow, Tommy is able to direct Big Bird out of the stall and into a green squeeze chute. Now comes the hard part. We try to coax him down the chute's corridor so that we can close the two ends. Big Bird refuses. He crashes against the sides and bucks again and again. With all our body weight, Kate (who's about my size), Tommy, and I lean against the openings at each end to try to secure the chute as much as possible. It shakes and rattles with Big Bird's bashings. So do we. I've never done anything like this before. I'm nervous.

Murray, watching from his stall with concern for his friend, moos loudly. From the woods come five female cows who answer his calls. They moo back and forth, adding to the commotion. Sadie and Waylon run at our feet, barking. The rooster hollers. The goat bleets. The hens, well I'm not sure what they are doing, but they aren't helping. There's Tommy yelling, "Hold it! Hold it!," Kate running back and forth, and I'm grinding my teeth. Everyone seems to be anxious and complaining. Except the horses, who appear to enjoy watching the ruckus.

Suddenly, Tommy yells, "Watch out!" Big Bird slams against the chute, knocking Kate down, and is free. I hustle out of his path, eyeing his sharp horns, and help Kate up. Tommy, Kate, and I turn to Dr. Anderson with the same question on our faces.

"I got him just before he bolted," she says.

Phew! I don't want to go through that again. I see Big Bird skulking off toward the female cows. They gather around him, lowly mooing, as if to say, "There, there, it's all over now." I wonder if the bovine ladies ever get together and roll their eyes at Big Bird's fearfulness.

We rest for a few minutes, wipe our sweaty faces, and sip water before we hop into the Kawasaki MULE, an open-top off-road vehicle. Waylon sits in Tommy's lap. Sadie, who's too big for the vehicle, runs after us. Dr. Anderson carries a dart gun, loaded with vaccine. We drive across the sanctuary in search of Cinnamon, a cow, Tommy tells me, who hates confinement and needles. *Don't they all?* I wonder, thinking of Big Bird. Tommy tells me that Cinnamon destroyed a stable when they tried to confine her before, but, he adds, "She really is a gentle cow."

In his denim shorts, checkered short-sleeved shirt, and baseball cap, Tommy looks like he should be driving across a golf course or stomping over old battlefields with a metal detector in hand. For a man who would rather spend his retirement looking for Civil War buttons than chasing cows, he looks relaxed. As we bump along the muddy ruts, Tommy turns to me and grins. His blond caterpillar mustache wiggles. "We got the MULE. Got the gun. Got the dog. Kind of reminds me of my hunting days." The sun glints off his eyeglasses as though he's winking at a joke.

"You ever miss it?" I ask.

"When I first got this land. I killed only two deer. When you live with them . . . they're here in the morning. They're here in the evening. I'd sit out in the stand and I just didn't want to kill them. I know them."

We drive for a half hour looking for Cinnamon. We find groupings of other cows here and there, relaxing under trees or grazing, but can't locate Cinnamon. I don't mind. I'm enjoying the warm sun, the breeze, the smell of mesquite trees, of dust and healthy animals.

We find Cinnamon sunning in the outer pasture in the company of two other cows. Reddish brown in color, Cinnamon is a Brahman cow with a large camel-like hump on her back. Tommy pulls to a stop several feet away. With one blow into the dart gun, Dr. Anderson makes a clean shot. Cinnamon jumps up and runs several meters with the dart sticking into her flank. We follow her until the dart falls off, then we pick it up and ride back to the horse stall.

Dr. Anderson has one last patient. Kate holds Lulu the hen, while the vet examines the large, hard abscess at the bottom of Lulu's right foot. Bumblefoot, an infection caused by staphylococcus bacteria, is common among chickens. With a scissor, Dr. Anderson pierces open the abscess and cleans it out. Lulu squirms and cries out a soft ooohooo ooohooo noise. "I know," Dr. Anderson murmurs to Lulu. "It's okay. I know. You can peck me." As the pus drains, Kate feels sick and hands Lulu to Tommy to hold. When drainage is complete, Dr. Anderson coats Lulu's foot with silver sulfadiazine cream, a topical antibiotic, and wraps a bandage around the wound. "Keep this bandage on for a week," she tells Tommy. "And keep her in her coop."

Lulu doesn't like this last order at all. As soon as Tommy carries her to her coop, Lulu tries to make a run for the door. But another hen gets in her way and squeezes out the door before Tommy shuts it. From inside the coop, we can hear the fifteen or so hens squabbling. "They'll calm down," Tommy says to me, "till dinner time."

I look at the clock on my cell phone. It's already late afternoon. Renee has been away, driving about town running errands. As I wait for her return, I walk over to Murray, standing alone in his stall. Big Bird is still off somewhere with a group of ladies who are probably consoling him. I stop a few feet away from Murray so he won't feel cornered. "Hey, Murray," I say, with my hand stretched out. Murray stands against the far wall, eyeing me with suspicion. "I'm not going to hurt you," I plead. "Come on, big boy." I stand there for fifteen minutes, arm reaching, murmuring nice things to Murray. He gets down on the ground, lowers his head as though for a nap, but keeps one eye open, watching me.

I give up. Renee has arrived now and walks toward me carrying a guitar. Silver bracelets jangle on her arms. "Aye-shur," she calls out, "wanna come on down with me to sing with the cows?"

Not *to* the cows, but *with* them. That's an invitation I've never had before.

I'm not into hippie stuff. Although I don't want to see animals hurt, I never aspired to commune with the cows. I look at Renee's big, enticing smile, though. Why not? We trudge along a dirt road to one of the outer pastures and find a group of mother cows with their babies and some aunts, too, I think. Big Bird is with them.

"Woop woop woop!" Renee calls. "Houdini! Lucky! Raaawdy Giiirl!"

Renee spreads out a blanket and we plop down. Two black cows walk right up to Renee and bump heads with her. "This is Rowdy Girl," Renee says, petting the cow with a diamond patch of white fur on her forehead. "And this here is her baby, Lucky. Everyone thinks I named the place after me, that I'm Rowdy Girl. She's my first girl. The one who started it all."

Renee plucks her guitar and starts singing, "Who's going next in the re-e-e-e-e-e-d trailer! Who's goin' on down the rooaaad?"

Hmm, I don't yet know the significance of this song, but it sounds rather mournful to me. Fortunately, Renee follows this song with a more cheery tune. As Renee sings, the other cows come closer. About twenty cows and calves take turns mooing with the song. It's as though they actually are singing with Renee.

As their mothers watch, two brown-and-white spotted calves walk up to me and nudge me. "They want to play with you," Renee tells me. The calves continue to bump their velvet heads against mine until they topple me over. I laugh.

Renee laughs along. "Ain't they just daaarlins'?" As the cows continue to gather around us, Renee says to me, "I never in a million years could of seen this coming. First sanctuary ever from a former cattle ranch."

But the sanctuary nearly didn't come to life. And Tommy and Renee's marriage almost died.

⌖

Tommy and Renee's ranch-style house overlooks much of the sanctuary. In their living room, I sit on the couch, flanked by two dogs. They drool on my lap as they snore away. Another dog squirms onto my lap. On the wall above us, where deer and elk heads used to hang, are landscape reproductions. Tommy has his feet up in his easy chair. Bullet the cat drapes over the back of the chair, licking Tommy's face. Renee, as frenetic as ever, fusses back and forth between the living room, the kitchen, and her office. The malty aroma of Assam tea curls up from my mug. My second night here and I feel like I know this place.

Renee grabs a bottle of Zeal, a nutritional drink, and joins us. Tommy and Renee married twice. "I met her in the early nineties," Tommy tells me. "She was a country music singer in a bar." I recall the kitchen poster of Renee from those days. Big, permed hair. Puffed neon-blue sleeves. Tight, metallic-silver pants and silver boots, like someone from a Flash Gordon comic.

After a few years into their first marriage, Renee and Tommy's opposite personalities led to a divorce. However, they kept seeing each other around town. Tommy was a chemist for Dow Chemicals, and Renee sold real estate. By then, Renee's hair had shrunk and her clothes had loosened, but her country-music-star personality still mesmerized Tommy. After ten years of running into each other in Pearland, Texas, Tommy and Renee remarried. There was one major difference this time, though: Renee had to move to Angleton and live on Tommy's cattle ranch. He had bought the ranch as supplemental income for his retirement. Renee moved in, but she didn't share her husband's enthusiasm for the ranch.

Renee reaches for her Zeal. When I earlier asked if she had any tea for my afternoon caffeine kick, she said, "Why don't you try Zeal? It's got all the an-tie-oxidants and vitamins and will give you all the energy boost you need." She sounded like a commercial, which shouldn't surprise me. She sells Zeal as a small side job. I dubiously eyed the bottle of Tropic Dream Zeal drink mix on the counter. "Uh, I'll stick with the tea, thanks."

Renee takes a long sip of her drink, smacks her lips as though to tell me *look what you missed out on*, and says, "When I got here, I just didn't want to have anything to do with the cows. I had no interest in them."

"So what happened?" I ask, blowing into my teacup.

"Tommy told me about a calf that needed a momma. She was a little bouncing thing, real rowdy, that's how she got her name Rowdy Girl. I bottle-fed her, twice every day. And it was like I took a pill and went down a rabbit hole. I was feeding her and all of a sudden I would go down this place in my mind where I could see all the other cows now. I could see their babies and I could see them. I never noticed them before. I started caring."

She takes another sip. "I named the cows. I named Rowdy—"

"I told you not to do that," Tommy interrupts.

"I know that," Renee replies to him. Then to me, "He kept telling me not to name them. I had to go back through the rabbit hole and be a rancher's wife again. But then the red trailer came."

Tommy made extra pocket change by breeding the cows and selling their calves. On the days the red trailer arrived, he and a friend would round up the calves, load them onto the trailer, and drive them away. Unable to bear children, Renee became acutely sensitive to the plight of the cows and the loss of their children.

"Aye-shur, it was horrible," she says. "The momma cows were bawlin'. I would go inside to get away, but I could still hear the moms screaming. Their babies were being taken away. And the babies—they just stood in the trailer, not knowing what was going on. The mommas would follow the trailer as far as they could. And when the trailer turned the corner, they turned the corner too, along the fence line. They stood by the road watching the trailer leave, screaming bloody murder. It was horrible. I just couldn't believe we were doing this. I would just shake my head and I would just scream, 'How can we be doing this, how can we be doing this?' And Tommy would say, 'You better suck it up and get used to it.'"

Tommy says, "That's when Renee went crazy."

A cat jumps onto Tommy's lap. Buddha. Tommy immediately wiggles around to make room for him. "What do you mean, 'crazy'?" I ask him, watching his arms instinctively wrap around Buddha.

Tommy looks at Renee. "You want to tell her?"

"No." She smiles. "I know you love telling this part."

I look at Tommy. He says, "She went out and put down little markers."

"To memorialize the animals," Renee adds.

Tommy lets out a long, long sigh. "Yeah, she went out there with sage. And I'd tell her, 'What are you doing out there?' She was moanin' all kinds of stuff—"

"I was chanting, with my sage, I was—You okay? You're making funny noises."

I can't help it. The laughter I try to hold back bursts free.

"I know." Renee smiles again. "I know. But you have to know. This was all new to me. I was feeling so much . . . all of a sudden. I was out there chanting. I was crying. I was begging for forgiveness."

Tommy looks up to the ceiling. "Didn't make me feel very good."

I ask Tommy, "How many times did the trailer come?"

"'Bout ten or twelve times. But it got worse."

"How did it get worse?"

Renee answers for Tommy. "I started calling him murderer."

I glance at Tommy with understanding. He looks at me and shrugs. Poor man. Tommy is the stark opposite of Renee. Where he is calm, Renee is charged. Where he is easygoing, Renee is determined.

All Tommy wanted at this stage of his life was to settle down and retire. Renee's newfound empathy broke his peace.

One of the dogs walks in from the kitchen and puts his paw on Renee. With her hand on his head, she says, "And I knew Tommy didn't like it. When I was saying this stuff to him, I knew that it was hurting his feelings. I could see it in his face, the way he was looking at me, like, 'How dare you go there with me,' because I called him a murderer. Because I knew he loved animals."

"But I countered her," Tommy says. "I said, 'Wait a minute. You've got a Chick-fil-A sandwich in your hand and you've got groceries in there with hamburgers and steaks, and you're telling me I'm murdering those cows? I know what I'm doing. You're the one that doesn't know what you're doing.'"

I turn to Renee. "So he was telling you that you were a hypocrite for getting upset. How did you react?"

"Every time he would say that to me it would cut through my heart because it was true. It was true."

"She loved Chick-fil-A sandwiches," Tommy says.

"I did. And I loved prime rib. And I loved all that bacon. Now my inside matches my outside. Both of us"—she nods at Tommy—"I feel whole now. But what happened back then was I started feeling very split. I loved my husband. I wanted to respect his livelihood, his choices about our retirement, what we were doing. But I just couldn't suck it up." When the red trailer came and carried calves away in December 2014, Renee reached a breaking point. "After that trailer went, I started watching all these slaughterhouse videos. I was in my office crying."

Tommy adds, "She'd be in there crying, and I'd be going, 'Renee quit watching that crap.' She'd be crying so loud I couldn't hear the TV."

"I couldn't stop," Renee says. "I would go deeper and deeper into the abuse. It's like I had to feel everything, because all my life, I hadn't felt anything. I forced myself to feel." As Renee's compassion for the cows grew, so did her anger towards Tommy. And his anger towards her. They fought. They screamed at each other almost daily. Divorce seemed inevitable. Again.

Renee says, "Tommy kept asking me, 'What do you want me to do? What do you want me to do?' He was mad at me because I was taking his livelihood. I was taking his identity."

Renee didn't know how to answer Tommy. As the weeks ticked by, Renee went online reading about animal sanctuaries. "One day," she says, "I looked outside and I saw the cows, and I thought, Gosh, all we have to do is change our perception." Instead of seeing a cattle ranch, Renee saw a sanctuary of her own. She went back inside, found Tommy, and said to him the last thing he expected. She asked him, 'Why don't you just sell the cows to me?'

Tommy rolls his eyes. "When she said that to me—I won't tell you exactly what I said—but I said something like, 'That's blankety blank crazy. You're stupid. There's nothing in Texas like that. That's something that happens in California or New York.'"

Despite Tommy's ridicule, Renee started a fund-raising campaign, and in six months she raised $36,000. With that money and a reluctant agreement by Tommy to lease the land to her for $1 for two years, a sanctuary was born. Their marriage was still on the brink, though. Renee says, "You can just imagine, me and Tommy are still together. We're not divorced, and I'm buying his cows. I had taken away his life. You can imagine the tension in this relationship."

Tommy caresses Buddha's feet. "I told myself I wasn't going to get divorced a third time—I was married once before Renee."

Even though Tommy resolved to fight for their marriage, the hurtful words he and Renee threw at each other cut deep. They lived under the same roof, but separately. On her laptop day and night, Renee read about Howard Lyman, a fourth-generation rancher who became an animal and environmental activist. Lyman never opened a sanctuary, but Renee hoped he might be able to provide advice as an ex-cattle rancher to an ex-cattle rancher's wife. She tried for weeks to contact him. Then on Christmas evening, a small miracle happened. Lyman answered her phone call.

"Hello. Mr. Lyman?" she asked into the phone.

"This must be Renee," he answered.

"How did you know?"

"Well, you called me and emailed me a couple of times now."

With the phone in her hand, Renee walked into the back of the house, away from the gathered family, and poured her heart out to Lyman. She cried over the cows. She cried over her marriage. After hearing her tale, Lyman said to her, "Renee, I'm going to tell you something. You're going to have to start loving your husband the way you do the cows."

⁂

I stand outside of Murray's stable, arm over the gate, trying to coax the steer to me. This is my eighth attempt over the past four days. For some reason, his past abuse touches me deeply, more so because he's not cute and cuddly. He's not the type of animal to normally arouse a person's compassion. He's sharp, angular, prickly. Like I was as a child. I really want to break through his mistrust. I have food this time, fresh grass. Murray backs away from me, huffing and snorting like a horse. He then watches me, as if in defiance. As if to say, "Seriously, do you think that old trick with food is going to work on me?" No, it doesn't work on Murray. But I know someone else it will work on.

I find Gizmo in the pigpen with his head on Alena Hidalgo's lap. She's homeschooled now, freed from the bullying at her high school. She tells me she's the happiest she's ever been since joining the FFA program. When Gizmo turned a year old, the sanctuary held a birthday party for him. Alena was the guest speaker. She was nervous about speaking, yet as she cried in front of a large audience describing the loss of her friends Kurtis and Chubbles, she brought the crowd to tears. For the first time since her troubles started, she experienced a sense of belonging. She no longer had to conform to what others expected of her. She no longer had to hide her love for all animals.

Alena has been visiting Gizmo every Friday afternoon since she first brought him to the sanctuary two years ago. She feeds Gizmo, brushes him, bathes him, and plays with him. Most of the time, they simply enjoy each other's company as they are doing now. Two other pigs, Roux and Penny, relax nearby. As with Gizmo, Penny was brought over by a former FFA student who couldn't bear having her slaughtered. The three pigs are good friends, though not as close, Alena tells me, as Gizmo was with Kurtis.

With fresh grass in hand, I feed Penny and Roux, who trot over to greet me and enjoy their fill. Gizmo stays with Alena. I walk away from the pigpen toward the little fenced-in yard to find Pepper, a silver, black, and white pygmy goat. Like all of the animals who have joined the sanctuary since it first opened, Pepper is a rescue. After his human dad died from a heart attack, Pepper needed a new home. Pepper joined the sanctuary just a week ago. Until he gets used to his surroundings, Tommy and Renee keep him in this small yard. He shares the yard with another newcomer, Ivy, a pink and gray pig.

"Hi, Pepper," I call out as I walk through the gate. "Hi, Ivy." They both walk up to me. Pepper's lips pull back, showing his teeth as though he's grinning. He butts me urgently with his head. Ivy is more timid. I crouch down and let her sniff my hand. She allows me to rub her head, behind her ears. Move too suddenly, though, and she will scurry away. Touch her face and she will squeal in dismay. Rub her belly and she will murmur *snoof, snoof* in delight. I've never met a more emotional being.

Pepper has two perpetual goals: to eat and get out of the pen. He tries to rush past me through the gate. I grab the dunderhead just in time. I can't let him out, but I can offer him food. I scoop a bucket of cereal—meant to be a rare treat—out of a bin. Oh boy, do Pepper and Ivy love Cheerios. They almost knock me over trying to get to it. I can't help it. I give them more than I should. I just love seeing them so excited. After a few more scoopfuls, I close the bin. "No more!" I command, more to myself than to them. Pepper quickly loses interest in me. He jumps up on a barrel to watch the other animals in the sanctuary. On top of his soapbox, he bleats loudly. Based on the tone of his bleats, I gather he doesn't think highly of the other animals.

I walk out of the yard. Off in the distance, I hear the rumble of Tommy's tractor engine. I look up and watch him drive across the field with Waylon in his lap. Sadie runs after them. Tommy sees me from afar and waves with a big grin on his face. Tommy and Renee's marriage survived their lowest point and they are now closer for it. Though Tommy would have preferred to retire at ease, he's committed to his new journey with Renee and the family of critters they have acquired. Renee and Tommy now have a common goal, and their new partnership is based on trust, compassion, and understanding.

Three hens walk by, clucking back and forth to one another as they make their way to a destiny unknown to me. When I first arrived, I didn't know one hen from another. Now I'm able to identify them individually. These three are always together. One is clearly the leader, perhaps the matron of the trio. The other two follow her about the yard, into the garage, into my car (after I forgot to close my door), always chatting, always inspecting things. I never knew chickens were so curious. Rearrange some cardboard boxes in the garage and these three are there, sniffing, pecking, jumping up on a table to get a better view. Seeing them walk past reminds me of Lulu.

Lulu, the chicken with the bandaged foot, shares her half of the chicken coop with fifteen or so hens. The other half of the coop holds a new group of chickens, who were previously used as bait to train cocks for fighting. The chickens first arrived in tiny shoeboxes. "They were so beat up, Aye-shur," Renee told me when she first introduced me to them. "Now look how good they look."

The coop is getting crowded. So is the rest of the sanctuary as more animals call this place home. With only three people working here—Tommy, Renee, and Kate—there are many repairs to be done. Fences need mending. Barns need building. I tell Patrick this over the phone, and he says he will return with me next time and help with the carpentry work.

After seeking permission from Renee, I find Lulu, who has been cooped up these past several days. "She needs some fresh air and sunlight, poor thing," Renee told me. I scoop Lulu into my arms. Holding a chicken was new to me when I got here. After four days at the sanctuary, I do it like a pro. I take Lulu into Ivy and Pepper's yard and let her down on the grass. Pepper and Ivy come out to meet their visitor. They watch for a few minutes as Lulu pecks at the ground, then wander away, seeing that Lulu doesn't come with Cheerios. Lulu walks about like she's looking for something in particular. I follow her.

Ah, she found it. On the other end of the yard is a patch of dry dirt. Lulu shuffles her feet in the dust for a few seconds and drops her bum down. She rolls on her back, kicks her feet in the air, and wriggles her fat little body from side to side as she stretches her wings. All the while, she coos. I've never seen a chicken take a dust bath before, but my god, she looks more blissful than anyone I've ever seen in my life.

Such a simple need. A little sunshine, the smell of sweet grass, some dust to roll in. And no one to hurt her.

<hr />

The last night.

In the thick warmth, I lie in bed shivering. And waiting. Just waiting. I know it's going to happen. The question that sits heavily as I lie here is When? Will it be in the next five minutes? Half hour? Or will I have to wait for two more hours?

The box fan drones and struggles against the heat in the open window. My bed is below the window, but the forced air blows right over me to another destination, as though I'm not even here. My armpits and palms are sticky. Still, I have the comforter pulled up to my chin. I'm hot and cold.

My nail-bitten fingers tap out the seconds. I count them as I learned during swim lessons. One one-thousand, two one-thousand, three one-thousand, four one-thousand.

I hear a hearty male laugh outside my window, then another. They are followed by the sweeter laugh of a girl. Teenagers. Only two floors up, I can hear their voices at the back of the apartment building. I can't identify them individually, but I have probably run into them in our building from time to time. Even though their exchanges are joyful, they scare me. I have seen what they do in the woods behind our building. Tonight is Saturday night. Time for cigarettes, drugs, and sex.

A small cough comes from the far wall. Then another cough and a rustle. I lift my head a little and peer over my blanket. My brother's bed faces perpendicular to mine, against the far wall. Kamran fell asleep almost as soon as his head touched the pillow. Now he stirs, mumbles something, and turns his back toward me. Is he awake? My fingers stop. I listen and wait. Then his gentle snores start up again. I put my head back down. Seventeen one-thousand.

I don't need to look over at the third bed, which is also perpendicular, but against the same wall as mine. Like my and Kamran's beds, it has a twin-size mattress and box spring, a metal frame, cheap tan sheets, and blue quilts. There are no headboards. My mom tried to make the room cozy for us by sewing a different colorful pillow for each bed. Mine is my favorite color, aqua blue, my brother's is forest green, and my sister's is orange. Tonight, though, the orange pillow is not on its rightful bed. In its place is a brown one with bleach stains. Sahar took her treasured orange pillow into the bedroom next door, which she is sharing with my parents and my second sister, who is younger still. Like last night, our guest will sleep in Sahar's bed.

The smell of grease from the fried *pakoras*—my favorite snack—lingers in the air. We had a family get-together tonight. Crowded into the small living room of our apartment, cousins, uncles, aunts, grandparents, and family friends all shared a large dinner in honor of our visitor.

My brother and sisters enjoyed those pakoras with our older cousins. But I stayed outside for hours today and missed out. There are probably still a few left in the kitchen. Mom always makes so much. She would rather have too much food than have people leave her table wanting. My mouth salivates as I think about dipping the pakoras in ketchup and tasting that sweet, tangy sauce with the spicy potato fritter. But I won't leave the bedroom, not while *he* is still out there.

Thirty-seven one-thousand. Thirty-eight one-thousand. To distract myself, I look up at the opposite wall above my brother. A *Jaws* movie poster bandages the three-foot-long crack in the basic beige–painted apartment walls. Ever since the movie came out, Kamran has been obsessed with sharks. He saves most of the quarters, dimes, and nickels he gets from odd jobs to collect all things shark. Shark books, shark drawings, shark models, shark posters. They are misunderstood creatures, he says, and one day he wants to be a marine biologist and save them. I don't know. I haven't seen the movie, but the shark in the poster sure looks scary to me. A pretty blonde swims, unsuspectingly, as the shark lurks beneath the surface. Is the shark going to pull her down? How long can she last underwater? How long can I?

Fifty-six one—The bedroom door slowly opens. I stiffen. Against my brother's snores, against the loud buzz of the fan, against the sounds of my parents settling down in the room next door, even against the yells of reveling teenagers outside, my ears have been trained, and I can still hear the soft pad of his footsteps on the parquet floor. Instead of the sweet ketchup, I now taste something sour. His pajamas rustle and my heart beats with each step as he makes his way closer and closer toward me.

As usual, I close my eyes and pretend to be asleep. The padding stops at my bed. I clench my hands so tightly that they hurt. I feel the pull of my blanket until I am exposed. I then feel the weight of his body as it climbs atop mine. Something wet drips onto my neck. His breath is hot in my ear as he tugs on my yellow nightgown, which clings to my knees. He pulls it above my waist. He breathes faster as his hands wander along my thighs.

I don't want it. Not again. "Stop it," I whisper.

Talup's hands keep moving. Did he hear? I say it again, a little louder: "Stop it." He freezes. This time he did hear. I think he's surprised. But my surprise is even greater than his. Never before, in all the years we both went through this scenario again and again and across two continents, had I uttered a single word of protest, let alone two. Every night before, I lay still, remained silent, and pretended to be someplace else. But not this night.

Stop it.

I had essentially said these words to Dave to protect Sylvester. And now, on this night, I'm saying them for me.

I hold my breath. Talup's heavy weight lifts off me. I don't look, but I hear his footsteps retreat to the empty bed. The springs of the thin mattress creak under his weight. I exhale and pull my nightgown back down. This will remain my favorite nightgown for a long time to come. Tonight and every night from now on, I'm on dry land.

⁂

On the warm grass, as I watch Lulu the chicken, Ivy the pig comes and sits besides me. Her snout sniffs the air.

"Well, Ivy," I say to her, "what should we do now?"

She looks up at me. *Snoof, snoof,* she replies.

I recall that Alena described playing chase with her pigs. I haven't played chase since a child, but I feel a little like a child here, among the animals. They unlock an innocence I haven't felt for many years. Perhaps ever.

I hop up. "Ivy!" I call out, "Come on girl!" I run a little away from her and hide behind the wooden shed that is her home. I look back toward her. "Ivy!" I call again.

Rook, she responds. She does a little jumping dance and runs after me. It actually works! I keep calling her name as I run around the shed and she chases me. Round and round we go, until I run out of breath. I plop on the ground, laughing. She stops too, walks up to me, sniffs my hand, says *roooook* and walks to the other side of the shed. I get up and follow her. A nest of hay rests under a small opening in the side of the wooden structure. Ivy plops down into her nest and squirms her body around several times until she finds the best spot. She tucks her nose into the warm hay, lets out a deep sigh, closes her eyes, and falls asleep. For the next half hour, I sit beside Ivy with my hand on her head. Sharing her serenity.

How do we achieve health? This question has plagued me ever since I first recognized my depressions, long before I became a doctor. Even after, the confines of medicine didn't give the answer. Although I agreed with it, the World Health Organization's definition of *health* as a "state of complete physical, mental, and social well-being" never gave guidance as to how to reach it. Sitting here watching Ivy, though, I come closer to an answer.

The path to health, especially mental and social health, lies in our empathetic relationships with others. During my depressions, I am completely alone. I fall into an isolated mental void, cut off into a seemingly endless spiral of distress, grief, and agony. But my relationships with others play a strong role in guarding me against these afflictions. And these connections, reinforced through kindness and understanding, arm me to better command my own fate. As I have seen with so many others, I am not alone in this. When we feel connected is when we are our strongest.

Empathy empowers. With empathy comes conviction, comes confidence, comes courage. Without empathy, most of the folks I met and learned about over these past few years would not have changed their own lives—or the lives of others—for the better. Without empathy for mother cows mourning the loss of their children, Renee might never have had the conviction to open a sanctuary. Without her empathy for Tommy and his for her, she might never have had the confidence to achieve it. Without empathy for Sylvester, I would not have braved Talup. Through Sylvester's abuse, I came to recognize my own for what it was. Through empathy, the stark divide between human and animal blurred, and, at some level, I understood that Sylvester's fight was my fight. My fight was his.

All forms of abuse share a commonality. They hide behind silence. They unmask through voice. My empathy for Sylvester taught me to speak up for him and that gave me the strength to change the course of my life as well.

Stop it.

It's amazing the power two little words can have. To me, they said I would longer doubt my self-worth. No longer obey another's rules. No longer assume the answers others give me. To Talup, they said I would no longer keep quiet. Two words changed my life. They were the hardest things I had ever said, but they set me free.

With empathy comes the empowerment to demand a better world. For ourselves and for others. One with less grief and more joy. But to achieve such a world, isn't it imperative to include animals? Shouldn't we extend our arms and bring animals into our circle of empathy?

We go to great lengths to separate ourselves from other animals. We tell ourselves animals don't laugh (rats do), don't get pessimistic (pigs do), don't use tools (crows do), don't understand time (scrub jays do), don't do math (chickens do), don't trick others (squirrels do), don't feel empathy (mice do), don't pass on culture (chimpanzees do), don't show interest in their dead (elephants do), don't console each other (voles do), don't use language (prairie dogs probably do), and don't love. Seriously? If we are honest, we will admit that what we say about other animals says more about us than the animals.

If there is a trait that truly distinguishes us from other animals, though, it's this: No other species is as capable of self-deceit as humans. We master the act. We paint over the stark, white negative spaces on the canvas, even if by doing so, we conceal the larger truth of the landscape. We ignore what affronts our worldview. We disbelieve what we can't ignore. We rationalize what we can't disbelieve. *These things happen. It's necessary. It's not as bad as we think.* And most dangerous of all, *it's normal.*

Normal whispers sweet nothings into our ears while it steals our empathy.

It is the same mind-set that encourages cruelty toward animals and toward other humans. Normalcy need not hold us prisoner, though. We can free ourselves to recognize that humans and animals largely share the same struggle—the need for safety, comfort, and a gentle hand. The good news is that the solution to our struggles is the same. Empathy for animals is the natural, inevitable extension of our empathy for each other.

Harvard psychologist Jerome Kagan noted that "although humans inherit a biological bias that permits them to feel anger, jealousy, selfishness, and envy, and to be rude, aggressive or violent, they inherit an even stronger biological bias for kindness, compassion, cooperation, love and nurture—especially toward those in need." Our neurological wiring creates a positive feedback loop that encourages our empathy to grow. In other words, the more we practice empathy, the stronger it becomes.

Our reach for animals is lengthening. We are increasingly recognizing the love and healing that friendships with animals can bring us. Humans now view wild animals that were traditionally vilified in a different light. Animals such as wolves, vultures, rats, bats, and even sharks are more popular today than they once were. Some researchers suggest that the ways in which Americans value wild animals are shifting toward a view that considers wildlife "as part of an extended family, and deserving of caring and compassion." The increasing media attention to the loss of species and the plight of animals raised for food and used in experiments reflect our increasing concern for them.

We are acknowledging the interconnectedness of our lives with other animals. Their well-being is not separate from ours. On the contrary, we share the same fate.

Moving forward, how we choose to be with animals will depend on how willing we are to be *with them*. Not as predator and prey, not as master and servant. But as kin, as partners, and as friends, strolling shoulder to shoulder along the dips and rises that stretch before us. We lose nothing when we do so. What we gain is our health, our happiness, our humanity. And friendships that are irreplaceable.

As I sit here beside Ivy, our sun slowly slumbers. One by one, the millions of suns from faraway worlds wink awake and greet me. I listen to everyone settling down for the night. In her sleep,

Ivy snorts. From the garage, Renee and Tommy chuckle over something. In the trees overhead, birds rustle. In their pond, the ducks quack. The chickens cluck, the cows moo, the horses neigh, the dogs snuffle. Immersed in this shimmering and humming, I am reminded of Mozart's "Piano Concerto 21." In the contented voices of humans and animals, I hear a symphony of beauty.

◦◦◦◦

Charger just arrived. A brown baby cow who looks like a teddy bear, Charger's human parents hadn't the heart to see him killed after their FFA son lost interest in him. Charger steps out of his trailer with unsteady feet after his long drive. "Moo-ooooh!" he says as he looks around his new home. He calls again. "Mooooo-ooooooh!" He invests his body and soul into his two-syllable moos.

From the east pasture, twenty cows answer Charger. Male, female, young, old. They make their way out of the trees and line up against the fence with curiosity. In succession, they stick their heads through the fence and touch Charger, nose to nose. Welcome, they say, to their new friend.

I leave Charger and the other cows and walk toward the main grounds. With my back against a fence, I settle down on the ground and close my eyes. I relax into the music of the cows and think about Sylvester. After my confrontation with Dave, we never again talked about his hurting Sylvester. But over many years, I had often wondered if he regretted how he treated Sylvester. Did he ever question normal? It was during our last moments with Sylvester when these questions were answered.

I was nineteen years old and reading on the front porch of my parents' home when Dave's car pulled into our driveway. Dave had often visited our home in Vienna, Virginia; but on that day, I immediately knew something was wrong. When he stepped out of his car, his long, lanky body didn't completely unfold.

When I met him by his car, I saw grief etched in his face. "Sylvester is sick," he told me, his voice faltering. "He has liver failure

and he's dying. The vet told me he only has a few more days."
He looked up at the bronzed plum tree leaves overhead. "I came
straight here."

I looked into the backseat of Dave's car and saw Sylvester huddled
on a blanket. My god, he was so skinny! I could see his rib cage and
his eyes were yellowed and sunken, his stomach bloated.

"I'm putting him to sleep tomorrow," Dave said. "Will you come
with me?"

The next afternoon I found Dave in the parking lot outside the
animal hospital. He waited for me so that we could take Sylvester in
together. I asked for a few moments with Sylvester first. I wanted one
last time with him before we entered the cold, sterile environment
of the hospital. I stepped inside Dave's car and kneeled on the floor.
Sylvester's eyes looked at mine and he thumped his tail against the
seat using the last reserves of his energy. I rested my head against
his and inhaled. The car smelled like him—his musky, warm scent.
I tried to ignore the smell of urine and feces and the acrid smell of
sickness. I buried my hands in his fur and stroked his soft belly. As
tears rolled out of my eyes, Sylvester licked my face. His last time to
comfort me. When all I wanted to do was comfort him.

When I stepped out of the car and nodded to Dave, he took a
deep breath, wrapped a blanket around Sylvester, and scooped him
into his arms. Sylvester was so weak, he put up none of his usual
resistance when taken to the vet. Dave cooed to Sylvester as he
carried him. "That's a good boy. Good boy. Vesty, my good boy."

We walked into the lobby where there were other visitors waiting
with a menagerie of animals—cats, hamsters, dogs, a cockatiel.
They hushed their voices when we entered and looked at us with
understanding. They knew what we were there for. There is a certain
look on people's faces when they go to euthanize their animals. It's
grief mixed with resolution, warring with dread.

We were led into an examination room where the veterinarian
and an assistant were waiting for us. They greeted us with kindness.
The metal examination table was cold and they offered a towel,
but we kept Sylvester in his soft blue-and-tan blanket. To distance

myself from the coming procedure, I became clinical. I watched as the vet took Sylvester's left hind leg and felt around for a good blood vessel. They had already drawn the syringe with pentobarbital and, despite my attempt at distraction, I winced when the needle pierced Sylvester's skin. The vet drew back a little on the syringe to check for blood. Sylvester's blood diffused into the pentobarbital. His life entered death. Satisfied he was in the vein, the vet pushed the syringe. I watched the syringe empty. Death entered life. It galloped the course of Sylvester's body—to his heart, lungs, arms, legs. When the messenger entered the base of the brain, it announced it was time to turn off the lungs' breathing, to stop the heart's pumping. It was time to shut down.

I stepped back and allowed Dave to have the last moments with Sylvester. His arms wrapped Sylvester's body and his hands cradled Sylvester's head. "It's all right, Vesty. Papa is here. Papa will always be with you," he whispered. Sylvester's head drooped. Dave lowered it on the blanket. Sylvester was gone.

Dave threw himself over Sylvester's body and shook and cried as if asking for forgiveness.

"We'll step out and give you time alone with him," The vet said. "Take as much time as you want."

I watched Dave as he caressed Sylvester's body. He ran his hands over his nose, his ears, his paws. He examined Sylvester's left back leg where the needle was placed and where there was now a bandage—I didn't even notice the vet placing the bandage. Dave looked at the bandage, confused. Then he raised the leg and kissed the wound. Tears I had held back threatened to pour out. I stepped outside into the waning afternoon to grieve in private.

Dave stayed a half hour with Sylvester's body. He would later cremate Sylvester and keep his ashes in an urn by his bed. When I went back in to check on Dave, the vet walked up to me privately and said, "I've had to put many animals down in front of their owners, but I never saw anyone cry as hard as your uncle."

Charger and the other cows continue to call back and forth, getting louder with excitement. From behind the fence against my back, I hear a different noise—the rustle and slow shuffling gait of arthritic legs. I feel a hesitant head nudge me through the wooden rails, the steer's horns are gentle against my arm. I get up, turn, and look into Murray's soft, brown eyes. They're not so different from Sylvester's.

Afterword

When I was a teenager, I heard a story, which I resort to whenever I feel overwhelmed with the enormity of the challenges facing us in making this world a better place. The story has evolved over time from its original. But the essence is this:

> Early one morning, I was walking along the shore after a storm had passed and found the vast beach littered with starfish as far as the eye could see, stretching in both directions.
>
> Off in the distance, I noticed another man standing, gazing at something in the sand. He then stooped and flung the object beyond the breaking surf.
>
> As I walked toward him, I could see that he was occasionally bending down to pick up a starfish and throw it into the sea. I called out, "Good morning! May I ask what it is that you are doing?"
>
> The man looked up and replied, "Throwing starfish into the ocean. The tide has washed them up onto the beach and they can't return to the sea by themselves. They will die unless I throw them back into the water."
>
> I replied, "But there must be thousands of starfish on this beach! You're only one man. I'm afraid you won't be able to make much of a difference."

The man bent down, picked up yet another starfish and threw it as far as he could into the ocean. Then he turned, smiled, and said, "I made a difference to that one!"

Silently, I sought and picked up a still-living star, spinning it far out into the wave. "I understand," I said, "call me another thrower." Only then I allowed myself to think, He is not alone any longer.

(Adapted from *The Star Thrower* by Loren Eiseley. Mariner Books, 1979.)

Perhaps no one person can save the world, but they can save a life . . . or two. And just think how much we can accomplish collectively.

For suggestions on how you can help make a difference, visit Dr. Akhtar's website at www.ayshaakhtar.com.

Notes

PROLOGUE

p. xix   *In 1946, the World Health Organization defined health as "a state of complete physical, mental and social well-being":* Constitution of the World Health Organization. Supplement, October 2006. http://www.who.int/governance /eb/who_constitution_en.pdf, accessed November 23, 2018.

p. xxi   *Edward O. Wilson introduced biophilia as ". . . the innately emotional affiliation of human beings to other living organisms":* Edward O. Wilson, *Biophilia* (Cambridge, MA: Harvard University Press, 1984).

p. xxiii   *"Our urge to make a connection with fellow creatures is so powerful that it takes a lot to override it":* Brian Fagan, *The Intimate Bond: How Animals Shaped Human History* (New York: Bloomsbury Press, 2015), Preface.

PART ONE: HEALING WITH ANIMALS

ONE: WHAT IS HOME?

p. 7   *Empathy derives from the German word* Einfühlung: R. Curtis and R. Elliott, "An introduction to *Einfühlung,*" *Art in Translation* 6, no. 4 (2014): 353–76.

p. 7   *Studies on animal behavior show . . . empathy:* Frans de Waal, *The Age of Empathy* (New York: Harmony Books, 2009).

p. 7   *In 1995, a team of neuroscientists recorded motor-evoked potentials:* L. Fadiga, L. Fogassi, G. Pavesi, et al. "Motor facilitation during action observation: a magnetic stimulation study," *Journal of Neurophysiology* 73, no. 6 (1995): 2608–11.

p. 8   *Since that study, others have supported the idea:* C. Keysers, B. Wicker, V. Gazzola, et al., "A touching sight: SII/PV activation during the observation and experience of touch," *Neuron* 42, no. 2 (2004): 335–46; and P. Ferrari and G. Rizzolatti, "Mirror neuron research: the past and the future," *Philosophical Transactions of the Royal Society B* 369 (2014): 2013.0169.

p. 8   *Both components of empathy:* K. Jankowiak-Siuda, K. Rymarczyk, and A. Grabowska, "How we empathize with others: A neurobiological perspective," *Medical Science Monitor* 17, no. 2 (2011): RA18–RA24.

p. 8   *The ability to empathize with others:* B. Bernhardt and T. Singer, "The neural basis of empathy," *Annual Review of Neuroscience* 35, no. 1 (2012): 1–23.

p. 9   *To understand how empathy affects the emotional experience of pain:* T. Singer, B. Seymour, J. O'Doherty, et al., "Empathy for pain involves the affective but not sensory components of pain," *Science* 303 (2004): 1157–62.

p. 9   *"Empathy . . . works by tapping into a brain mechanism":* L. Nelson, "I feel your pain. Empathy lights up the same parts of the brain as personal injury," *Nature,* February 20, 2004.

p. 9   *Singer's study added further proof:* J. Decety, "The neurodevelopment of empathy in humans," *Developmental Neuroscience* 32, no. 4 (2010): 257–67; J. Decety and M. Svetlova, "Putting together phylogenetic and ontogenetic perspectives on empathy," *Developmental Cognitive Neuroscience* 2, no. 1 (2012): 1–24.

p. 9   *Researchers from the Department of Psychology:* R. Franklin Jr., A. Nelson, M. Baker, et al., "Neural responses to perceiving suffering in humans and animals," *Social Neuroscience* 8, no. 3 (2013): 217–27.

p. 9   *In* The Empathic Civilization: Jeremy Rifkin, *The Empathic Civilization* (New York: Penguin, 2009), 10.

p. 10   *As Kristin Dombek describes . . . empathetic accuracy:* Kristin Dombek, *The Selfishness of Others: An Essay on the Fear of Narcissism* (New York: Farrar, Straus and Giroux, 2016).

p. 10   *"She's part of Texas Task Force One":* Kevin Reece, "Cy-Fair Firefighters Say Goodbye to Last 9/11 Search-and-Rescue Hero," KHOU News, June 7, 2016, https://www.khou.com/article/news/local/animals/cy-fair-firefighters-say-goodbye-to-last-911-search-and-rescue-hero/285-234723483, accessed October 27, 2018.

p. 10   *According to Merriam-Webster's Dictionary, one definition of* family: Merriam-Webster's Online Dictionary, https://www.merriam-webster.com/dictionary/family, accessed October 28, 2018.

p. 10   *Statistically, a family is no longer a mother, father, and their biological children:* Lisa Belkin, "A 'Normal' Family," *The New York Times,* February 23, 2011, https://parenting.blogs.nytimes.com/2011/02/23/a-normal-family/, accessed October 27, 2018.

p. 11   *Since at least 2001, most US households have included companion animals:* "Pets by the Numbers," Humane Society of the United States, http://www.humanesociety.org/issues/pet_overpopulation/facts/pet_ownership_statistics.html, accessed May 26, 2018.

p. 11   *China is . . . behind the United States in cat and dog guardianship:* Marianna Cerini, "China's Economy Is Slowing, but Their Pet Economy Is Booming," *Forbes,* March 23, 2016, https://www.forbes.com/sites/mariannacerini/2016/03/23/chinas-economy-is-slowing-but-their-pet-economy-is-booming/#2d5e49b04ef7, accessed October 27, 2018.

p. 11   *Between 2006 and 2014, the number of companion animals in India grew:* Manali Shah and Poorva Joshi, "Here Is Why Urban India Is Bringing Pets Home Faster Than Ever Before," *Hindustan Times,* January 12, 2016, https://www.hindustantimes.com/fashion-and-trends

/animal-instict-here-is-why-urban-india-is-bringing-pets-home-faster-than-ever-before/story-vPwK5yRIOPH98EGRBlvNzM.html, accessed October 27, 2018.

p. 11   *More than 1,800 people, almost half of them elderly, died:* Ali Berman, "Hurricane Katrina Prompted a Shift in Pet Rights," Mother Nature Network, August 19, 2015, http://www.mnn.com/family/pets/stories/why-hurricane-katrina-was-shift-pets-rights, accessed September 13, 2016.

p. 12   *People who survive disasters:* M. Hunt, H. Al-Awadi, and M. Johnson, "Psychological sequelae of pet loss following hurricane Katrina," *Anthrozoos* 21, no. 2 (2008): 109–21.

p. 12   *After Hurricane Mitch hit Honduras and Nicaragua in 1998:* T. Caldera, L. Palma, U. Penayo, et al., "Psychological impact of the hurricane Mitch in Nicaragua in a one-year perspective," *Social Psychiatry and Psychiatric Epidemiology* 36, no. 3 (2001): 108–14.

p. 12   *Six months after Hurricane Andrew struck Florida in 1992:* F. Norris, J. Perilla, J. Riad, et al., "Stability and change in stress, resources, and psychological distress following natural disaster: Findings from Hurricane Andrew," *Anxiety, Stress, and Coping* 12, no. 4 (1999): 363–96.

p. 12   *The Centers for Disease Control . . . found that even seven weeks after Katrina:* R. Voelker, "Post-Katrina mental health needs prompt group to compile disaster medicine guide," *JAMA* 295, no. 3 (2006): 259–60.

p. 12   *Mary Foster . . . captured one of the most iconic moments:* Mary Foster, "Evacuation of Pets a Priority after Katrina," Associated Press, August 24, 2010.

p. 12   *When the little boy . . . and his parents were boarding a bus headed for Houston:* Associated Press, "Sad Story of Little Boy and his Dog Grips U.S.," NBC News, September 6, 2005, http://www.nbcnews.com/id/9223167/ns/health-pet_health/t/sad-story-little-boy-his-dog-grips-us/, accessed September 12, 2016.

p. 13   *It was likely that rescuers found animals in two out of every three homes:* Wayne Pacelle, *The Bond: Our Kinship with Animals, Our Call to Defend Them* (New York: William Morrow, 2011), 183.

p. 15   *When Katrina made landfall north of Miami:* "The Storm: 14 Days, a Timeline," *Frontline*, PBS, http://www.pbs.org/wgbh/pages/frontline/storm/etc/cron.html, accessed September 13, 2016.

p. 16   *One of the most frequent reasons people give for leaving their animals behind during disasters:* M. Hunt, K. Bogue, and N. Rohrbaugh. "Pet ownership and evacuation prior to hurricane Irene," *Animals* (Basel) 2, no. 4 (2012): 529–39.

p. 17   *Among primary school children from Slavonia:* L. Arambasic, G. Kereste, G. Kuterovac-Jagodic, et al., "The role of pet ownership as a possible buffer variable in traumatic experiences," *Studia Psychologica* 42, nos. 1–2 (2000): 135–46.

p. 17   *In a study of 365 low-income African American women:* S. Lowe, J. Rhodes, L. Zwiebach, et al., "The impact of pet loss on the perceived social support and psychological distress of hurricane survivors," *Journal of Traumatic Stress* 22, no. 3 (2009): 244–47.

p. 17   *Likewise, the loss of animals during Katrina caused greater negative impact:* M. Hunt, K. Bogue, and N. Rohrbaugh, "Pet ownership and evacuation prior to hurricane Irene," *Animals* (Basel) 2, no. 4 (2012): 529–39.

p. 17   *As compared with people who did not lose their animals during Katrina:* M. Hunt, H. Al-Awadi, and M. Johnson, "Psychological sequelae of pet loss following hurricane Katrina," *Anthrozoos* 21, no. 2 (2008): 109–21.

p. 17   *After 2008's Hurricane Ike, loss of animals among survivors in Galveston, Texas:* S. Lowe, S. Joshi, P. Pietrzak, et al., "Mental health and general wellness in the aftermath of hurricane Ike," *Social Science and Medicine* 124 (2015): 162–70.

p. 17   *That love can shield us from stress, anxiety, and depression:* M. Cordaro, "Pet loss and disenfranchised grief: Implications for mental health counseling practice," *Journal of Mental Health Counseling* 43 (2012): 283–94; N. Doherty and J. Feeney, "The composition of attachment networks through the adult years," *Personal Relationships* 11 (2004): 469–88; and P. Sable, "Pets, attachment, and well-being across the life cycle," *Social Work* 40, no. 3 (1995): 334–41.

p. 17   *People with companion animals feel that the animals are important to their well-being:* C. Rogers, "The critical need for animal disaster response plans," *Journal of Business Continuity & Emergency Planning* 9, no. 3 (2016): 262–71.

p. 17   *Perhaps most importantly, animals are reliable presences:* Caroline Schaffer, DVM, "Human-animal bond considerations during disasters," Integrated Medical, Public Health, Preparedness and Response Training Summit: Learning Together for a Nation Prepared, Dallas, TX, April 8, 2009, http://virginiasart.org /wordpress/wp-content/uploads/2012/05/Human-animal_bond_considerations _during_disasters_-_schaffer_caroline.pdf, accessed on September 9, 2016.

p. 18   *Almost half of the people . . . lost a companion animal:* Francis Battista, "The Forgotten Victims of Disaster," CNN.com, August 28, 2015, http://www .cnn.com/2015/08/28/opinions/battista-animals-katrina-aftermath/, accessed September 13, 2016; Louisiana SPCA, "Animal Rescue Facts," Katrina Dogs and Animal Rescue Stories, http://www.la-spca.org/about /katrina-dogs-animal-rescue-stories/rescuefacts, accessed September 14, 2016; Fritz Institute, "Fritz Institute–Harris Interactive Katrina Survey Reveals Inadequate Immediate Relief Provided to Those Most Vulnerable," news release, April 26, 2006, http://www.fritzinstitute.org/prsrmPR-FI -HIKatrinaSurvey.htm, accessed May 27, 2018.

p. 18   *They had good reason not to evacuate:* L. Zottarelli, "Broken bond: An exploration of human factors associated with companion animal loss during Hurricane Katrina," *Sociological Forum* 25, no. 1 (2010): 110–22.

p. 18   *Only 15 to 20 percent of lost animals were ever reunited with their human families:* Louisiana SPCA, "Animal Rescue Facts," Katrina Dogs and Animal Rescue Stories, http://www.la-spca.org/about/katrina-dogs-animal-rescue-stories /rescuefacts, accessed September 14, 2016.

p. 18   *One-fifth to one-third of human evacuation failures during disasters:* S. Heath and R. Linnabary, "Challenges of Managing Animals in Disasters in the U.S.," *Animals* (Basel) 5, no. 2 (2015): 173–92.

p. 18   *Of those who did leave, many remained homeless:* S. Heath, P. Kass, A. Beck, et al., "Human and pet-related risk factors for household evacuation failure during a natural disaster," *American Journal of Epidemiology* 153, no. 7 (2001): 659–65; S. Heath, S. Voeks, and L. Glickman, "Epidemiologic features of pet evacuation failure in a rapid onset disaster," *Journal of the American Veterinary Medical Association* 218, no. 12 (2001): 1898–1904.

p. 19   *Grief is even lonelier when an animal dies:* K. Thompson, D. Every, S. Rainbird, et al., "No pet or their person left behind: Increasing the disaster resilience of vulnerable groups through animal attachment, activities and networks," *Animals* (Basel) 4, no. 2 (2014): 214–40.

p. 19   *An animal's death can cause . . . depression:* N. Field, L. Orsini, R. Gavish, et al., "Role of attachment in response to pet loss," *Death Studies* 33, no. 4 (2009): 334–55; M. Hunt, H. Al-Awadi, and M. Johnson, "Psychological sequelae of pet loss following hurricane Katrina," *Anthrozoos* 21, no. 2 (2008): 109–21.

p. 20   *Among those who lose animals:* N. Field, L. Orsini, R. Gavish, et al., "Role of attachment in response to pet loss," *Death Studies* 33, no. 4 (2009): 334–55.

p. 20   *Researchers found that people's distress . . . was worse among those who abandoned them:* M. Hunt, H. Al-Awadi, and M. Johnson, "Psychological sequelae of pet loss following hurricane Katrina," *Anthrozoos* 21, no. 2 (2008): 109–21.

p. 20   *Saving Rooty was one rescue that stood out:* Stewart Cook, "I Saved a 300-Pound Pig From Hurricane Katrina," *The Dodo,* September 9, 2015, https://www .thedodo.com/rooty-300-pound-pig-rescue-hurricane-katrina-1330659378 .html, accessed October 15, 2015.

p. 22   *Americans donated more than $40 million:* S. Heath and R. Linnabary, "Challenges of Managing Animals in Disasters in the U.S.," *Animals* (Basel) 5, no. 2 (2015): 173–92; S. Ivry, "An Outpouring for Other Victims, the Four-Legged Kind," *The New York Times,* November 14, 2005.

p. 22   *It also authorized the use of funds for . . . "pets and service animals":* Ali Berman, "Hurricane Katrina Prompted a Shift in Pet Rights," Mother Nature Network, August 19, 2015, http://www.mnn.com/family/pets/stories/why-hurricane-katrina-was-shift-pets-rights, accessed September 13, 2016; and Public Law 109–308, 109th Cong. (2006), https://www.gpo.gov/fdsys/pkg/PLAW-109 publ308/pdf/PLAW-109publ308.pdf, accessed May 28, 2018.

p. 22   *PETS legislation has had a positive, measurable effect:* M. Hunt, K. Bogue, and N. Rohrbaugh. "Pet ownership and evacuation prior to hurricane Irene," *Animals* (Basel) 2, no. 4 (2012): 529–39.

p. 26   *Research has repeatedly shown that family-violence victims:* F. Ascione, "Battered women's reports of their partners and their children's cruelty to animals," *Journal of Emotional Abuse* 1 (1997): 119–33; C. Marcus, "Victims of Domestic Violence; Women Suffer for Sake of Their Pets," *Sun Herald,* March 9, 2008; A. Volant, J. Johnson, E. Gullone, et al., "The relationship between domestic violence and animal abuse," *Journal of Interpersonal Violence* 23, no. 9 (2008): 1277–95; G. Goodman, "The relationship between intimate partner violence and other forms of family and social violence," *Emergency Medicine Clinics of North America* 24, no. 4 (2006): 889–903; S. Agrell, "Pets Help Abused Women—But May Make Them Vulnerable," *Globe and Mail* (Toronto), June 12, 2008; B. Gallagher, M. Allen, and B. Jones, "Animal abuse and intimate partner violence: Researching the link and its significance in Ireland—A veterinary perspective," *Irish Veterinary Journal* 61 (2008): 658–67: S. Ross, "Abuse victims who refuse to leave for fear of their pets being harmed," *The Scotsman*, October 20, 2008; P. Owen, "Abuse Victims Often Fear for Pets," *Worcester Telegram & Gazette*, October 17, 2015, http://dev.telegram.com /article/20151017/NEWS/151019223; A. Gray, A. Fitzgerald, and B. Barrett, "Fear for pets can put abused women at further risk," *The Conversation*, June 26, 2017; Ascione, "Battered women's reports of their partners and their children's cruelty to animals," *Journal of Emotional Abuse* 1 (1997): 119–33; J. Quinlisk, "Animal Abuse and Family Violence," in Frank Ascione and Phil Arkow (eds.), *Child Abuse, Domestic Violence, and Animal Abuse: Linking the Circles of Compassion for Prevention and Intervention* (West Lafayette, IN.: Purdue University Press, 1999), 168–75.

p. 26   *In a survey of 107 battered women:* C. Flynn, "Women's best friend: Pet abuse and the role of companion animals in the lives of battered women," *Violence Against Women* 6, no. 2 (2000): 162–77.

p. 26   *In 2012, a woman . . . caused them to overhaul their practice:* "Heroic Dog Saves Woman from Abuser, Incites Change in Shelter Policy," *Life with Dogs*, January 12, 2012, http://www.lifewithdogs.tv/2012/01/heroic-dog-saves-owner-from-abusive-spouse-incites-change-in-shelter-policy/, accessed July 7, 2017.

p. 27   *Fitzgerald found that the presence of animals can both help battered women and heighten their risks of danger:* A. Fitzgerald, "'They Gave Me a Reason to Live': The Protective Effects of Companion Animals on the Suicidality of Abused Women," *Humanity and Society* 31 (2007): 355–78.

p. 28   *In 2015, with funding from RedRover:* Hilary Hanson, "Why This Domestic Violence Center's Pet Shelter Is Crucial for Both Animals and People," *Huffington Post*, May 22, 2015, https://www.huffingtonpost.com/2015/05/22 /domestic-violence-center-pets_n_7421378.html.

p. 30   *The US Code of Federal Regulations defines* homelessness *as lacking "a fixed, regular and adequate nighttime residence":* "42 U.S. Code § 11302—General Definition of Homeless Individual," Cornell Law School, Legal Information Institute, https://www.law.cornell.edu/uscode/text/42/11302?qt-us_code _temp_noupdates=3#qt-us_code_temp_noupdates, accessed July 11, 2017.

p. 30   *On a single night in 2017, according to the US Department of Housing and Urban Development (HUD), 553,742:* Meghan Henry, Rian Watt, Lily Rosenthal, and Azim Shivji, Abt Associates, *The 2017 Annual Homeless Assessment Report (AHAR) to Congress*, U.S. Department of Housing and Urban Development, December 2017, https://www.hudexchange.info/resources/documents/2017 -AHAR-Part-1.pdf.

p. 32   *The dogs . . . ."eat before I do.":* Leslie Irvine, *My Dog Always Eats First: Homeless People and Their Animals* (Boulder, CO: Lynne Rienner Publishers, 2013), 54.

p. 32   *"People think because you're homeless, you can't take care of a dog"*: Leslie Irvine, *My Dog Always Eats First: Homeless People and Their Animals* (Boulder, CO: Lynne Rienner Publishers, 2013), 55.

TWO: FINDING OUR VOICES

p. 40   *In fact . . . children who learn a second language can maintain greater attention*: Susan S. Lang, "Learning a Second Language Is Good Childhood Mind Medicine, Studies Find," *Cornell Chronicle*, May 12, 2009.

p. 42   *Levinson looked "more like an evil sorcerer than a child psychologist"*: Conversation with Stanley Coren.

p. 42   *The case Levinson presented was that of a young boy who had become withdrawn*: B. Levinson, "The dog as 'co-therapist.'" *Mental Hygiene* 46 (1962): 59–65; B. Levinson, "Pet psychotherapy: Use of household pets in the treatment of behavior disorder in childhood," *Psychological Reports* 17 (1965): 695–98.

p. 43   *Cherishing his own dogs . . . Freud let them have the run of his office*: Melinda Beck, "Beside Freud's Couch, a Chow Named Jofi," *The Wall Street Journal*, December 21, 2010.

p. 43   *Jofi was originally brought into the office to help Freud relax*: Stanley Coren, "How Therapy Dogs Almost Never Came to Exist," *Psychology Today*, February 11, 2013.

p. 43   *Jeeter . . . was the first dog given permission to appear in court*: William Glaberson, "By Helping a Girl Testify at Trial, a Dog Ignites a Legal Debate," *The Seattle Times*, August 9, 2011; Christine Clarridge, "Courthouse Dogs Calm Victims' Fears about Testifying," *The Seattle Times*, September 22, 2012.

p. 43   *They may never have done so if it hadn't been for Jeeter*: Christine Clarridge, "Courthouse Dogs Calm Victims' Fears about Testifying," *The Seattle Times*, September 22, 2012.

p. 44   *"It's hard to explain," said the twins' mother*: Christine Clarridge, "Dogs Lend Comfort to Kids in Court," *The Seattle Times*, May 12, 2009.

p. 45   *African grey parrots . . . from social isolation when held in captivity in separate cages*: D. Aydinonat, D. Penn, S. Smith, et al., "Social isolation shortens telomeres in African grey parrots (*Psittacus erithacus erithacus*)," *PLOS One* (2014), https://doi.org/10.1371/journal.pone.0093839.

p. 45   *In her book, Animal Madness*: Laurel Braitman, *Animal Madness: How Anxious Dogs, Compulsive Parrots, and Elephants in Recovery Help Us Understand Ourselves* (New York: Simon and Schuster, 2014), 85.

p. 46   *As Beston contemplated their nature, he took aim against the dominant view held by philosopher Rene Descartes*: Henry Beston, *The Outermost House* (New York: Henry Holt and Company, 1928), 24–25.

p. 47   *Nearly 90 percent of the characters in young children's books*: Stephen R. Kellert, *Birthright: People and Nature in the Modern World* (New Haven, CT: Yale University Press, 2012), 26–28.

p. 47   *Animals in stories are used to teach children critical issues*: Stephen R. Kellert, *Birthright: People and Nature in the Modern World* (New Haven, CT: Yale University Press, 2012), 26–28.

p. 47   *When psychologist Boris Levinson . . . used the boy's identification with a cat to heal him:* B. Levinson, "Pet psychotherapy: Use of household pets in the treatment of behavior disorder in childhood," *Psychological Reports* 17 (1965): 695–88.

p. 50   *In 1792, the Retreat in York, England, brought in animals: The Health Benefits of Pets,* National Institutes of Health OMAR Workshop, September 10–11, 1987, https://consensus.nih.gov/1987/1987healthbenefitspetsta003html.htm.

p. 50   *Even famed nurse Florence Nightingale recognized the beneficial role animals play in healing:* J. Shiller, RN, "Nightingale's Cats," (n.d.), http://www.countryjoe .com/nightingale/cats.htm, accessed July 13, 2016.

p. 50   *In her seminal text . . . wrote "a small pet animal is often an excellent companion for the sick, for long chronic cases especially":* Florence Nightingale, *Notes on Nursing: What It Is, and What It Is Not* (New York: D. Appleton and Company 1860).

p. 51   *In the late 1970s . . . Friedmann made a startling discovery:* E. Friedmann, A. Katcher, J. Lynch, et al., "Animal companions and one-year survival of patients after discharge from a coronary care unit," *Public Health Reports* 95 (1980): 307–12.

p. 52   *Studies have since indicated that contact with animals can reduce our risk:* G. Levine, K. Allen, L. Braun, et al., "Pet ownership and cardiovascular risk. A scientific statement from the American Heart Association," *Circulation* 127 (2013): 2353–63; E. Friedmann, S. Thomas, P. Stein, et al., "Relation between pet ownership and heart rate variability in patients with healed myocardial infarcts," *American Journal of Cardiology* 91 (2003): 718–21; E. Friedmann, S. Thomas, "Pet ownership, social support, and one-year survival after acute myocardial infarction in the Cardiac Arrhythmia Suppression Trial (CAST)," *American Journal of Cardiology* 76 (1995): 1213–17; L. Jennings, "Potential benefits of pet ownership in health promotion," *Journal of Holistic Nursing* 15 (1997): 358–72; E. Friedmann and H. Son, "The human-companion animal bond: How humans benefit," *Veterinary Clinics of North America: Small Animal Practice* 39 (2009): 293–326; A. Beetz, K. Uvnas-Moberg, H. Julius, et al., "Psychosocial and psychophysiological effects of human-animal interactions: The possible role of oxytocin," *Frontiers in Psychology* 3, Article 234 (2012).

p. 55   *The first mention of symptoms correlating with PTSD:* Richard A. Gabriel, *No More Heroes: Madness and Psychiatry in War* (New York: Macmillan, 1988); Steve Bentley, "A Short History of PTSD: From Thermopylae to Hue Soldiers Have Always Had a Disturbing Reaction to War," *The VVA Veteran,* March/April 2005; Paul Lashmar, "The True Madness of War," *The Independent* (UK), September 2, 1998, https://www.independent.co.uk/arts-entertainment/the -true-madness-of-war-1195452.html.

p. 55   *During the mid- and late 19th . . . were called Soldier's Heart and Da Costa Syndrome:* "The Soldier's Heart," *Frontline,* PBS, March 1, 2005, https://www .pbs.org/wgbh/pages/frontline/shows/heart/.

p. 55   *Doctors noticed something strange among many of the soldiers . . . after they were exposed to exploding shells:* Caroline Alexander, "The Shock of War," *Smithsonian Magazine,* September 2010, https://www.smithsonianmag.com/history /the-shock-of-war-55376701/.

p. 55   *In World War II, combat stress reaction, also known as "battle fatigue," replaced the term shell shock:* Matthew J. Friedman, "History of PTSD in Veterans. Civil War to DSM-5," US Department of Veteran Affairs, https://www.ptsd.va.gov /understand/what/history_ptsd.asp, accessed October 28, 2018; C. Wooley, "Where are the diseases of yesteryear?" *Circulation* 53 (1976): 749–51.

p. 56   *At first, the DSM classified* trauma *as an event existing "outside the range of usual human experience":* L. Jones and J. Cureton, "Trauma redefined in the *DSM-5*: Rationale and implications for counseling practice," *Professional Counselor,* http://tpcjournal.nbcc.org/trauma-redefined-in-the-dsm-5-rationale-and -implications-for-counseling-practice/, accessed July 30, 2017; C. North, A. Suris, R. Smith, et al., "The evolution of PTSD criteria across editions of DSM," *Annals of Clinical Psychiatry* 28 (2016): 197–208.

p. 56   *The most recent iteration of the DSM . . . narrowed the defining borders somewhat:* American Psychiatric Association, *Diagnostic and Statistical Manual of Mental Disorders,* 5th ed. (Washington, DC: American Psychiatric Publishing, 2013); A. Pai, A. Suris, and C. North, "Posttraumatic stress disorder in the DSM-5: controversy, change and conceptual considerations," *Behavioral Science* 7 (2017): 7.

p. 56   *Anywhere between 11-30 percent . . . will have experienced PTSD in their lifetimes:* National Center for PTSD, "How Common Is PTSD?" US Department of Veteran Affairs, https://www.ptsd.va.gov/public/ptsd-overview/basics/how -common-is-ptsd.asp, accessed July 30, 2017.

p. 56   *Roughly twenty American veterans . . . commit suicide every day:* Leo Shane III and Patricia Kime, "New VA Study Finds 20 Veterans Commit Suicide Each Day," *Military Times,* July 7, 2016.

p. 60   *Studies have shown that we generally perceive scenarios containing animals as more friendly:* E. Friedmann and H. Son, "The human-companion animal bond: How humans benefit," *Veterinary Clinics of North America: Small Animal Practice* 39 (2009): 293–326.

p. 60   *In 1944, Cpl. Bill Wynne came upon a stray dog while stationed in New Guinea:* Rebecca Frankel, "Dogs at War: Smoky, a Healing Presence for Wounded WWII Soldiers," *National Geographic,* March 22, 2014.

p. 60   *Patients at the Army Air Corps Convalescent Hospital in Pawling, New York:* M. Birch, L. Bustad, S. Duncan, et al., "The Role of Pets in Therapeutic Programmes" in I. Robinson (ed.), *The Waltham Book of Human-Animal Interaction* (Oxford, United Kingdom: Pergamon, 1995), 57, 58.

p. 61   *Currently, only half of veterans with PTSD seek healthcare:* Holloway Marston and Alicia Kopicki, "The impact of service dogs on postraumtic stress disorder in the veteran population," *The Military Psychologist,* April 2015.

p. 61   *Studies on those with PTSD find that a variety of animals:* M. O'Haire, N. Guerin, and A. Kirkham, "Animal-assisted intervention for trauma: A systematic literature review," *Frontiers in Psychology* 6 (2015): 1121.

p. 61   *In one study, psychologists noted an 82 percent reduction in symptoms:* D. Mims and R. Waddell, "Animal assisted therapy and trauma survivors," *Journal of Evidence-Informed Social Work* 13, no. 5 (2016): 452–57.

p. 63   *Psychologist Andrea Beetz proposes that oxytocin plays a key role:* A. Beetz, K. Uvnas-Moberg, H. Julius, et al., "Psychosocial and psychophysiological effects of human-animal interactions: The possible role of oxytocin," *Frontiers in Psychology* 3, Article 234 (2012).

p. 63   *In an article for the APA:* Tori DeAngelis, "The two faces of oxytoxin," *American Psychological Association* 39 (February 2008): 30, http://www.apa.org/monitor /feb08/oxytocin.aspx, accessed September 27, 2016.

p. 63   *In a famous study led by neuroeconomist Paul Zak:* P. Zak, A. Stanton, and S. Ahmadi, "Oxytocin increases generosity in humans," *PLOS ONE* 2, no 11 (2007): e1128, doi:10.1371/journal.pone.0001128.

p. 64   *In further studies, Zak and his colleagues found that oxytocin increases:* Paul Zak, "Dogs (and Cats) Can Love," *The Atlantic,* April 22, 2014.

p. 64   *Beetz and her colleagues found that many of the beneficial effects of oxytocin:* A. Beetz, K. Uvnas-Moberg, H. Julius, et al., "Psychosocial and psychophysiological effects of human-animal interactions: The possible role of oxytocin," *Frontiers in Psychology* 3, Article 234 (2012).

p. 64   *Two researchers from South Africa were among the first to test . . . after interactions with animals:* J. Odendaal and R. Meintjes, "Neurophysiological correlates of affiliative behavior between humans and dogs," *Veterinary Journal* 165 (2003): 296–301.

p. 64   *Brain imaging reveals . . . activates in dogs similarly in response to hand signals indicating food and to the smells of familiar humans:* Gregory Berns, "Dogs Are People, Too," *The New York Times,* October 5, 2013.

p. 65   *He tested if oxytocin increases when humans engage with animals:* Paul Zak, "Dogs (and Cats) Can Love," *The Atlantic,* April 22, 2014.

THREE: HUMANIZING OURSELVES

p. 72   *An excerpt from a 1980 article in* Cats Magazine *titled "Tom: A Cat and His Patients":* David Lee, "Tom: A Cat and His Patients," *Cats Magazine,* July 1980.

p. 75   *The second largest poured-concrete building in the world:* Jennifer Feehan, "Doors Locked on Empty Prison Cells," *The Blade,* June 27, 2004.

p. 76   *The institution admitted its first patients on July 10, 1915:* 7th Annual Report of the Ohio Board of Administration for the Fiscal Year ended June 30, 1918, to the Governor of the State of Ohio (Mansfield, OH: Ohio State Reformatory Press, 1918).

p. 76   *Once admitted to the hospital, a patient would be measured:* J. Crist, "Psychiatric examinations at Lima State Hospital," *Ohio State Medical Journal* 63 (1967): 899–901.

p. 77   *They snored soundly believing . . . "one of the most modern and best-equipped institutions of its kind":* "State Hospital May Turn over Wards to the U.S.," *Lima News* (Ohio), June 10, 1917.

p. 78   *In 1937, the institution's superintendent . . . therapy's remarkable ability to "cure" patients:* Elisabeth Fisher, "Insulin Treatment for Insane Employed Here," *Lima News* (Ohio), July 18, 1937.

p. 80   *When faced with adversity, children often turn to their animals for support:* University of Cambridge, "Children often have a closer relationship with their pet than their siblings," *Science Daily*, May 13, 2015.

p. 81   *In the past 150 years, all the US presidents brought animal companions:* The Data Team, "A Key White House Post Remains Unfilled: First Pet," *The Economist*, July 17, 2017.

p. 81   *Researchers found that strangers . . . if they had animals with them:* L. Hart, B. Hart, and B. Bergin, "Socializing effects of service dogs for people with disabilities," *Anthrozoos* 1 (1987): 41–44.

p. 82   *A study of more than 2,500 people in the United States and in Australia:* L. Wood, K. Martin, H. Christian, et al., "The pet factor—Companion animals as a conduit for getting to know people, friendship formation and social support," PLOS ONE 10, no. 4 (2015): e0122085.doi:10.1371/journal.pone.0122085.

p. 82   *One investigator refers to this as "triangulation":* Julie Beck, "How Dogs Make Friends for Their Humans," *The Atlantic*, November 30, 2015.

p. 82   *In 2008, a male researcher was able to get women's phone numbers:* N. Gueguen and S. Ciccotti, "Domestic dogs as facilitators in social interaction: An evaluation of helping and courtship behaviors," *Anthrozoos* 21 (2008): 339–49.

p. 82   *Similarly, in a study of college students . . . psychotherapists as more trustworthy if they had a dog with them:* M. Schneider and L. Harley, "How dogs influence the evaluation of psychotherapists," *Anthrozoos* 19 (2006): 128–42.

p. 82   *As early as 1699, John Locke advised giving children animals to care for:* John Locke, *The Educational Writings of John Locke*, John William Adamson (ed.) (1912; repr., London: Edward Arnold, 1922), 91.

p. 83   *Sarah Josepha Hale . . . animals are a "great preventative against the thoughtless cruelty and tyranny they are so apt to exercise toward all dependent beings":* Katherine C. Grier, *Pets in America* (Chapel Hill, NC: University of North Carolina Press, 2006), 177.

p. 83   *"Empathy is the fundamental people skill":* Daniel Goleman, *Emotional Intelligence*, 10th ed. (New York: Bantam, 2006), 43.

p. 83   *In a study published in 2014 . . . asked them to rate sixty photos of women making neutral facial expressions:* Y. Zang, F. Kong, Y. Zhong, et al., "Personality manipulations: Do they modulate facial attractiveness ratings?" *Personality and Individual Differences* 70 (2014): 80–84.

p. 84   *Its findings support a growing series of studies that have revealed that we like people who are ethical:* Scott Barry Kaufman, "Is kindness physically attractive?" *Scientific American*, October 9, 2014; V. Swami, A. Furnham, T. Chamorro-Premuzic, et al., "More than just skin deep? Personality information influences men's ratings of the attractiveness of women's body sizes," *Journal of Social Psychology* 150 (2010): 628–47.

p. 84   *As early as five months of age, our attraction to kindness is evident:* J. Hamlin, K. Wynn. "Young infants prefer prosocial to antisocial others," *Cognitive Development* 26 (2011): 30–39.

p. 84   *Preadolescent children who extended kindness to others:* K. Layous, S. Nelson, E. Oberle, et al., "Kindness counts: Prompting prosocial behavior in preadolescents boost peer-acceptance and well-being," *PLOS ONE* 7 (2017): e51380, https://doi.org/10.1371/journal.pone.0051380.

p. 84   *School programs, such as social-emotional learning programs, have proven successful:* Daniel Goleman, "Wired for Kindness: Science Shows We Prefer Compassion, and Our Capacity Grows with Practice," *Washington Post,* June 23, 2015.

p. 84   *In a yearlong school program . . . children who learned empathy through animal companionship also showed greater empathy toward other humans:* F. Ascione and C. Weber, "Children's attitude about the humane treatment of animals and empathy: One year follow-up of a school based intervention," *Anthrozoos* 4 (1996): 188–95.

p. 84   *The stronger the bond a child has with an animal, the greater her empathy and social competence:* R. Poresky and C. Hendrix, "Differential effects of pet presence and pet-bonding on young children," *Psychological Reports* 67 (1990): 51–54.

p. 85   *Other school-based programs show that children learn empathy . . . by being with animals:* J. Sprinkle, "Animals, empathy, and violence: Can animals be used to convey principles of prosocial behavior to children?" *Youth Violence and Juvenile Justice* 6 (2008): 47–58; A. Beetz, K. Uvnas-Moberg, H. Julius, et al., "Psychosocial and psychophysiological effects of human-animal interactions: The possible role of oxytocin," *Frontiers in Psychology* 3, Article 234 (2012).

p. 87   *During their six-week investigation, reporters Richard Widman and Theodore Whelan and photographer William Wynne interviewed patients:* David L. Hopecraft, "Jury Probe Ordered into Lima Hospital," *Plain Dealer* (Cleveland), August 7, 1971.

p. 87   *They detailed accounts of widespread brutality at the institution:* Edward P. Whelan and Richard C. Widman, "Medication Was Denied Diabetic, Says Lima Aide," *Plain Dealer* (Cleveland), May 25, 1971; "50 Exclusive Stories Showed Lima Horror," *Plain Dealer* (Cleveland), August 7, 1971; Edward P. Whelan and Richard C. Widman, "Aide Forced Homosexual Acts, Lima Patients' Statements Say," *Plain Dealer* (Cleveland), May 20, 1971; Edward P. Whelan and Richard C. Widman, "State Patrol Sifts Files on Deaths at Lima State," *Plain Dealer* (Cleveland), May 29, 1971; Edward P. Whelan and Richard C. Widman, "Beatings Led to Lima Patient's Suicide, Says Fired Attendant," *Plain Dealer* (Cleveland), May 21, 1971; Edward P. Whelan and Richard C. Widman, "Lima's Inmates Exist Amid Fear, Brutality," *Plain Dealer* (Cleveland), May 14, 1971; Edward P. Whelan and Richard C. Widman, "Lima Inmate Tells of Two Beatings," *Plain Dealer* (Cleveland), May 19, 1971; Edward P. Whelan and Richard C. Widman, "Abuse Killed 2 Patients, Lima Aide Says," *Plain Dealer* (Cleveland), May 27, 1971.

p. 88   *A grand jury indicted twenty-six male and five female Lima State Hospital employees:* Richard C. Widman and Edward P. Whelan, "31 Lima Indictments Made," *Plain Dealer* (Cleveland), November 23, 1971.

p. 88   *A subsequent federal court order led to a litany of reforms at the hospital:* Davis v. Watkins, 384 F. Supp. 1196 (N.D. Ohio 1974).

p. 90   *A juvenile inmate . . . "how much a dog can love you depends on you":* K. Davis, "Perspectives of youth in an animal-centered correctional vocational program: A qualitative evaluation of Project Pooch," 2007, www.pooch.org /documents/project-pooch-qualitative-eval.pdf.

p. 92   *Additionally, the presence of animals increases not only the morale of the inmates:* T. Harkrader, T. Burke, and S. Owen, "Pound puppies: The rehabilitative use of dogs in correctional facilities," *Corrections Today* (2004): 74–79.

p. 92   *In one prison program, researchers assessed the inmates' social skills and social sensitivity:* A. Fournier, E. Geller, and E. Fortney, "Human-animal interaction in a prison setting: Impact on criminal behavior, treatment progress, and social skills," *Behavior and Social Issues* 16 (2007): 89–105.

p. 93   *One such program in Washington State reported that the state's average three-year recidivism rate is 28 percent:* R. Huss, "Canines (and cats!) in correctional institutions: Legal and ethical issues relating to companion animal programs," *Nevada Law Journal* 14 (2014): 25–62.

p. 93   *Other programs have shown similar findings:* E. Strimple, "A history of prison inmate-animal interaction programs," *American Behaviorial Scientist* 4 (2003): 70–78.

p. 94   *"In the past, I never had that really deep-down compassion-type feeling for any kind of animal . . .":* "Pets and people: A new look at an old alliance," *Carnation Research Digest* 17 (Fall 1981): 3–6.

p. 94   *"I had never felt compassion":* "Lima's pet therapy program proves successful to patients," *Mental Horizons* (December 1978).

p. 95   *"I used to argue with the attendants . . . Now I just come in and talk to the bird, and I just don't yell at anyone anymore":* Kathy Gray Foster, "A Means of Escape: Pet Therapy in Prison," *Columbus Dispatch*, December 5, 1982.

p. 95   *"I'll tell you . . . If those fish can live in peace with each other, I can":* Janet Filips, "Lima's Menagerie Helps the Inmates Conquer Depression," *Dayton Journal Herald*, June 1981.

p. 95   *Researchers had thirty adults inhale oxytocin and then examine photos of people's eyes:* G. Domes, M. Heinrichs, A. Michel, et al., "Oxytocin improves 'mind reading' in humans," *Biological Psychiatry* 61, no. 6 (2007): 731–33.

p. 95   *Two-thirds of human communication is nonverbal:* Allan and Barbara Pease, "The Definitive Book of Body Language," *The New York Times*, September 24, 2006.

PART TWO: BREAKING WITH ANIMALS

FOUR: THE MAKING OF A MURDERER

p. 104   *When Ringling Brothers . . . defenders mourned the "end of an era":* Susan Zalkind, "'The End of an Era': Ringling Bros Circus Closes Curtain on Elephant Shows," *The Guardian* (UK), May 2, 2016; Kate Good, "Exposed! Ringling Brothers and Barnum and Bailey Circus," *One Green Planet*, August 22, 2014, http://www .onegreenplanet.org/animalsandnature/ringling-brothers-barna-bailey -cruelest-show-on-earth/, accessed January 21, 2017.

p. 105   *One major limitation of examinations of human-animal violence is that they are rather superficial:* R. Gleyzer, A. Felthous, and C. Holzer III, "Animal cruelty and psychiatric disorders," *Journal of the American Academy of Psychiatry and the Law* 30, no. 2 (2002): 257–65.

p. 105   *I had already reviewed the litany of published studies:* A. Akhtar, *Animals and Public Health: Why Treating Animals Better Is Critical to Human Welfare* (Hampshire, UK: Palgrave Macmillan, 2012), 27–51; A. Akhtar, "The need to include animal protection in public health policies," *Journal of Public Health Policy* 34 (2013): 549–59.

p. 106   *Keith Jesperson . . . is serving a life sentence without parole in the Oregon State Penitentiary:* Motion and Affidavit for Order Authorizing Issuance of Warrant of Arrest, signed by Dennis M. Hunter, Clark County Prosecuting Attorney, March 25, 1995; Superior Court of the State of Washington. State of Washington v. Keith Hunter Jesperson, October 19, 1995; Superior Court of the State of Washington. State of Washington v. Keith Hunter Jesperson, December 19, 1995; Superior Court of the State of Washington. State of Washington v. Keith Hunter Jesperson, January 12, 1996; Superior Court of the State of Washington. State of Washington v. Keith Hunter Jesperson, February 15, 1996.

p. 106   *Jesperson . . . sent a letter to reporters bragging about his murders:* Copy of letter retrieved from State of Washington court documents.

p. 106   *Jesperson's five-year killing spree ended only when he murdered a woman whom the police could tie him to directly:* John Painter Jr., "Long-Haul Trucker Admits Being Killer," *The Oregonian*, August 4, 1995; John Painter Jr., "Could He Be Happy Face Killer?" *The Oregonian*, August 6, 1995.

p. 110   *John M. Macdonald published the first study to suggest that certain behaviors in childhood could indicate later violence:* J. MacDonald, "The threat to kill," *American Journal of Psychiatry* 120 (1963): 125–30.

p. 111   *The APA did not recognize animal cruelty as a sign of a psychiatric disorder until 1987:* R. Gleyzer, A. Felthous, and C. Holzer III, "Animal Cruelty and Psychiatry Disorders," *Journal of the American Academy of Psychiatry and the Law* 30, no. 2 (2002): 257–65.

p. 111   *Ressler joined the FBI in 1970:* Robert K. Ressler and Tom Schactman, *Whoever Fights a Monster* (New York: St. Martin's Press, 1992), 26, 29; Daniel Goleman, "Clues to a Dark Nurturing Ground for One Serial Killer," *The New York Times*, August 7, 1991.

p. 111   *Ressler originated and developed the FBI's first research program of violent offenders:* Don DeNevi and John H. Campbell, *Into the Minds of Madmen* (Amherst, NY: Prometheus Books, 2004), 181.

p. 111   *In total, they interviewed thirty-six convicted serial and sexual murderers:* Robert K. Ressler, Ann W. Burgess, and John E. Douglas, *Sexual Homicide: Patterns and Motives* (New York: Free Press, 1992), xiii.

p. 112   *More than one out of three killers revealed that they had been cruel to animals:* Robert K. Ressler, Ann W. Burgess, and John E. Douglas, *Sexual Homicide: Patterns and Motives* (New York: Free Press, 1992), 29.

p. 112   *In 2001, psychologist Frank Ascione . . . reviewed the existing data and concluded:* F. Ascione, "Animal abuse and youth violence," *Juvenile Justice Bulletin* (September 2001): 1–15.

p. 112   *A "socially unacceptable behavior that intentionally causes unnecessary pain, suffering or distress to, and/or death of, an animal":* F. Ascione, "Children who are cruel to animals: A review of research and implications for developmental psychopathology," *Anthrozoos* 6 (1993): 2226–47.

p. 112   *Although his definition is one of the most frequently used, it has been criticized as being too narrow:* C. Flynn, "Examining the links between animal abuse and human violence," *Crime, Law and Social Change* 55 (2011): 453–68.

p. 113   *Parents tend to significantly underestimate their children's involvement in cruelty toward animals:* D. Offord, M. Boyle, and Y. Racine, "The epidemiology of antisocial behavior in childhood and adolescence," in K. Rubin and D. Pepler (eds.), *The Development and Treatment of Childhood Aggression* (Hillsdale, NJ: Lawrence Erlbaum Associates, 1991), 31–54; F. Ascione, "The abuse of animals and human interpersonal violence: Making the connection," in F. Ascione and P. Arkows (eds.), *Child Abuse, Domestic Violence, and Animal Abuse: Linking the Circles of Compassion for Prevention and Intervention* (West Lafayette, IN: Purdue University Press, 1999), 50–61; B. Boat, "The relationship between violence to children and violence to animals. An ignored link?" *Journal of Interpersonal Violence* 10 (1995): 229–35.

p. 113   *Alan Brantley stated, "We believe that the real figure was much higher":* R. Lockwood and A. Church, "Deadly Serious: An FBI Perspective on Animal Cruelty," *HSUS News*, Fall 1996, 27–30.

p. 113   *Regardless of the limitations . . . a history of animal abuse remains one of the most consistent findings among violent adults:* S. Tallichet and C. Hensley, "Exploring the link between recurrent acts of childhood and adolescent animal cruelty and subsequent violent crime," *Criminal Justice Review* 29 (2004): 304–16; C. Flynn, "Examining the links between Animal Abuse and Human Violence," *Crime, Law and Social Change* 55 (2011): 453–68; and F. Ascione, "Animal abuse and youth violence," *Juvenile Justice Bulletin* (September 2001): 1–15.

p. 113   *Childhood animal cruelty . . . is a harbinger of adult violence:* Eric W. Hickey, *Serial Murderers and Their Victims*, 7th ed. (Belmont, Calif.: Wadsworth Publishing, 2015), 142; S. Tallichet and C. Hensley, "Exploring the link between recurrent acts of childhood and adolescent animal cruelty and subsequent violent crime," *Criminal Justice Review* 29 (2004): 304–16.

p. 117   *"Manipulation. Domination. Control . . . These are the three watchwords of violent serial offenders":* John Douglas and Mark Olshaker, *Mind Hunter: Inside the FBI's Elite Serial Crime Unit* (New York: Pocket Books, 1995), 108.

p. 117   *Sigmund Freud noted . . . "The child does not yet show any trace of the pride which afterwards moves the adult . . .":* As cited in F. Ascione, *Children and Animals: Exploring the Roots of Kindness and Cruelty* (West Lafayette, IN: Purdue University Press 2005), 70.

p. 118   *Seven-to-ten-year-old children named on average two companion animals each:* C. Siebert, "The Animal-Cruelty Syndrome," *The New York Times*, June 7, 2010.

p. 119   *Psychologist Dr. Randall Lockwood . . . "are often driven to suppress their own feelings of kindness":* C. Siebert, "The Animal-Cruelty Syndrome," *The New York Times*, June 7, 2010.

p. 120 *Both girls and boys abuse animals:* F. Ascione, *Children and Animals: Exploring the Roots of Kindness and Cruelty* (West Lafayette, IN: Purdue University Press 2005), 70.

p. 120 *One theory is that witnessing infrequent or milder forms of animal abuse may lead to greater empathy:* B. Daly and L. Morton, "Empathic correlates of witnessing the inhumane killing of an animal: An investigation of single and multiple exposures," *Society & Animals* 16 (2008): 243–55.

p. 120 *The younger children are when they witness animal abuse . . . more likely they are to abuse animals themselves:* C. Hensley and S. Tallichet, "Learning to be cruel? Exploring the onset and frequency of animal cruelty," *International Journal of Offender Therapy and Comparative Criminology* 49 (2005): 37–47.

p. 120 *Children who grow up witnessing animals abused or neglected:* S. Vollum, J. Buffington-Vollum, and D. Longmire, "Moral disengagement and attitudes about violence toward animals," *Society & Animals* 12 (2004): 209–35.

p. 121 *Those who abuse animals or other humans are frequently from troubled families:* F. Tapia, "Children who are cruel to animals," *Child Psychiatry and Human Development* 2 (1971): 70–77; C. Siebert, "The Animal-Cruelty Syndrome," *The New York Times*, June 7, 2010; F. Ascione, "Animal abuse and youth violence," *Juvenile Justice Bulletin* (September 2001): 1–15.

p. 128 *A study looked at the most sadistic serial killers:* J. Levin, A. Arluke, "Reducing the Link's False Positive Problem," in A. Linzey (ed.), *The Link between Animal Abuse and Human Violence* (Eastbourne, United Kingdom: Sussex Academic Press, 2009), 164–71.

p. 134 *Margaret Mead noted: "One of the most dangerous things that can happen to a child is to kill or torture an animal and not be held responsible":* As cited in Eric W. Hickey, *Serial Murderers and Their Victims*, 7th ed. (Belmont, CA: Wadsworth Publishing, 2015), 142.

p. 135 *Piers Beirne argues, empathy for animals and humans is probably strongly linked:* Piers Beirne, *Confronting Animal Abuse. Law, Criminology, and Human-Animal Relationships* (Lanham, MD: Rowman & Littlefield Publishers, 2009), 187.

p. 136 *On November 23, 1996 . . . police arrested two McNary High School students for bludgeoning to death a tabby cat:* Kaly Soto, "Teen Accused in Abuse of Cat Remains on Team," *Statesman Journal* (Salem, OR), November 25, 1996; Janet Davies, "Teens Accused of Bludgeoning Cat Are Indicted on Felony Animal Abuse," *Statesman Journal* (Salem, OR), December 5, 1996.

p. 137 *Smythe told reporters: "Let's put this in perspective":* Kaly Soto, "Teen Accused in Abuse of Cat Remains on Team," *Statesman Journal* (Salem, OR), November 25, 1996.

p. 137 *Among the letters was Jesperson's:* Keith Jesperson, "Animal Abuse Should Set Off Alarm, Killer Says," *Statesman Journal* (Salem, OR), December 7, 1996.

FIVE: IT'S JUST AN ANIMAL

p. 141 *"Crime doesn't happen in a vacuum":* R. Simmons, "Dog Eat Dog: The Bloodthirsty Underworld of Dogfighting," *OC Dog Newspaper*, December 26, 2005.

p. 144   *A study of 261 incarcerated . . . found that 43 percent committed animal cruelty:* S. Tallichet, C. Hensley, A. O'Bryan, et al., "Targets for cruelty: Demographic and situational factors affecting the type of animal abused," *Criminal Justice Studies* 18 (2005): 173–82.

p. 144   *Another study found animal cruelty to be especially prevalent among the most violent criminals:* K. Schiff, D. Louw, and F. Ascione, "Animal relations in childhood and later violent behavior against humans," *Acta Criminologica* 12 (1999): 77–86.

p. 144   *The Massachusetts Society for the Prevention of Cruelty to Animals:* A. Arluke, J. Levin, C. Luke, et al., "The relationship of animal abuse to violence and other forms of antisocial behavior," *Journal of Interpersonal Violence* 14 (1999): 963–75.

p. 144   *The Chicago Police Department found similar results:* B. Degenhardt, *Statistical Summary of Offenders Charged with Crimes against Companion Animals July 2001–July 2005*, Chicago Police Department.

p. 144   *The FBI recently made major changes to how it tracks animal abuse:* Lisa Gutierrez, "FBI Begins Tackling Animal Abuse Like It Does Murder and Rape," *Kansas City Star*, January 26, 2016; Colby Itkowitz, "A Big Win for Animals: The FBI Now Tracks Animal Abuse Like It Tracks Homicides," *Washington Post*, January 6, 2016.

p. 145   *In 2007, Vick was convicted of the brutal treatment and killing of dogs:* C. Brown, "Dogfighting Charges Filed against Falcons' Vick," *The New York Times*, July 18, 2007; M. Maske, "Falcons' Vick Indicted in Dogfighting Case," *Washington Post*, July 18, 2007; Associated Press, "Michael Vick Sentenced to 23 Months in Jail for Role in Dogfighting Conspiracy," December 10, 2007.

p. 147   *A metabolic bone disease due to a lack of calcium in the diet:* Kenneth A. Harkewicz, "Three Common Ailments of Tortoises in Captivity," *Reptile Magazine*, http://www.reptilesmagazine.com/Reptile-Health/Disease-Management/Three -Common-Ailments-Of-Tortoises-In-Captivity/, accessed December 1, 2017; Mary Hopson, "Metabolic Bone Disease," The Turtle Puddle, https://www .turtlepuddle.org/health/mbd.html; Richard W. Woerpel and Walter J. Rosskopf Jr., "Care of Water Turtles," Chadwell Animal Hospital, http://chadwell animalhospital.com/care-water-turtles/, accessed December 1, 2018.

p. 150   *The 2015 appeals case concerned defendant Curtis Basile and a dog under his care:* People v. Basile, 2015 NY Slip Op 05623.

p. 151   *In addition to other crimes, animal cruelty is associated with antisocial behaviors:* R. Gleyzer, A. Felthous, and C. Holzer III, "Animal cruelty and psychiatric disorders," *Journal of the American Academy of Psychiatry and the Law* 30, no. 2 (2002): 257–65.

p. 151   *Using the results from the National Epidemiological Survey on Alcohol and Related Conditions:* M. Vaughn, Q. Fu, M. DeLisi, et al., "Correlates of cruelty to animals in the United States: Results from the national epidemiologic survey on alcohol and related conditions," *Journal of Psychiatric Research* 43 (2009): 1213–18.

p. 152   *The researchers interviewed 193 adolescents entering outpatient substance abuse treatment centers:* M. Gordon, T. Kinlock, and R. Battjes, "Correlates of early substance abuse and crime among adolescents entering outpatient substance abuse treatment," *American Journal of Drug and Alcohol Abuse* 30 (2004): 39–59.

p. 152 *Animal cruelty . . . occurs disproportionately in households with interhuman violence:* S. Degue and D. Dilillo, "Is animal cruelty a "red flag" for family violence? Investigating co-occurring violence toward children, partners, and pets," *Journal of Interpersonal Violence* 24 (2009): 1035–56; J. Quinlisk, "Animal Abuse and Family Violence," in F. Ascione and P. Arkow (eds.), *Child Abuse, Domestic Violence, and Animal Abuse: Linking the Circles of Compassion for Prevention and Intervention* (West Lafayette, IN: Purdue University Press, 1999), 168–75; M. Volant, J. Johnson, E. Gullone, et al., "The relationship between domestic violence and animal abuse: An Australian study," *Journal of Interpersonal Violence* 23, no. 9 (2008): 1277–95; C. Simmons and P. Lehmann, "Exploring the link between pet abuse and controlling behaviors in violent relationships," *Journal of Interpersonal Violence* 22 (2007): 1211–22.

p. 152 *60 percent of those who either witnessed or committed violence against animals:* F. Walsh, "Human-animal bonds II: The role of pets in family systems and family therapy," *Family Process* 48 (2009): 481–99.

p. 152 *In a study in North Carolina, investigators compared police reports . . . with animal cruelty reports:* "UNCC research links animal abuse, crimes against people," *Community Policing Digest* 3 (1998): 3–4.

p. 156 *Oregon says an animal is "any nonhuman mammal, bird, reptile, amphibian or fish":* 2017 ORS 167.310, "Definitions for ORS 167.310 to 167.351," https://www.oregonlaws.org/ors/167.310, accessed November 29, 2017.

p. 156 *Missouri defines them as "every living vertebrate except a human being":* "Vernon's Annotated Missouri Cruelty to Animal Statutes. Title XXXVIII. Crimes and Punishment; Peace Officers and Public Defenders. Chapter 578. Miscellaneous Offenses," Michigan State University College of Law, Animal Legal and Historical Center, https://www.animallaw.info/statute/mo-cruelty-consolidated-cruelty-statutes.

p. 156 *Texas's definition:* Texas Penal Code § 42.092. Cruelty to Nonlivestock Animals. https://codes.findlaw.com/tx/penal-code/penal-sect-42-092.html.

p. 156 *The AWA is the "only Federal law in the United States that regulates the treatment of animals":* US Department of Agriculture, *Animal Welfare Act and Animal Welfare Regulations*, https://www.aphis.usda.gov/animal_welfare/downloads/AC_BlueBook_AWA_FINAL_2017_508comp.pdf, accessed November 29, 2017.

p. 156 *New York defines animals:* New York Agriculture and Markets, Article 26, Law § 350–380*2, https://www.nysenate.gov/legislation/laws/AGM/A26.

p. 157 *The penalty for a misdemeanor:* Stacy Wolf, "Animal Cruelty: The Law in New York," ASPCA, 2003, http://www.potsdamhumanesociety.org/files/cruelty/ASPCA_NYlaws.pdf, accessed June 5, 2018.

p. 157 *So is potentially any "domesticated animal normally maintained in or near the household of the owner or person who cares for such other domesticated animal":* New York Agriculture and Markets, Article 26, Law § 350–380*2, https://www.nysenate.gov/legislation/laws/AGM/A26.

p. 168   *Thanks to a million-dollar donation from Bob Barker:* U.Va. News Staff, "Bob Barker Donates $1 Million for Creation of Animal Law Program at U.Va.," *UVA Today,* January 13, 2009, https://news.virginia.edu/content /bob-barker-donates-1-million-creation-animal-law-program-uva.

p. 168   *In a 2013 divorce proceeding in New York:* Shannon Louise TRAVIS, v. Trisha Bridget MURRAY, 977 N.Y.S.2d 621 (Sup. Ct. 2013), Michigan State University College of Law, Animal Legal and Historical Center, accessed December 1, 2017. https://www.animallaw.info/case/travis-v-murray; Law Offices of Jay D. Raxenberg, "Who Gets Doggy Custody?," https://www.divorcelawlongisland. com/2014/02/19/who-gets-doggy-custody/, accessed June 5, 2018.

p. 168   *In January 2016, Alaska became the first state to enact "pet custody" legislation:* Christopher Mele, "When Couples Divorce, Who Gets to Keep the Dog? (Or Cat.)," *The New York Times,* March 23, 2017.

p. 169   *In 2017, police in Boston urged the public's help in locating a lost dog:* Emily Sweeney, "State Police Searching for Missing Dog at Logan Airport," *Boston Globe,* June 14, 2017; and Travis Anderson, "Dog Spotted Last Week on the Pike Still Missing; Cops Seeking Public's Help in Locating the Puppy," *Boston Globe,* October 23, 2017.

p. 169   *In 2013, attorney and president of the Nonhuman Rights Project:* David Grimm, "Judge Rules Research Chimps Are Not 'Legal Persons,'" *Science,* July 30, 2015.

p. 169   *Two of the chimpanzees, Tommy and Kiko, were privately owned:* Our Clients, Nonhuman Rights Project, https://www.nonhumanrights.org/litigation/, accessed December 1, 2017.

p. 169   *Jaffe expressed sympathy for Wise's arguments:* Matter of Nonhuman Rights Project, Inc. v. Stanley, 2015 NY Slip Op 25257, 49 Misc 3d 746 (Sup. Ct. New York County 2015).

p. 171   *The terrier, he said, was "acting irrational" and scratched his arms:* Leigh Egan, "Man Says He Stabbed Pet Dog in Self-Defense, but Prosecutor Says Suspect Only Had Small, Minor Scratches," Crime Online, August 1, 2017, https://www .crimeonline.com/2017/08/01/man-says-he-stabbed-pet-dog-in-self-defense -but-prosecutor-says-suspect-only-had-small-minor-scratches/; Rebecca Rosenberg, "Man Who Viciously Killed Pet Dog Now Volunteers at Animal Charity," *New York Post,* July 31, 2017, https://nypost.com/2017/07/31 /man-who-viciously-killed-pet-dog-now-volunteers-at-animal-charity/.

SIX: DO WE HURT WITH ANIMALS?

p. 174   *Each year, more than 64 billion animals are raised and killed for food globally:* Aysha Akhtar, "The need to include animal protection in public health policies," *Journal of Public Health Policies* 34 (2013): 549–59; A. Akhtar, M. Greger, H. Ferdowsian, et al., "Health professionals' roles in animal agriculture, climate change, and human health," *American Journal of Preventive Medicine* 36 (2009): 182–87.

p. 174   *The transformation of animal agriculture is so dramatic:* J. Pearson, M. Salman, B. Jebarak, et al., "Global risks of infectious animal diseases," Council for Agricultural Science and Technology, *Issue Paper* no. 28 (2005).

p. 175   *This unprecedented change in the human relationship with animals:* A. Akhtar, *Animals and Public Health: Why Treating Animals Better Is Critical to Human Welfare* (Hampshire, United Kingdom: Palgrave Macmillan, 2012), 86–131.

p. 175   *Presented data showing how animal agriculture . . . and infectious diseases like salmonella, E. coli, and bird flus:* J. Leibler, J. Otte, D. Roland-Holst, et al., "Industrial food animal production and global health risks: Exploring the ecosystems and economics of avian influenza," *EcoHealth* 6 (2009): 58–70; Food and Agriculture Organization of the United Nations, *Livestock's Long Shadow: Environmental Issues and Options,* 2006; A. Akhtar, M. Greger, H. Ferdowsian, et al., "Health professionals' role in animal agriculture, climate change, and human health," *American Journal of Preventive Medicine* 36 (2009): 182–87.

p. 175   *The evidence is so strong, the American Public Health Association called for a moratorium on factory farms:* K. Thu (ed.), "Understanding the Impacts of Large-Scale Swine Production," Proceedings from an Interdisciplinary Scientific Workshop (Des Moines, IA, June 29–30, 1995); Food and Agriculture Organization of the United Nations, *Livestock's Long Shadow: Environmental Issues and Options,* 2006; American Public Health Association, Precautionary Moratorium on New Concentrated Animal Feed Operations, Policy no. 20037, November 18, 2003.

p. 176   *The undercover investigators videotaped farm employees beating sick chickens with spiked clubs:* Jonathan Chew, "Ex-McDonald's Suppliers Plead Guilty to Abusing Chickens," *Fortune,* October 30, 2015.

p. 176   *"Ag-gag" laws . . . criminalize journalists and animal protection groups:* Richard A. Oppel Jr., "Taping of Farm Cruelty Is Becoming the Crime," *The New York Times,* April 6, 2013.

p. 176   *Ag-gag "illustrates just how desperate these industries are to keep this information from getting out":* Cody Carlson, "The Ag Gag Laws: Hiding Factory Farm Abuses from Public Scrutiny," *The Atlantic,* March 20, 2012.

p. 177   *Methods that clearly don't work, given how often bird and swine flu epidemics sweep across industrial farms in the United States:* J. Graham, J. Leibler, L. Price, et al., "The animal-human interface and infectious disease in industrial food animal production: Rethinking biosecurity and biocontainment," *Public Health Reports* 123 (2008): 282–99; For information on one of the more recent outbreaks, see Associated Press, "Bird Flu Outbreak Is Nation's Worst in Years," March 22, 2017.

p. 179   *Birds' beaks are sensitive, highly innervated and able to feel pain and other sensations:* Humane Society of the United States, An HSUS Report: The Welfare of Animals in the Egg Industry, http://www.humanesociety.org/assets/pdfs/farm/welfare_egg.pdf, accessed December 13, 2017.

p. 182   *Psychologist Joshua Correll studied how skin color affects real-life decisions:* J. Correll, B. Park, J. Judd, et al., "The influence of stereotypes on decision to shoot," *European Journal of Social Psychology* 37 (2007): 1102–07.

p. 182   *There is mounting evidence that empathy can be modulated by our categorization of another:* J. Decety and M. Svetlova, "Putting together phylogenetic and ontogenetic perspectives on empathy," *Developmental Cognitive Neuroscience* 2 (2012): 1–24; J. Decety, "The neuroevolution of empathy," *Annals of the New York Academy of Sciences* 1231 (2011): 35–45.

p. 182   *A study published in 2011 . . . showed that how we identify social groups:* M. Cikara, M. Botvinick, and S. Fiske, "Us versus them: Social identity shapes neural responses to intergroup competition and harm," *Psychological Science* 22 (2011): 306–13.

p. 182   *Portraying the "out-group" as animal-like and less capable of emotions:* A. Bandura, "Selective moral disengagement in the exercise of moral agency," *Journal of Moral Education* 31 (2002): 101–19.

p. 183   *A study conducted at Brock University:* K. Costello and G. Hodson, "Exploring the roots of dehumanization: The role of animal-human similarity in promoting immigrant humanization," *Group Processes & Intergroup Relations* 13 (2009): 3–22.

p. 183   *Robert Burton provides a compelling case that most of what we think we know is not based on conscious rational thought:* Robert A. Burton, *On Being Certain: Believing You Are Right Even When You're Not* (New York: St. Martin's Press, 2008).

p. 183   *"The more committed we are to a belief, the harder it is to relinquish . . .":* Robert A. Burton, *On Being Certain: Believing You Are Right Even When You're Not* (New York: St. Martin's Press, 2008), 12.

p. 184   *Today, though, we don't need to hurt animals:* For information on options to animal research, see: Wyss Institute, "Human Organs-on-Chips," https://wyss .harvard.edu/technology/human-organs-on-chips/; C. Gohd, "EPA Releases Strategy to Reduce Animal Testing on Vertebrates," Futurism.com, March 15, 2018; A. Akhtar, "The flaws and human harms of animal testing," *Cambridge Quarterly of Healthcare Ethics* 4 (2015): 407–19; Barnaby J. Feder, "Saving the Animals: New Ways to Test Products," *The New York Times*, September 12, 2007; Christiana Reedy, "Animal Testing Isn't Working but Better Alternatives Are on the Way," Futurism.com, July 10, 2017.

p. 185   *A group of psychologists found that the simple identification of animals as "food" has a significant effect on how we think of those animals:* B. Bratanova, S. Loughman, and B. Bastian, "The effect of categorization as food on the perceived moral standing of animals," *Appetite* 57, no. 1 (2011): 193–96.

p. 185   *People have started to learn that pigs can be pessimistic or optimistic . . . and rats enjoy being tickled:* L. Asher, M. Friel, K. Griffin, et al., "Mood and personality interact to determine cognitive biases in pigs," *Biology Letters* 12 (2016): 20160402, DOI: 10.1098/rsbl.2016.0402; K. Hagen and D. Broom, "Emotional reactions to learning in cattle," *Applied Animal Behavior Science* 85 (2004): 203–13; Emma Young, "Only Hungry Chickens Heed the Dinner Call," *New Scientist*, November 15, 2006; B. Yang, P. Zhang, K. Huang, et al., "Daytime birth and postbirth behavior of wild *Rhinopithecus roxellana* in the Qinling Mountains of China," *Primates* 57 (2016): 155–60; Emily Underwood, "Watch These Ticklish Rats Laugh and Jump for Joy," *Science*, November 10, 2016.

p. 185   *A seminal study looked at how different ways of presenting information influence altruism:* D. Small, G. Lowenstein, and P. Slovic, "Can Insight Breed Callousness? The Impact of Learning about Identifiable Victim Effect on Sympathy," University of Pennsylvania, 2005.

p. 185   *A study looking at people's willingness to eat meat:* J. Kunst and S. Hohle, "Meat eaters by disassociation: How we present, prepare and talk about meat increases willingness to eat meat by reducing empathy and disgust," *Appetite* 105 (2016): 758–74.

p. 188   *According to the US Department of Agriculture . . . "producers must demonstrate to the Agency that the poultry has been allowed access to the outside":* United States Department of Agriculture, Meat and Poultry Labeling Terms, https://www.fsis .usda.gov/wps/wcm/connect/e2853601-3edb-45d3-90dc-1bef17b7f277/Meat_and _Poultry_Labeling_Terms.pdf?MOD=AJPERES, accessed December 15, 2017.

p. 188   *The definition of outside is shaky and up to interpretation by the producers:* Francis Lam, "What Do 'Free Range,' 'Organic' and Other Chicken Labels Really Mean?" Salon, January 20, 2011.

p. 188   *The organic label is even more vague:* Lynne Curry, "Certified 'Organic' Livestock Are Supposed to Have Outdoor Access: In Practice, They Don't," *New Food Economy*, November 9, 2017, https://newfoodeconomy.org/usda-organic -animal-welfare-rule-livestock-poultry-practices/, accessed March 13, 2018.

p. 189   *As biologist Jonathan Balcombe wrote "Just thirty years ago it was scientific heresy to ascribe such emotions . . .":* Jonathan Balcombe, *Second Nature: The Inner Lives of Animals* (New York: Palgrave Macmillan, 2010), 4.

p. 192   *Psychologist Rachel MacNair first proposed that the act of inflicting trauma on another causes:* Rachel MacNair, *Perpetration-Induced Traumatic Stress: The Psychological Consequences of Killing* (New York: Authors Choice Press, 2005).

p. 193   *Analysis of WWII soldiers found that most soldiers did not fire their weapons:* Dave Grossman, *On Killing: The Psychological Cost of Learning to Kill in War and Society* (New York: Back Bay Books, 1995).

p. 194   *Slaughterhouses have high employee turnover rates:* A. Fitzgerald, "A social history of the slaughterhouse: From inception to contemporary implications," *Human Ecology Review* 17 (2010): 58–69.

p. 194   *Two psychologists who conducted in-depth interviews with slaughterhouse employees noted:* K. Victor, A. Barnard, and D. Phil, "Slaughtering for a living: A hermeneutic phenomenological perspective on the well-being of slaughterhouse employees," *International Journal of Qualitative Studies on Health and Well-Being* 11 (2016): 10.3402/qhw.v11.30266.

p. 194   *In one confession, he describes a night on the kill floor:* Virgil Butler, "A Night in Tyson's Hell," *The Cyberactivist* blog, September 23, 2003, http://cyberactivist .blogspot.com/2003/09/, accessed December 17, 2017.

p. 195   *"The industry has become quite adept at recruiting the most marginalized populations that are quite vulnerable":* Jean Lian, "Silence on the Floor. The Recent Meat Recall at XL Foods, Inc. in Brooks, Alberta Is Not Wanting in Superlatives," *OHS Canada Magazine*, January 10, 2013.

p. 195   *Temple Grandin found that the most common psychological approach:* T. Grandin, "Commentary: Behavior of slaughter plant and auction employees toward animals," *Anthrozoos* 1 (1988): 205–13.

p. 195   *"The worst thing, worse than the physical danger, is the emotional toll . . .":* Gail Eisnitz, *Slaughterhouse: The Shocking Story of Greed, Neglect, and Inhumane Treatment Inside the U.S. Meat Industry* (Amherst, NY: Prometheus Books, 1997), 87.

p. 196   *Signs of PITS . . . occur frequently in slaughterhouse workers:* J. Dillard, "A slaughterhouse nightmare: psychological harm suffered by slaughterhouse employees and the possibility of redress through legal reform," *Georgetown Journal on Poverty Law & Policy* 15 (2008): 391–408; Gail Eisnitz, *Slaughterhouse: The Shocking Story of Greed, Neglect, and Inhumane Treatment Inside the U.S. Meat Industry* (Amherst, NY: Prometheus Books, 1997).

p. 196   *A large study of almost one thousand employees in Brazil:* C. Hutz, C. Zanon, and H. Brum Neto, "Adverse working conditions and mental illness in poultry slaughterhouses in southern Brazil," *Psicologia: Reflexão e Crítica* 26, no. 2 (2013): 296–304.

p. 196   *Among employees who routinely kill animals in shelters and laboratories:* V. Rohlf and P. Bennett, "Perpetration-induced traumatic stress in persons who euthanize nonhuman animals in surgeries, animal shelters, and laboratories," *Society & Animals* 13 (2005): 201–19.

p. 196   *Although it's been a hush topic:* Helen Kelly, "Overcoming Compassion Fatigue in the Biomedical Lab," *ALN Magazine*, August 4, 2015; Andy Coghlan, "Lab Animal Careers Suffer in Silence," *New Scientist*, March 29, 2008; "The Double Trauma of Animal Experimentation," *Queen's Animal Defence* blog, April 12, 2013.

p. 196   *A team of former laboratory workers created a support group for researchers traumatized by their work:* See *Laboratory Primate Advocacy Group* blog, http://www.lpag.org.

p. 198   *Ninety-seven percent of pigs are imprisoned in factory farms:* Lynne Rossetto Kasper, "Inside Factory Farms: Where 97% of Pigs Are Raised," *The Splendid Table*, podcast, May 6, 2015, https://www.splendidtable.org/story/inside-the-factory-farm-where-97-of-us-pigs-are-raised, accessed December 17, 2017.

p. 199   *A team of sociologists examined whether socially sanctioned violence can "spill over" into other spheres of life:* L. Baron, M. Straus, and D. Jaffee, "Legitimate violence, Violent attitudes, and rape: A test of the cultural spillover theory," *Annals of the New York Academy of Sciences* 528 (1988): 79–110.

p. 200   *Finney County . . . experienced a 130 percent increase in violent crimes:* Donald Stull and Michael Broadway, *Slaughterhouse Blues: The Meat and Poultry Industry in North America* (Toronto: Wadsworth, 2004), 135–42.

p. 200   *"I've got the short temper . . .":* K. Victor, A. Barnard, and D. Phil, "Slaughtering for a living: A hermeneutic phenomenological perspective on the well-being of slaughterhouse employees," *International Journal of Qualitative Studies on Health and Well-Being* 11 (2016): 10.3402/qhw.v11.30266.

p. 201   *"Every sticker I know carries a gun . . . you're killing several thousand beings a day":* Gail Eisnitz, *Slaughterhouse: The Shocking Story of Greed, Neglect, and Inhumane*

Treatment Inside the U.S. Meat Industry (Amherst, NY: Prometheus Books, 1997), 88.

p. 201   *To test the Sinclair Effect, Fitzgerald compiled information from the FBI's Uniform Crime Report database:* A. Fitzgerald, L. Kalof, and T. Dietz, "Slaughterhouses and increased crime rates: An empirical analysis of the spillover from 'The Jungle' into the surrounding community," *Organization & Environment* 22 (2009): 158–84.

p. 202   *A more recent study in Australia tested levels of aggression in slaughterhouse workers:* E. Richards, T. Signal, and N. Taylor, "A different cut? Comparing attitudes toward animals and propensity for aggression within two primary industry cohorts—farmers and meatworkers," *Society & Animals* 21 (2013): 395–413; Tory Shepherd, "Slaughterhouse Workers Are More Likely to Be Violent, Study Shows," News.com.au, January 24, 2013, http://www.news.com.au/national /slaughterhouse-workers-are-more-likely-to-be-violent-study-shows/news-story/f16165f66f38eb04a289eb8bd7f7f273, accessed December 17, 2017.

p. 205   *In 1981, a psychologist published a review of the emotional reactions of therapists who worked with Holocaust survivors:* Aaron Reuben, "When PTSD Is Contagious," *The Atlantic* December 14, 2015.

p. 205   *A survey by* The Guardian *revealed that almost 80 percent of humanitarian workers:* Holly Young, "Guardian Research Suggests Mental Health Crisis Among Aid Workers," *The Guardian*, November 23, 2015.

p. 205   *Vicarious traumatization causes high risk of burnout:* C. Pross, "Burnout, vicarious traumatization and its prevention," *Torture* 16 (2006): 1–9.

p. 205   *The more time journalists spend combing through violent images and videos:* A. Feinstein, B. Audet, and E. Waknine, "Witnessing images of extreme violence: a psychological study of journalists in the newsroom," *The Royal Society of Medicine* 5 (2013): 1–7.

p. 205   *It came, then, as a real surprise when some investigators learned that drone pilots suffer:* James Dao, "Drone Pilots Are Found to Get Stress Disorders as Much as Those in Combat Do," *The New York Times*, February 22, 2013; Julie Watson, "Emotional Toll Taxes Military Drone Operators Too," Associated Press, September 29, 2014; Dan Gettinger, "Burdens of War: PTSD and Drone Crews," *Center for the Study of the Drone at Bard College*, April 21, 2014; Denise Chow, "Drone Wars: Pilots Reveal Debilitating Stress Beyond Virtual Battlefield," *Science*, November 5, 2013; Pratap Chatterjee, "A Chilling New Post-Traumatic Stress Disorder: Why Drone Pilots Are Quitting in Record Numbers," Salon, March 6, 2015.

p. 206   *Defined as "perpetrating, failing to prevent, bearing witness to, or learning about acts that transgress deeply held moral beliefs and expectations":* Laura Copland, Staff Perspective: On moral Injury. Uniformed Services University, https://deploy mentpsych.org/blog/staff-perspective-moral-injury, accessed June 10, 2018; B. Litz, N. Stein, E. Delaney, et al., "Moral injury and moral repair in war veterans: a preliminary model and intervention strategy," *Clinical Psychology Review* 29 (2009): 695–706.

p. 206   *"A predator [drone] pilot has been watching his target[s] . . ."*: Pratap Chatterjee, "A Chilling New Post-Traumatic Stress Disorder: Why Drone Pilots Are Quitting in Record Numbers," Salon, March 6, 2015.

p. 206   *Studies on media exposure to tragedies like the Boston Marathon bombings and 9/11 show*: E. Holman, D. Garfin, and R. Silver, "Media's role in broadcasting acute stress following the Boston Marathon bombings," *Proceedings of the National Academy of Sciences of the United States of America* 11 (2014): 93–98; M. Otto, A. Henin, D. Hirshfeld-Becker, et al., "Posttraumatic stress disorder symptoms following media exposure to tragic events: Impact of 9/11 on children at risk for anxiety disorders," *Journal of Anxiety Disorders* 21 (2007): 888–902.

PART THREE: JOINING WITH ANIMALS
SEVEN: STANDING WITH ANIMALS

p. 211   *In August 2004, six cows . . . made a dash for freedom*: Mark Kawar, "Cows Make a Stand: Freedom Is Fleeting for Cattle in Plant Escape," *Omaha World Herald*, August 5, 2004.

p. 212   *News spread rapidly among the slaughterhouse employees*: Timothy Pachirat, *Every Twelve Seconds* (New Haven, CT: Yale University Press, 2011), 2.

p. 218   *I first meet James Guiliani at his pet store*: James's story comes from a mixture of personal communication and excerpts from James Guiliani and Charlie Stella, *Dogfella: How an Abandoned Dog Named Bruno Turned This Mobster's Life Around* (Boston: Da Capo Press, 2015).

p. 224   *It can be an emotional response to someone else's distress that results in anger rather than grief*: M. Hoffman, "Empathy and Prosocial Activism," in N. Eisenberg, J. Reykowski, and E. Staub (eds.), *Social and Moral Values: Individual and Societal Perspectives* (Hillsdale, NJ: Lawrence Erlbaum Associates, Inc., 1989), 65–85.

p. 224   *College students . . . who feel more empathetic anger concerning various social issues*: ASU News, "Empathetic Anger Is a Motivator for Student Advocacy, May 7, 2014, http://www.news.appstate.edu/2014/05/07/empathic-anger/, accessed January 12, 2017.

p. 225   *Tug too hard on our heartstrings, though, and that can lead to ineffective altruism*: For discussion concerning empathy, morality, and altruism, see: J. Decety and J. Cowell, "Empathy, justice, and moral behavior," *AJOB Neuroscience* 6 (2015): 3–14; Peter Singer, "Against Empathy," *Boston Review*, August 26, 2014; Caroline Mimbs Nyce, "Against Empathy, Cont.," *The Atlantic*, March 25, 2016; Nathan J. Robinson, "Empathy: Probably a Good Thing," *Current Affairs*, October 20, 2017.

p. 226   *For these and other reasons the use of empathy as a moral guide . . . is often criticized*: Peter Singer, "Against Empathy," *Boston Review*, August 24, 2014; and Caroline Mimbs Nyce, "Against Empathy, Cont.," *The Atlantic*, March 25, 2016.

p. 228   *"One can't truly empathize with the vulnerability and struggle of another . . ."*: Jeremy Rifkin, *The Empathic Civilization* (New York: Penguin Group, 2009), 159.

p. 228   *Business leaders with good self-awareness . . . have more committed employees and are more successful*: Leslie Brokaw, "Self-Awareness: A Key to Better

Leadership," *MIT Sloan Management Review*, May 7, 2012; Chinwe Esimai, "Great Leadership Starts with Self-Awareness," *Forbes*, February 15, 2018; K. Hofslett Kopperud, Ø. Martinsen, I. Sut, et al., "Engaging leaders in the eyes of the beholder: On the relationship between transformational leadership, work engagement, service climate, and self-other agreement," *Journal of Leadership and Organizational Studies* 21 (2013): 29–42.

p. 230   *Syrian Association for Rescuing Animals (SARA) who risk their lives every day "for the outcasts, for the needy, for the forgotten ones"*: Personal communication.

p. 230   *And like the Cat Man of Aleppo*: Rachel Nuwer, "Syria's Cat Calamity: War Is Hell for Ppets, Too," *Newsweek*, December 16, 2015; Nadim Salem and Ammar Cheikh Omar, "'Cat Man of Aleppo' Forced to Start Again—from Scratch," NBC News, May 14, 2017.

p. 231   *But Matsumura . . . returned and has not left since*: Sarah Ridley, "Last Man Standing. Fukushima Animal Lover Stayed Behind After Nuclear Disaster to Feed Abandoned Pets," *Daily Mirror* (UK), March 15, 2015.

p. 231   *He's been tested for radiation contamination and the results*: Kyung Lah, "Resident Defiant in Japan's Exclusion Zone," CNN, January 27, 2012.

p. 231   *The worst scene he remembered was of a mother cow who was just skin and bones*: Kyung Lah, "Resident Defiant in Japan's Exclusion Zone," CNN, January 27, 2012.

p. 231   *"I couldn't leave the animals behind"*: Ema O'Connor, "This Man Lives Alone in a Radioactive Town to Care for the Abandoned Animals," Buzzfeed, March 19, 2015.

EIGHT: FRIENDS

p. 236   *The FFA is the largest technical and career student-education program in the United States*: Future Farmers of America, https://www.ffa.org/about/media-center/ffa-fact-sheet, accessed March 3, 2018.

p. 238   *The FFA's mission is to make "a positive difference in the lives of students . . ."*: Future Farmers of America, https://www.ffa.org/home, accessed March 3, 2018.

p. 260   *We tell ourselves animals don't laugh . . . don't use language*: J. Panksepp and J. Burgdorf, "'Laughing'" Rats and the Evolutionary Antecedents of Human Joy?" *Physiology and Behavior* 79 (2003): 533–47; L. Asher, M. Friel, K. Griffin, et al., "Mood and personality interact to determine cognitive biases in pigs," *Biology Letters* 12 (2016) 20160402; DOI: 10.1098/rsbl.2016.0402; Ed Yong, "Scientists Have Found Another Crow That Uses Tools," *The Atlantic*, September 14, 2016; N. Clayton, T. Bussey, and A. Dickinson, "Can animals recall the past and plan for the future?" *Nature Reviews Neuroscience* 4 (2003): 685–91; R. Rugani, L. Fontanari, E. Simoni, et al., "Arithmetic in newborn chicks," *Proceedings of the Royal Society B* 276 (2009): 2451–60; Natalie Angier, "Nut? What Nut? The Squirrel Outwits to Survive," *The New York Times*, July 5, 2010; D. Langford, S. Crager, Z. Shehzad, et al., "Social modulation of pain as evidence for empathy in mice," *Science* 312 (2006): 1967–70; Charles C. Choi, "Chimps Pass on Culture Like Humans Do," *Live Science*, June 7, 2007; Shaoni Bhattacharya, "Elephants May Pay Homage to Dead Relatives," *New Scientist*,

October 26, 2005; "Voles console stressed friends," *Nature* 529 (2016): 441; Ferris Jabr, "Can Prairie Dogs Talk?" *The New York Times*, May 12, 2017.

p. 261   *"Although humans inherit a biological bias that permits them to feel anger . . .":* Jerome Kagan, "On the Case for Kindness," in Anne Harrington and Arthur Zajonc (eds.), *The Dalai Lama at MIT* (Cambridge, MA: Harvard University Press, 2006).

p. 261   *Animals such as wolves . . . are more popular today than they once were:* K. George, K. Slagle, R. Wilson, et al., "Changes in attitudes toward animals in the United States from 1978 to 2014," *Biological Conservation* 201 (2016): 237–42.

Acknowledgments

First off, I want to thank all of the folks who opened up their lives and shared their stories with me. While most of the names in the book are true, some have been changed to protect identities. I have had a wonderful agent, Beth Vesel, who provided great insight on how to improve the book. Jessica Case, my editor, has been incredibly supportive of the book from the beginning and gave me a chance that many other editors, who argued that there was no audience for a book like this, wouldn't. Jessica knew better. I am also lucky to have a publicist, Tanya Farrell, who not only loves the book, but also is 100 percent behind its central messages.

This book took five years from a glimmer of an idea to completion. One of my dearest friends, Greg Goodale, has been with me throughout, acting as a sounding board, exploring ideas with me. He was always there, giving me the confidence boost to continue when I most needed it. No one could ask for a better friend. My sister Jabeen, a writer herself, helped me punch up the book. Juliette White had the miserable task of transcribing hours and hours of interviews for me.

My husband Patrick and my feline Silos are the two reasons why I love being home more than anywhere else in the world. Patrick is such a fun, amusing person. Living with him is like living with the casts of *Monty Python*, *Seinfeld*, and *It's a Mad, Mad, Mad, Mad World* all rolled into one. No one makes me laugh more than he does. He also built me a beautiful book-filled library, which inspired me to write even on gray, dark days. My Silos has captured my heart and soul with his feline ways. He tells me each day when it's time to take a break and play with him. I love that little cat so much. Lastly, of course, is Sylvester, who made me a stronger person.

And, since I work for the US government, I must give the obligatory disclaimer: the opinions I express in this book are mine.

Index